Engaging Reflection in Practice

Engaging Reflection in Practice
A Narrative Approach

Christopher Johns

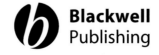

Blackwell
Publishing

© 2006 Christopher Johns

Blackwell Publishing Ltd,
Editorial offices:
Blackwell Publishing Ltd, 9600 Garsington Road, Oxford OX4 2DQ, UK
    Tel: +44 (0)1865 776868
Blackwell Publishing Inc., 350 Main Street, Malden, MA 02148-5020, USA
    Tel: +1 781 388 8250
Blackwell Publishing Asia Pty Ltd, 550 Swanston Street, Carlton, Victoria 3053, Australia
    Tel: +61 (0)3 8359 1011

First published 2006 by Blackwell Publishing Ltd

ISBN-13: 978-14051-4973-0
ISBN-10: 1-4051-4973-6

Library of Congress Cataloging-in-Publication Data
Johns, Christopher.
   Engaging reflection in practice : a narrative approach / Christopher Johns.
      p. ; cm.
   Includes bibliographical references and index.
   ISBN-13: 978-1-4051-4973-0 (pbk. : alk. paper)
   ISBN-10: 1-4051-4973-6 (pbk. : alk. paper)   1. Nursing–Study and teaching.
2. Nursing–Philosophy.   3. Self-evaluation.   4. Self-knowledge, Theory of.   I. Title.
   [DNLM: 1. Philosophy, Nursing.   2. Holistic Nursing.   3. Self Assessment
(Psychology)   4. Writing. WY 86 J65e 2006]

   RT73.J64 2006
   610.73076–dc22

                                                                  2006009952

A catalogue record for this title is available from the British Library

Set in 10/12.5pt Palatino
by Graphicraft Limited, Hong Kong
Printed and bound in Singapore
by Utopia Press Pte Ltd

For further information on Blackwell Publishing, visit our website:
www.blackwellnursing.com

Contents

Foreword by Michael Kearney   vii
Preface   ix
Acknowledgments   xi

Part 1
Chapter 1   Revealing the essence of reflective practice   3

Chapter 2   A reflective model for clinical practice   12

Chapter 3   Knowing desirable practice   20

Chapter 4   Exploring narrative dialogue   36

Chapter 5   Weaving the narrative   52

Part 2
Chapter 6   The heron & the tree and other stories   65

Appendix   *Summary of therapies*   265
References   266
Index   274

Foreword

The easing of suffering is at the core of the health-care mandate, and as Balint has so eloquently argued[1], we, *ourselves*, are the most potent medicine we can prescribe to ease our patients' suffering.

One way of understanding suffering more deeply, and what we need to do to alleviate it in our patients and their families, is by reflecting on the nature of health. The renowned Buddhist teacher, the late Chogyam Trungpa offers the following insight: 'Although the usual dictionary definition of "health" is, roughly speaking, "free from sickness", we should look at health as something more than that. According to the Buddhist tradition, people inherently possess Buddha-nature; that is, they are basically and intrinsically good. From this point of view, health is intrinsic. That is, health comes first: sickness is secondary. Health IS'.[2] If this is correct, then suffering can be understood as the experience of disconnection from our innate inner wholeness, and healing, rather than being something we do for our patients, becomes something patients can be encouraged to do for themselves; an act of deeply remembering (in the sense of re-connecting with) what already is.

How can we enable this to happen for our patients? By what we do, by how we do what we do, and by who we are as persons. 'What we do' describes our skills and knowledge, our effectiveness as practitioners in whatever area our expertise is. In lessening suffering and creating security and trust, efficient treatment and care foster within the patient conditions that are conducive to healing. 'How we do what we do' is about the quality of the care we offer. As Saunders observed, 'The way that care is given can reach the most hidden place and open space for unexpected development'.[3]

'Who we are as persons' is, however, what matters most in our task as enablers of healing for others. I am referring here to the quality of our presence. Like the effect of a magnetic field on iron filings, the quality of our subjectivity impacts dynamically on the subjectivity of our patients (just as theirs does with ours). It seems to me that the question is not whether or not we are such fields of healing, but what kind of healing fields we are and choose to be? In other words, what is the quality of the life we, each of us, bring to our clinical encounters? What is the quality of *our* life? This matters because this is

[1] Balint, M. (2000) *The Doctor, His patient and The Illness*, Churchill Livingstone, Edinburgh.
[2] Trungpa, C. (1985) in Wellwood, J. (editor), *Awakening the Heart*, New Science Library, p. 126.
[3] Saunders, C. (1996) in Kearney, M., *Mortally Wounded*, Touchstone, New York, p. 14.

precisely what we bring to the bedside, and what our patients experience in our presence.

Hindu teacher Sri Madhava Ashish suggests that in our quest to become effective healers, the first move needs to be one of pausing, of stepping back, of self-reflection. He writes, 'When you want to help a person towards healing you must, in some way, retreat into yourself to the level from which the healing flows'.[4] In other words the first move towards another in suffering must, paradoxically, be a backwards one. As we do this, and as we go inwards, we may notice an inability to 'make it all better' and experience feelings such as inadequacy and sadness. With this comes insight into a shared humanity and a negation of the power differential between the caregiver and the patient. Simultaneously, we begin to tap into sources of deep intuitive wisdom which carry us in a compassionate flow back towards the one who suffers. Being a healer entails an attitude of working cooperatively and respectfully with the different aspects of this dynamic process.

In this important book Chris Johns outlines just how this can happen by engaging reflection in practice. With wisdom and compassion he teaches how being mindful eases suffering and creates the space where healing may happen.

Michael Kearney, MB, FRCPI
Palliative Care Physician, Santa Barbara, California
June, 2006

---

[4] Ashish, Sri. (1992) Personal Communication.

Preface

In the human encounter everything is unique, although seemingly familiar nothing is certain. The moment is always a mystery. Hence reflection is the exploration of uncertainty and narrative the revelation of mystery.

When I commenced work as General Manager of Burford Community Hospital and Head of Burford Nursing Development Unit in 1989, I was inspired by the idea of reflective practice as a way to structure clinical practice and facilitate practitioner performance. At that time, my understanding of reflective practice was influenced by Margaret Clarke's paper *Action and reflection* (Clarke 1986) although her ideas were more philosophical than practical. I also had a 0.2 whole-time equivalent (WTE) contract with Oxford Polytechnic as a lecturer-practitioner both to supervise student nurses and provide their module theoretical input. I decided to structure the theoretical learning through reflection as a way to link practice with theory. This approach had meaning for the students because they were required to meet their learning objectives through reflection.

Burford had a strong history of practice development through the pioneer work of Alan Pearson between 1982 and 1985, based on the ideas he set out in his book *The Clinical Nursing Unit* (1983). Arriving in 1989, many of his ideas had eroded. For example, the philosophy for practice was based on Lydia Hall's nursing theory (1964), yet no practitioners could articulate this in any meaningful way.

In response, I facilitated a new collaborative vision for clinical practice grounded in holistic and reflective values within the role of a community hospital served by local general practitioners.

Yet, what does it mean to be a holistic and reflective practitioner?

Since that time, my work has been dedicated to exploring these questions through my teaching, research and publications. And so, in 2000, nine years after leaving Burford, I was again posing these questions when I commenced to write my narrative *Being Mindful, Easing Suffering* (Johns 2004b), simply because I claimed to be a reflective and holistic practitioner working as a complementary therapist and nurse in a hospice.

In my narrative *The heron & the tree*, I explore these claims further by reflecting on my clinical practice between September 2002 and September 2004, continuing my journey towards understanding and realising holistic and reflective practice as a lived reality, what I term the artistry of *engaged* reflection as the hallmark of professional practice.

The narrative weaves together two movements. The first movement is finding meaning in the process of reflection as a way of being within practice characterised by being mindful. Reflective structures offer guidance to sign-post the way. The second movement is to appreciate that reflective practice is ultimately concerned with enabling the practitioner to realise desirable clinical practice. Again reflective structures throw light on the nature of the desirable practice.

The narrative reveals the beneficial impact of hospice care and complementary therapies for patients and their families facing imminent death within the culture of a hospice. Every story reveals the emergence of my 'healing' ability and using 'healing' energy. I use the word 'healing' here in the holistic sense of intent to bring the other's energy into best shape for self-healing to take place, not in any traditional medical 'curing' sense. Flemons and Green (2002b: 188) note:

> 'The thing about the word *healing*, it comes from the same root as the word whole, and so to heal is to make whole.' (their italics)

In this sense, my stories are primarily stories of connection between myself as a therapist and as a Buddhist, with people who receive my care. I have been careful to change all names of people mentioned in my reflections to respect their privacy, although many of these persons would have liked me to use their real names so that others could learn through our healing work.

I also write to explore the artistry of narrative writing. As I guide others to construct narratives through academic programmes at the University of Luton (for example, see the work of Jarrett and Johns 2005), it seemed vital to walk the talk and construct my own narrative if I am to better guide others. So, wrapped around the narrative is my narrative of writing it, a background in five chapters against which I position myself. The background is selective, developing reflective and holistic ideas that I have previously written about (Johns 2002, Johns 2004a).

The book is arranged in two parts. Part 1 composes 5 chapters that present my narrative of writing a narrative. In chapters 1–3, I set out the background in terms of reflective and holistic ideas. In chapter 1, I explore the nature of reflective practice. In chapter 2, I explore the reflective model that frames the hospice's clinical practice. In chapter 3, I set out a holistic vision for my clinical practice, notably the idea of 'easing suffering' and the way a holistic vision might be 'known' using the Being Available Template. In chapters 4 and 5, I organise the text through six layers of dialogue that represent how I actually went about constructing the narrative, rather than a theoretical treatise of how to construct narrative. Part 2 is chapter 6, in which I present my narrative *The heron & the tree*. These first chapters are not essential reading. They can be skipped, skimmed over or read after reading *The heron & the tree*.

Acknowledgements

To all the patients, families and practitioners with whom I have engaged within the narrative and who made this book possible. All names have been changed to protect identity. To my teachers, whose words enlighten the text and inspire me to touch my well of goodness and ride the windhorse. To Beth and Katharine at Blackwell Publishing who have produced this fine book.

The publisher and authors would also like to thank the organisations and persons listed below for permission to reproduce material from their publications:

Hazeldene Foundation for quotes from *Earth Dance Drum* by Blackwolf Jones and Gina Jones, copyright 1996, reprinted by permission of Hazeldene Foundation, Center City, MN.

The Random House Group Ltd for quotes from *The Powerbook* by Jeanette Winterson, published by Jonathan Cape.

Kate Rusby.

Suzanne Vega.

Windhorse Publications for quotes from *Exploring Karma and Rebirth*, Nagapriya, 2004.

Every effort has been made to obtain necessary permission with reference to copyright material. The publisher and author apologise if, inadvertently, any sources remain unacknowledged and will be glad to make the necessary arrangements at the earliest opportunity.

Part 1

Chapter 1   Revealing the essence of reflective practice   3

Chapter 2   A reflective model for clinical practice   12

Chapter 3   Knowing desirable practice   20

Chapter 4   Exploring narrative dialogue   36

Chapter 5   Weaving the narrative   52

Chapter 1

Revealing the essence of reflective practice

To begin, I position myself within reflective practice. The notion of *engaged* reflection is inspired by Thich Nhat Hanh's (1987) idea of *Engaged* Buddhism as something lived rather than a philosophical idea. Hence reflection is purposeful activity toward realising my vision of practice as a lived reality.

Simply, and yet profoundly, reflective practice is concerned with learning through everyday experiences towards realising desirable practice. Insights are gained through reflection that can be acted on in subsequent experiences within a reflexive spiral of realisation. Such learning is both deliberative and intuitive, and can take place within or after practice. The basic idea of reflection-on-experience is that practitioners can reveal and resolve the contradictions between their visions of holism and their actual practice. No easy task – for clinical practice is fashioned by deeply embedded social norms governed by tradition, authority and embodiment that resist change.

Efforts to define reflection reflect a need to grasp and know 'it' as a concept. For this reason, I prefer to refer to 'description' rather than 'definition'. Such gestures may feel semantic, but reflect a deeper truth than any definition of reflection could reveal. At least for the purposes of this book, I am keen to pursue a more holistic description of reflection simply to try and more accurately capture the nature of reflection as holistic. This makes sense when I view or grasp practice as watching a complete or whole performance. The mind takes in the whole rather than reducing it into bits. Hence reflection begins as a story and only later do the reflective cues begin to pull it apart, yet never losing sight of the wholeness of the situation.

The essence of reflection is captured by the idea of Bimadisiwin:

> Bimadisiwin is a conscious decision to become. It is time to think about what you want to be. The dance cannot be danced until you envision the dance, rehearse its movements and understand your part. It is demanding for every step needs an effort in becoming one with the vision. It takes discipline, hard work and time. Decide to be an active participant in your life journey. It is rewarding. Embrace the joy your vision brings you, it is yours to hold forever. It is freeing, for it frees the spirit. It releases you to become as you believe you must.
>
> (Blackwolf & Gina Jones 1996:47)

Blackwolf Jones is of the Obijway nation and offers a timeless wisdom. Such words invite the imagination as if a flower opening to the morning sun. The idea of caring as a dance captures its performance, the fluid and knowing movement of moving my hands across someone's feet is poetry in motion. Yet to be a skilful dancer requires effort, discipline, commitment, patience, compassion and wisdom. Blackwolf and Gina Jones (1996:47) offer the following inspirational mantra:

> Believe in the vision of you
> Practice this vision
> Become the vision

Let these words stir the mind and heart. Listen to my own, more prosaic, description of reflective practice:

> Reflection is being mindful of self, either within or after experience, as if it is a window through which the practitioner can view and focus self within the context of a particular experience, in order to confront, understand and move toward resolving contradiction between one's vision and their actual practice.
>   Through the conflict of contradiction, the commitment to realise one's vision, and understanding why things are as they are, the practitioner can gain new insights into self and be empowered to respond more congruently in future situations within a reflexive spiral towards developing practical wisdom and realising one's vision as a lived reality. The practitioner may require guidance to overcome resistance or to be empowered to act on understanding.

> (Johns 2004a)

From this description of reflection, I want to emphasise some ideas.

Ideas about reflection

Being mindful

I want to fuzz a distinction between reflection either within or after experience by appealing to the idea of being mindful, i.e. being mindful is paying attention to self within the reflective moment, a moment that might be at home after work or within work itself. Reflection-on-experience is still being mindful, whether hours, days or weeks after the actual event.

I have previously suggested a typology of reflective practices shifting from *doing reflection* as some technique to *being reflective* as a way of being within practice (Johns 2004a, 2005). *Doing reflection* is typified by reflection-on-experience; something I do after an event, for example by writing a reflective account or relating the experience in clinical supervision. In contrast, *being reflective* is typified by what I term mindful practice; being attentive to self within each unfolding moment with the intent to realise my vision of desirable practice.

The Pali word for mindfulness is *sati*. Buddhadasa Bhikkhu (1997:154) notes that sati is:

> reflective awareness: the mind's ability to recall, know and contemplate itself. *Sati* allows us to be aware of what we are about to do. It is characterised by speed and agility.

Being mindful is having a virtual space between self and the situation where the situation can be appreciated for what it really is and where I can contemplate how best to respond given the particular circumstances. Clinical practice is never predictable and must always be interpreted within the unfolding moment. The practitioner may have experienced many similar situations, yet the particular situation is unique, it has never happened before. The nature of 'what is best' is always the focus for the reflective practitioner to appreciate. Being mindful I pay attention and cultivate my presence in order to be fully available within each unfolding moment. It is appreciating the call of a robin amidst the din of a busy hospital. Being mindful is Buddha nature.

> The root word *Budh* means to wake up, to know, to understand; and he or she who wakes up and understands is called a Buddha. It is as simple as that. The capacity to wake up, to understand, and to love is called Buddha nature.

> (Thich Nhat Hanh 1987:13)

Reflection is my commitment to wake up and understand.

Reflection-on-experience

I want to emphasise that being reflective is nurtured through the discipline of reflection-on-experience. If one evening I reflect on an experience, then the next day I am more sensitive to any ideas and insights gained from that reflection. These ideas and insights are like seeds planted in my mind to germinate as appropriate.

Contradiction

I want to emphasise that contradiction is the learning impetus even though the practitioner may not be conscious of any obvious contradiction. To not experience contradiction is to suggest a perfect harmony between my vision and my reality. However, one can never master a discipline. As Senge (1990:11) puts it:

> The more you learn, the more acutely you become aware of your ignorance.

Sangharakshita (1990:35) gives an intriguing spin on contradiction:

> Why is there this terrible gulf, this terrible chasm, between our theory and our practice, our understanding and our operation? Why are most of us most of the time unable to act in accordance with what we know is true, what we know is right? Why do we fail so miserably again and yet again? The answer to this question is to be sought in the very depths of human nature.

The practitioner's reflective effort is then to consider how *this terrible chasm* can be eased when faced with a similar situation. The imagination rises to various possibilities and their consequences. Yet to be realistic, I must also consider whether I am able to respond differently by appreciating what factors might constrain me. Of course, my ability to see myself is limited by what Patti Lather (1986a,b) describes as 'false consciousness'. Hence I may benefit from a guide to challenge me to pull away the masks of false consciousness and help me reveal myself to myself, and infuse me with courage to act on my insights. The proof of learning is revealed in subsequent reflections.

The trigger for reflection is generally regarded as 'uncomfortable' feelings such as anger, frustration, anxiety, distress and guilt (Boyd & Fales 1983). However, contradiction may not arouse such feelings or even that such feelings necessarily indicate contradiction although I do acknowledge that uncomfortable feelings are most likely to stem from a sense of contradiction. A sense of unease draws the experience into consciousness. As Paramanda (2001:58) notes:

> Whenever we begin to feel frustrated in what we are doing, we should slow down and pay closer attention to it. Frustration takes us away from ourselves; we become alienated from our experience.

Positive feelings may also trigger reflection where any underlying contradiction may be less apparent. However, the reliance on feelings as triggers for reflection reflects a lack of mindfulness. As I become increasingly mindful, then every experience, whether traumatic, joyful or simply mundane, becomes available for reflection. This is very evident within my narrative.

Harnessing energy

I want to emphasise that reflection is concerned with harnessing energy for taking action. Prigogine's theory of dissipate structures (1980), as cited by Newman (1994) in her theory of Health as Expanded Consciousness, provides a compelling theoretical understanding for appreciating energy conversion through reflection. In my sketch the straight curly lines represent effective self-organisation until they hit a crisis, represented by a mass of curly lines. In crisis, normal patterns of self-organisation fail, resulting in anxiety (negative energy). Being open systems, people can exchange or convert this energy with the environment and create positive energy for taking action based on a reorganisation of self as necessary to resolve the crisis and emerge at a higher level of consciousness; that is, until the next crisis.

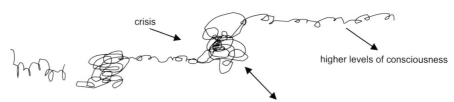

crisis

higher levels of consciousness

conversion of negative energy to positive energy

Recognition of crisis may seem obvious, but it is usually reflected in a subtle sense of breakdown and not easy to discern within my normal patterns of thinking. As such, a guide may be a vital transformative catalyst. The word crisis might be replaced with 'chaos'. Wheatley (1999:119) notes that:

It is chaos' great destructive energy that dissolves the past and gives us the gift of a new future. It releases us from the imprisoning patterns of the past by offering us its wild ride into newness. Only chaos creates the abyss in which we can recreate ourselves.

Reflection is the vehicle for this ride. Hold on!

Action-oriented

I want to emphasise that reflection is always action-oriented towards realising vision as a lived reality. In other words, reflection is not a neutral thing but a political and cultural movement towards creating a better, more caring and humane world. As such, the ideals of a critical social science are enshrined. Notably that reflection is:

(1) A process of enlightenment or understanding as to why things are as they are (self in context)
(2) A process of empowerment to take action as necessary based on understanding
(3) A process of emancipation whereby action actually transforms situations for a vision to be realised (in the understanding that visions actually shift in the process of realisation)

Fay (1987) highlighted the limitations of rationality to bring about change due to three key aspects of culture; tradition, power and embodiment, that offers a typology of resistance. The exploration of contradiction between what on one hand is desirable and on the other hand is 'current reality' (as interpreted through reflection) inevitably is a reflection on resistance and the focus for subsequent action. Hence the idea of reflection as action to overthrow oppression is a powerful metaphor, accepting that nursing is an oppressed group in terms of having authority to realise its own therapeutic potential.

The language of a critical social science may be intimidating with its rhetoric of oppression and misery yet it can be argued that nursing, as a largely female workforce, has been subjugated by patriarchal attitudes that render it politically passive and thus unable to fulfil its caring destiny. If so, then realising a holistic vision requires an analysis and eventual overthrow of oppressive political and cultural systems. The link between oppression and patriarchy is obvious, considering nursing as women's work, and the suppression of women's voices in 'knowing their place' within the patriarchal order of things. Images of 'behind the screens' where women conceal their work, themselves, and their significance (Lawler 1991) and images of emotional labour being no more than women's natural work, therefore unskilled and unvalued within the heroic stance of medicine (James 1989) are powerful signs of this oppression steeped in power, tradition and embodiment. Maxine Greene (1988:58) inspires me:

Concealment does not simply mean hiding; it means dissembling, presenting something as other than it is. To 'unconceal' is to create clearings, spaces in the midst of things where decisions can be made. It is to break through the masked and the falsified, to reach toward what is also half-hidden or concealed. When a woman, when any human being, tries to tell the truth and act on it, there is no predicting what will happen. The 'not yet' is always to a degree concealed. When one chooses to act on one's freedom, there are no guarantees.

I feel my excitement tingle as I read and write these works. Reflection opens up a clearing where caring can be visible, can be valued, can be acknowledged as skilled, where action can be planned to confront the bullies and tyrants of the land, where my voice is no longer quiet and stuttering, where my demeanour is no longer passive.

In my narrative I talk about creating and holding space where healing can take place. So it is with practitioners. Indeed, this is how they can learn to create clearings for their patients, often in a hostile care environment that has little sympathy for their plight. It is what holism seeks. The commitment to the truth also seems vital in Greene's words. Anything less would be futile. Yet how comfortable are people in their illusions of truth? Is it better to conform than rock the boat? Is it better to sacrifice the ideal for a quiet life and patronage of more powerful others? Is it better to keep your head down than have it shot off above the parapet for daring to reveal the truth? Reflection offers nurses (and other health care workers, including men) a voice to reveal what has been concealed, and those norms that compose the taken-for-granted. Greene (1988:58) favours this idea:

> If the 'world' refers to interpreted experiences or to commonsense constructs of what is taken to be real, it would indeed 'split open' if people were to listen, to pay heed'.

Yet, having a voice is one thing, having it heard is another thing. Having it acted on is another thing entirely. Perhaps one could get despondent but the vision of holism is powerful, and virtue and integrity are powerful motivators towards its realisation.

Being in-place

Linked to the previous point I want to sow an image of realising desirable practice as a journey from *Knowing your place* – a place determined and controlled by more powerful others to – *Being in-place* – the place where I need to be to realise my vision as a lived reality (Mayeroff 1971).

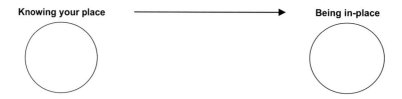

Try this exercise:

- In each circle write a description of 'knowing your place' and 'being in-place'

- Identify what factors constrain you from being in-place
- Now identify positive actions you can take to be in-place
- Reflect each day on the difference positive action makes
- Repeat the exercise at least weekly and mark along the line your progress toward being in-place

I shall assume that not *being in-place* is a deeply disturbing idea that creates a strong sense of internal conflict. I may pretend I am in a 'good enough place' as some sort of compromise to survive a hostile world. However, it is not necessarily easy to shift to being in-place. Deeply embodied forces rally to uncomfortably remind me to know my place. Perhaps all I can do is chip away at the edges, but if so, I can imagine being a sculptor chipping away slowly but purposefully at the granite slab toward creating a beautiful thing. For without doubt caring is a beautiful thing.

Qualities

I want to emphasise that becoming a reflective practitioner requires discipline, skill, commitment, time and patience. As Nagapriya (2004:52) suggests:

> We can't completely change ourselves overnight because our more deeply ingrained patterns of thinking, feeling, speaking and behaving require *constant attention over a prolonged period of time* if they are to be changed. There is no quick fix. (my italics)

As such, reflection might be described as the discipline of *constant attention over a prolonged period of time towards internalising reflection as a way of being.*

For example, my experience of working with students on the Masters in Clinical Leadership programme I guide at the University of Luton, whereby reflection is the core learning process, suggests it takes these students between 12–18 months to internalise reflection as a natural way of being with their practice. Or, put another way, to be mindful of self as being the clinical leader they desire to be moment to moment. From this appreciation, the occasional reflective effort would seem of little learning value.

Holographic reflection

I want to emphasise the holographic nature of reflection as a learning process. This is illustrated in Figure 1.1, where reflection may start as a reflection on self within the context of a particular situation but can be framed within ever broader contexts of social and political life until we come to the ultimate questions – what does it mean to be human and (in response) what sort of community life should we create and sustain? As Wheatley (1999:35) notes:

> None of us exists independent of our relationships with others.

From this perspective, it can be appreciated that action I take, no matter how apparently mundane, will ripple through the different levels and have an affect. In chaos theory it is described as the 'butterfly effect' – the idea that when a butterfly flutters its wings in Tokyo a hurricane can occur in Mexico.

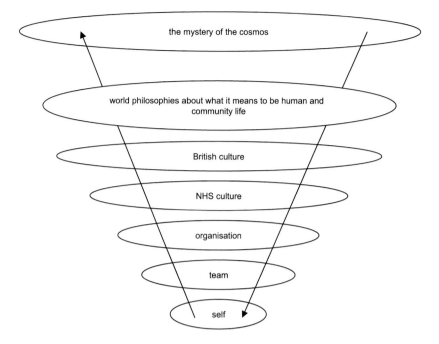

Figure 1.1   Holograph of reflective learning.

I know from experience that to smile at a colleague when before there was indifference will ripple through that person and change the dynamic between us. Just to ask a question in a meeting where before my voice was muted will shift the dynamic of the meeting. To hold the hand of someone dying will transform that person's experience of dying and those who observe.

Remember, actions have consequences, and that if practitioners like myself act with integrity to respond in caring ways it will always have a positive impact (Wheatley 1999). Caring is the main attractor, yet to be significant caring needs to be invested with meaning.

> By far the most powerful force of attraction in organisations and in our individual lives is meaning.

> (Wheatley 1999:132)

Practical wisdom

I want to emphasise the idea of practical wisdom as the focus for learning in contrast with theoretical learning; a type of wisdom termed by Aristotle as *phronesis*, of particular use in dealing with ethical and political matters. Fay (1987:181) notes:

> Aristotle insisted that practical wisdom is different from theoretical wisdom, most especially in that it does not result in knowledge which is determinate and universal; indeed it does not result in propositional knowledge at all but in discriminations and action.

It is the wisdom of expertise that requires complex judgements specific to the particular situation at hand. It is beyond the application of rules and procedures, for these always need to be interpreted for their value within the specific clinical situation. Through reflection, I may sense patterns of responding and tentatively draw propositions from this understanding as a form of sense-making that will inevitably inform my future practice; what might be understood as insights.

In more contemporary reflective literature, Schön (1987) differentiated reflective knowing and technical rationality. Schön strongly advocated the primacy of intuitive or reflective knowing for professional practice in contrast with technical rationality. Reflective knowing is the knowing that practitioners use in their practice or professional artistry, whilst technical rationality is rule-based propositional knowledge. It is only through reflection that propositional knowledge can be applied meaningfully to practice. As such, we should talk of expert-based practice rather than evidence-based practice; evidence being just one type of knowledge to inform the practitioner.

Summary

Reflective practice is revealed as both a mindful way of being within practice and a process to reflect-on-experience to appreciate and resolve contradiction with the intent of realising my vision of practice as a lived reality. There can be no more meaningful approach to practice and learning simply because it is grounded in who I am and my practice.

Chapter 2

A reflective model for clinical practice

The hospice where I practice uses the Burford Nursing Development Unit (NDU) Model: Caring in Practice to guide clinical practice (Johns 1991, 1994, 2004a). Before I commenced working at the hospice in my volunteer role as a complementary therapist and nurse, I had worked with the hospice staff to implement the Burford model. It replaced a systems model based on 12 activities of living (Roper, Logan & Tierney Model of Nursing 1980) that practitioners felt was not congruent to guide their holistic vision for practice. A review revealed they generally didn't use the Roper, Logan, & Tierney model in any meaningful way. It was a hindrance to realising holistic practice but they felt obliged to use it despite its inadequacy simply because it was the model! It was as if the model had imposed a demand.

The Burford model's explicit assumptions

The Burford model was attractive to hospice practitioners because it is based on a holistic vision for practice as reflected in its reflective and holistic assumptions:

(1) Caring in practice is grounded in a valid vision for practice
(2) The practitioner is mindful of easing suffering and nurturing growth as she goes about her practice moment to moment
(3) The core therapeutic of nursing practice is the practitioner being available – a working-with relationship focused to enable the other to find meaning in their health-illness experience, to make best decisions and help take appropriate action to ease suffering and meet their life needs
(4) Growth is a mutual process of realisation
(5) Practitioners accept responsibility for working toward creating the Learning Organisation (Senge 1990)
(6) Caring in practice is a responsive and reflexive form in context with the environment in which it is practised

The assumption *Growth is a mutual process of realisation* acknowledges the way reflective practice contributes towards creating a dynamic learning environment whereby every experience becomes a learning opportunity for both patients and practitioners to grow through the experience. The assumption *Caring in practice is a responsive and reflexive form in context with the environment in which it is practised* acknowledges that, **at** an organisational level, reflective practice offers a dynamic review of the organisation itself to facilitate effective

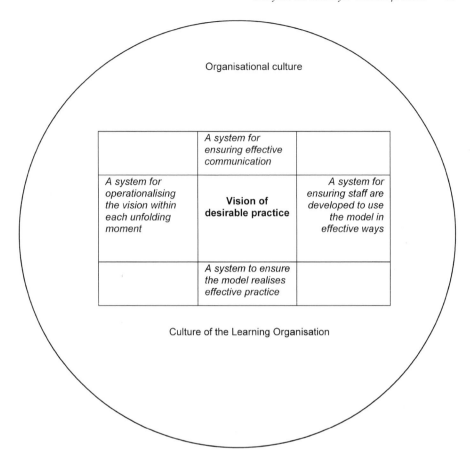

Figure 2.1   Structural view of a reflective framework for clinical practice.

practice. The organisation becomes like the organic body, always changing and learning in response to situations, developing to become more effective, more resilient, more satisfying. I address the assumption concerned with creating the Learning Organisation below. The assumptions concerned with easing suffering and being available are explored in chapter 3.

The Burford model's reflective systems

Four reflective systems are considered necessary to realise the vision as a lived reality (Figure 2.1) set against a background of the organisational culture.

A system for operationalising the vision within each unfolding moment

To answer the question '*What information do I need to nurse this patient and family?*' nine reflective cues enable me to tune into the person and family requiring care, and myself, from the perspective of the hospice's holistic values within each unfolding moment:

- Who is this person?
- What meaning does this illness/meaning have for the person?
- How is this person feeling?
- How has this event affected their usual life pattern and roles?
- How do I feel about this person?
- How can I help this person?
- What is important for this person to make their stay in the hospice comfortable?
- What support does this person have in life?
- How does this person view the future for themselves and others?

The cues intend to tune me into the person (s) receiving care. As such, I internalise the cues as a natural lens to view situations. They are *not* intended as a formulaic response to assess the patient. Each cue is significant to pattern the holistic response to the person.

'Who is this person?' challenges me to see the person first rather than as a patient with an array of symptoms, a medical diagnosis, receiving various treatments, labelled with a prognosis, etc. The cue is an explicit reminder to guard against a descent into the medical model. As such, it is vital. As the first cue it also intends to remind me to be mindful and curious – who *is* this person that I am connecting with?

'What meaning does this health event have for the person?' cues me to listen and be empathic to the person's experience; i.e., what does the health-illness event *really* mean for the person? Understanding the person's experience opens up the possibility for me to tune into and synchronise with the person's wavelength and to flow with the person on the ebb and flow of their health-illness experience, helping the person find a new, more harmonious, wavelength in tune with well-being.

'How is this person feeling?' guides me to inquire into the person's particular concerns and anxieties. As you can imagine, being admitted into a hospice can be a very emotional experience.

'How has this event affected their usual life pattern and roles?' guides me to explore with the person the way illness has disrupted their life pattern and ways their life pattern might be shifted in tune with a greater comfort, harmony and well-being. Such issues as sleep, nutrition, bowels, fatigue, pain, finance, mobility come to the fore.

'How do I feel about this person?' guides me to be mindful of my attitude and reaction towards the person and reflect on any resistance I might have to being available to the person. It is a vital cue in that my relationship with the person is a unique human–human encounter, where my humanness is my most vital therapeutic tool.

'How can I help this person?' summarises the first four cues and prompts me to negotiate care processes and goals with the patient and my colleagues

so that we can work together to realise them in the most beneficial and resourceful way.

'What is important for this person to make their stay in the hospice comfortable?' pays attention to caring detail on the premise that 'the little things are important' and give powerful messages of recognising and respecting the person's individuality and cultural world.

'What support does this person have in life?' draws my attention to any ongoing care outside the immediate care environment by framing the person within his or her social and cultural world. I draw any family, friends, community into the caring gaze.

'How does this person view the future?' prompts me to open a dialogue about what the future might hold, especially fears of dying and death.

   The pattern of these nine reflective cues ripple through the narrative for the discerning reader to appreciate.

A system for ensuring effective communication

The information gained from using the cues and working with the patient and family is written as an unfolding narrative. On review, the nursing process had no value either as a comprehensive record of care or enabling the continuity of care. Indeed, the nursing process was considered a hindrance to effective practice because most aspects of holistic practice could not be predetermined.

   Clearly writing narratives with patients needs to be both meaningful and practical. Clearly I can't write long stories because no one would read them – however meaningful they might be. Finding practical solutions to practice narratives led to a renaissance of chart keeping to map unfolding care processes (see Johns 2004a: Chapter 8).

A system for ensuring that staff are developed to use the model in effective ways

To effectively use the reflective cues and write patient narratives requires considerable skill, especially if practitioners have been socialised into reductionist approaches to clinical practice. Learning is a process of un-learning ways that may have become deeply embodied and resistant to change.

   The most effective developmental approach is clinical supervision or guided reflection. So, my narrative can be viewed as a continuous process of learning through reflection to become an effective reflective and holistic practitioner using the Burford model.

A system to ensure the model realises effective practice

As a responsible practitioner, I must take responsibility for ensuring my own effectiveness. Guided reflection creates an opportunity for this, both on an individual and collective level. Other organisational reflective opportunities are clinical audit and reflective standards of care. This approach to quality assurance is based on a structure, process, and outcome approach whereby a group of practitioners write standards around discrete aspects of clinical practice that can be monitored. The approach is reflexive in that the standards are modified in light of feedback so that they are an adequate representation of clinical practice. It becomes a dynamic approach to practice development. The standards are 'owned' by the practitioners and use monitoring criteria that become part of everyday clinical practice. In this way, quality is not imposed but 'lived'. Although this approach requires an attitude of practitioner responsibility to quality and practice development, commitment and resources, if successful the benefits are profound (see Johns 2004a:Chapter 9).

The Learning Organisation

Clinical practice does not take place in a vacuum. It is always set against an organisational culture that exerts a strong influence in enabling practitioners to realise desirable practice. My claim is that the understanding and commitment to establishing the Learning Organisation is vital to accommodate reflective practice, and that reflective practice itself is vital to create the Learning Organisation. Senge (1990:3) describes the Learning Organisation as:

> One where people continually expand their capacities to create the results they truly desire, where new and expansive patterns of thinking are nurtured, where collective aspiration is set free, and where people are continually learning how to learn together.

The learning organisation comprises five inter-relating disciplines:

- Shared vision
- Team learning
- Mental models
- Systems thinking
- Personal mastery

Shared vision

A shared vision gives purpose and direction to practice and learning. The practice of building a shared vision involves the skills of unearthing shared beliefs and values about the nature of practice that fosters genuine commitment (rather than compliance). In mastering this discipline, leaders learn the counterproductiveness of trying to dictate a vision, no matter how heartfelt. I assume that a shared vision is vital for practitioners to work together across professional boundaries toward realising common purpose. As suggested in the description of reflective practice, vision of desirable practice is necessary to focus reflective action towards resolving contradiction between desirable actual practice. To be valid, a vision for practice needs to address four cornerstones.

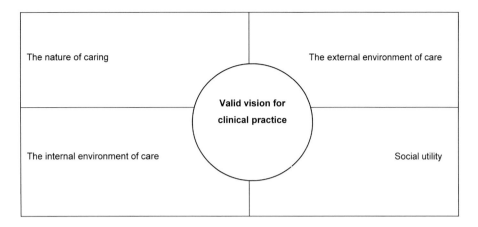

The nature of caring is concerned with the values and beliefs practitioners hold regarding care of persons. The internal environment is concerned with the relationships between practitioners to support patient care. Ask yourself – what is the congruent pattern of relationship that reciprocates the holistic relationship with patients and families? It can *only* be a relationship invested in dialogue and consensus, that acknowledges and values each person's view, that is mutually and genuinely supportive. Such patterns can be written within the vision as a constant reminder. For example, at Burford Community Hospital we wrote in our vision:

> Our caring is enhanced when we work in relationship with our (multi) professional colleagues on the basis of mutual respect and care for each other within our respective roles. This means being free to share our feelings openly but appropriately, acknowledging that as persons, we are stressed and have differences of opinions at times. This is the basis of the therapeutic team that is essential; to reciprocate and support our caring to patients.

> (Johns 2004a:49)

Fine words – but they need to be lived as a reality. It requires each practitioner to have an assertive voice; a voice that is connected to the patient's and their own experience, informed, ethical, passionate, respected, and heard.

The external environment is concerned with the role of the unit within society, i.e., what does the unit exist to do? Social utility is about responding to and influencing societal expectations, and wider professional issues such as research and teaching, for example, reflective practice and becoming a Learning Organisation.

Team learning

Whilst the ideal of a shared vision is irresistible, in practice issues of professional rivalry and dominance can interfere with its realisation. Hence the significance of team learning as a way of talking and listening to each other, in conversations, in dialogue. To *work together* demands a culture of mutual respect for each other's role within the team reflected in the idea of team learning. The discipline of team learning starts with 'dialogue'; the capacity of members of a team to suspend their individual assumptions and enter into a genuine 'thinking together' and recognising the patterns of interaction in teams that undermine learning. Reflection opens a clearing for practitioners to express and nurture their voice so it can be heard and respected (Belenky et al. 1986, Johns & Hardy 2005) in the mutual effort towards creating the conditions of dialogue.

Mental models

Mental models are deeply ingrained assumptions or images that influence how the practitioner understands the world and how they take action. The discipline of working with mental models starts with turning the mirror inward; learning to unearth our internal images and assumptions of the world, to bring them to the surface and hold them rigorously to scrutiny. It also includes the ability to carry on 'learningful' conversations that balance inquiry and advocacy, where people expose their own thinking effectively and make their thinking open to the influence to others (Senge 1990:8/9).

Systems thinking

The discipline of systems thinking is being able to perceive the whole pattern of things and the ways systems or parts inter-relate with each other, even when apparently invisible. Wheatley (1999:118) suggests that:

> When we concentrate on individual moments or fragments of experience, we see only chaos. But if we stand back and look at what is taking shape, we see order. Order always displays itself as patterns that develop over time.

Through reflective feedback loops, systems are constantly fine-tuned towards creating the conditions whereby vision can be most effectively and resourcefully realised. Hence feedback loops seek to find the balance between creativity and stability.

Personal mastery

Personal mastery is the discipline of continually clarifying and deepening our personal vision, of focusing our energies, of developing patience, and of seeing reality objectively. People with a high level of personal mastery are able to consistently realise the results that matter most to them – in effect; they approach life as an artist would approach a work of art. Personal mastery is perhaps the most significant discipline because it reflects the individual's quest to realise desirable practice through reflective practice. In doing so, the practitioner must focus vision, explore and shift mental models, collaboratively engage with others and critique systems for their congruence in supporting desirable practice. The holistic nature of personal mastery is reflected in Senge's words (1990:141):

> It (personal mastery) goes beyond competence and skills, though it is grounded in competence and skills. It goes beyond spiritual unfolding or opening, although it requires spiritual growth. It means approaching one's life as a creative work, living life from a creative as opposed to reactive viewpoint.

My narrative reflects my creative and spiritual unfolding toward realising holistic practice. Indeed, the narrative illuminates that holistic practice *is* creative and spiritual.

Leadership

A transformational leadership is vital to create and sustain the Learning Organisation (see Johns 2004a: chapter 10). Reflective practice has a strong congruency with the notion of transformational leadership in contrast with the transactional leadership that generally characterises health care organisations (Johns 2004a). Transformational leadership is concerned with holding and realising a valid vision of practice, investment in practitioners and creating collaborative caring ways of relating congruent with the vision itself. Such leaders have a primary concern with the process of relationship rather than outcomes. If the process is right then the right outcomes creatively emerge. Chantal Cara (1999), from her study on nurses' perspective on how management can promote caring practice, notes that when leadership promotes working relationships congruent with caring values then practitioners can be more caring. When they don't, it leads to demoralisation and loss of caring. As Cara notes (1999:27):

> This research reveals that both the environment and managers can create a significant influence on caring practice.

Summary

I have set out The Burford NDU Model: caring in practice as the background for my clinical practice. If practitioners seek to be holistic and reflective then the models they choose to guide practice need to be congruent. Otherwise they become a contradiction and a hindrance.

In chapter 3, I set out my understanding of holistic practice so the reader can appreciate the way I approach my practice. In particular, I explore the two Burford model assumptions concerned with easing suffering and being available.

Chapter 3

Knowing desirable practice

When you are you, you see things as they are, and you become one with your surroundings. There is your true self. There you have true practice.

(Susuki 1999:83)

Reflection is not an end in itself but a continuous movement to realise a vision as a lived reality, which for myself and health practitioners everywhere is grounded in holism. Yet, whilst many practitioners espouse holism as desirable, understanding what holism means and realising it as a lived reality seems problematic. The idea of holistic practice is very different from being a holistic practitioner. You cannot become a holistic practitioner by reading theories on holism. Indeed not! No, you need to live holism and reflect on your practice and learn through it. As Yoko Beck (1989:123) so astutely observes:

> Suppose we want to know how a marathon runner feels; if we run two blocks, or two miles, or five miles, we will know something about running these distances, but we won't yet know anything about running a marathon. We can recite theories about marathons; we can describe tables about the physiology of marathon runners; we can pile up endless information about marathon running; but it doesn't mean we know what it is. We can only know when we are the one doing it. We only know our lives when we experience them directly . . . this we can call running in place, being present as we are, right here and now.

Whilst I agree with Yoko Beck, it would seem necessary to grasp some idea of the nature of holistic practice if it is to guide my approach to practice. For example, a marathon is run over 26 miles. Hence to run a marathon I would need to know that. I think of holistic practice as 'whole' practice, that the whole is greater than the summation of its parts. I nurse a whole person not its parts. Indeed the parts distract me from the whole person. Holism is the basis for human caring as a unique human–human encounter from the perspective of the patient's needs. As such, the meanings the patient attributes to their health-illness experience are paramount. These thoughts resonate with Kramer (1990), who emphasises the relationship between care receiver and giver:

> The holistic view holds the individual ultimately responsible for health, and individuals are deemed both capable and responsible for choosing experiences that will enhance health. In this holistic view, the health care provider is not in a detached power relation to the patient. Rather, both are active and committed participants in enhancing growth toward health.

(cited in Johns 1994:24)

Kramer asserts that the holistic relationship is characterised by a 'working-with' relationship between caregiver and care receiver towards *enhancing growth towards health*. This raises the question –'what is health'? As the person faces death, this may mean quality of life rather than cure. That may mean having a pint of Guinness every evening in the pub or smoking fags. Perhaps the person does not want to or is unable to take responsibility for their health or grow through the dying experience.

From this perspective, holism is an attitude the caregiver has towards care, to open a potential space for growth that may or may not be accepted by the patient. In other words, holism is not deterministic.

So I ask – how might I know holism in my practice?

The Being Available Template: the he(art) of holistic practice

This question has intrigued me since 1990 when I sought to understand the nature of holistic practice through analysing reflective accounts shared by practitioners within guided reflection relationships who espoused a holistic intent (Johns 1998). If guided reflection intended to enable practitioners to become effective practitioners then how could that be known? Finding no adequate schemes in the nursing literature my solution was to construct my own – *The Being Available Template*.

The Being Available Template asserts that the core characteristic of holistic practice is:

> The practitioner being available to help the person(s) requiring care to find meaning in their health-illness experience, to help the person make best decisions about their life and health, and to respond with appropriate action to help the person meet their health needs.

My analysis suggested that the extent the practitioner *can* be available is influenced by six inter-related dimensions (Figure 3.1). I was aware that reducing holistic practice into six observable bits might be a contradiction, hence I was anxious to assert its core irreducible characteristic.

Vision

> To speak too much of grief is to blunt its edge. It might even make us deaf to the cry that sparked the discourse about suffering in the first place. A cold, calculating intelligence cannot grasp the rough contours of grief. Diagnostic techniques, whether in the hands of medical professionals or political authorities, frequently maul its fragile core.

> (Schwarcz 1997:119)

Vision is at the heart of clinical practice, at the heart of the Learning Organisation, and at the heart of reflective practice. If I do not have a meaningful vision, how can I focus my actions to practise skilfully? To give

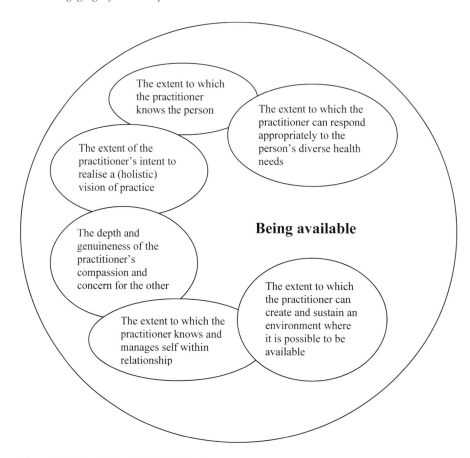

Figure 3.1   The Being Available Template.

my definition of palliative care validity you might expect it to be influenced by the World Health Organization's (2005) definition of palliative care (see Box 3.1).

The WHO definition does not explicitly state holistic practice. Instead it prefers to pay attention to parts. However, it does emphasise the idea of easing suffering; an idea I deeply resonate with. Suffering lies at the heart of my vision for palliative care. In speaking of suffering, of caring, of palliative care, I do not want to intellectualise it, to conceptualise it, sterilise it, take the edge off its sharpness. Suffering is something felt. I want to capture something of its mystery, its horror and indeed its beauty, for suffering awakens the self to its human plight and the possibilities for living.

My vision of palliative care is to ease suffering. First, I must enable people to find meaning in their suffering amidst the chaos of lives torn apart by life-threatening illness. Yet what is suffering and how does it manifest? How can I best ease suffering? Such questions are at the heart of caring and provide an inquisitive background to my narrative.

Box 3.1   World Health Organization definition of palliative care (2005).

An approach that improves the quality of life of patients and their families facing the problems associated with life-threatening illness, through the prevention and relief of suffering by means of early identification and impeccable assessment and treatment of pain and other problems, physical, psychosocial and spiritual.

Palliative care
- Provides relief from pain and other distressing symptoms
- Affirms life and regards dying as a normal process
- Intends neither to hasten or postpone death
- Integrates the psychological and spiritual aspects of patient care
- Offers a support system to help patients live as actively as possible until death
- Offers a support system to help the family cope during the patient's illness and in their own bereavement
- Uses a team approach to address the needs of patients and their families, including bereavement counselling if indicated
- Will enhance quality of life, and may also positively influence the course of illness
- Is applicable early in the course of illness, in conjunction with other therapies that are intended to prolong life, such as chemotherapy or radiation therapy, and includes those investigations needed to better understand and manage distressing complications

Box 3.2   The Four Noble Truths.

- The truth of suffering which we see all around us and also experience within ourselves
- The cause of suffering
- The cessation of suffering that leads to enlightenment
- The path that leads to the cessation of suffering

Buddhist influence

I am a Buddhist. As such, I am influenced by the Dharma or Buddhist philosophy and teachings. Easing suffering is at the heart of Buddhist practice enshrined within the Four Noble Truths, see Box 3.2 (Sangharakshita 1990).

The truth of suffering

The first Noble Truth is concerned with acknowledging the existence of suffering. This may seem obvious – especially working with people experiencing cancer and palliative care – but the idea of 'suffering' itself is rarely expressed in the caring literature. Acknowledging suffering is also to recognise my own suffering and the way this impinges on my practice. There is a synchronicity between my suffering and the other's. Indeed my practice can be viewed as a process of mutual growth; to ease the suffering of both self and other towards enlightenment. I cannot imagine a more appropriate vision to guide my practice. So simple, so powerful.

The cause of suffering

The second Noble Truth is concerned with knowing the cause of suffering. Whilst people's suffering may ripple on the surface of who they are, expressed in what they say or how they present themselves, the causes go much deeper into the very core of their being. As a therapist I need to read the surface signs and probe, tuning into who this person is. In doing so, I help the other person see themselves. This may be traumatic especially when the person faces or turns away from the reality of dying. It requires great sensitivity on my part. There can be no imposition of values or judgement but simply to tune in and flow with the other on their unfolding journey. It is being one with the person yet mindful of being separate. I appreciate that dying is a family affair and that the role of professionals is to find a place within the family that honours the primacy of the family. As Eifried (1998:33) notes:

> Patients are assisted in their search for meaning when nurses recognise patients' suffering and *stand alongside them* in response to the call to care.

Stand alongside them mirrors Heidegger's idea of 'dwelling consciousness', what Wheatley (1999:141) describes as *moving past cognition into a realm of sensation*. Wheatley notes:

> When we dwell with a group or a problem we move quietly into our senses, away from our sharpened analytical skills. Now I allow myself to pick up impressions, to notice how something feels, to sit with a group and call upon my intuition. I try to encourage myself and others to look for images, words, patterns that surface as we focus on an issue.

The nature of dwelling with a patient or family; quietly reading the signs, tuning into our senses and the surface patterns, exploring depth, moving within the complex unfolding whole towards harmony. I can define holistic practice as *the art of creating and holding space to dwell within and ease suffering*. To *dwell with* is to become one with, a fusing of spirits in mutual endeavour. The word *clearing* is appealing because it suggests a place free from the entanglement of the jungle, yet not separate from the jungle (as a metaphor for the world). A place of sanctuary.

The ease of suffering

The third Noble Truth acknowledges that suffering needs to be eased in order to grow and reach higher levels of consciousness, leading eventually to enlightenment. Suffering is a mystery and, as such, my response to it is essentially intuitive. How could it be otherwise? Whether patients and families overtly express it or not, an existential or spiritual need is always present in palliative care simply because these people face death. It behoves the practitioner, whether doctor, complementary therapist or nurse, to be mindful of this need and create the space where such need can be honoured and dwelt with.

Whilst I may have dwelt with many people who face death I know I can never truly empathise with their predicament. As the narrative reveals, I have tried to put myself there, in their shoes facing their death. Yet such knowing is elusive, perhaps impossible. I ask myself – 'how would I feel faced with the certainty of my immediate death?' What would I think? Of course I can specu-late. I sense a ripple of fear but beyond that I cannot tell. And so, with people facing death I must learn to be mindful of who I am. Mindful of being open to the possibilities; mindful of my own stuff so I can dwell with them with compassion, and without intrusion, without imposition, and without fear. Only by being mindful can I be wise, to *not know* and see everything as it is rather than as a projection of my previous knowing. Being mindful is having faith, and the narrative is a journey of finding and exploring faith.

> Whatever takes us to our edge, to our outer limits, leads us to the heart of life's mystery, and there we find faith. In the process, however, we may have to confront many old habits.
>
> (Salzberg 2002:92)

In *confronting old habits* I must be self-aware to go deep inside in order to understand my reality and the journey I need to make in order to realise my vision. Along this path will be many boulders that must be confronted and shifted in order to move on. As Rachel Reiman (1996:70) says:

> Whatever we have denied may stop us and dam the creative flow of our lives . . . avoiding pain, we may linger in the vicinity of our wounds . . . without reclaiming that which we have denied, we cannot know our wholeness or have our healing.

This is not easy work. I may need some guidance.

The path that leads to the cessation of suffering

The fourth Noble Truth can be realised by following The Noble Eight-Fold Path to ease suffering (see Figure 3.2). The entrance to the path is the realisa-tion of suffering for whatever reason. People suffer, feeling:

> That something is not quite right, not quite enough. So we are always trying to feel the gap, to make things right, to find that extra bit of pleasure or security . . . if we enjoy pleasure we are afraid to lose it, we strive for more pleasure or try to contain it. If we suffer pain we want to escape it. We experience dissatisfaction all the time.
>
> (Chogyam Trungpa 2002:152)

Dying often brings to the surface reflections on the past, unresolved con-flicts, guilt, unfulfilled dreams, cutting across the taken-for-grantedness of life to challenge people's sense of immortality, that induces fear and insecurity besides obvious physical discomfort. It is a similar story for relatives. What does it mean to die well? Is that a valid focus for palliative care? If so, the suffering of the other is the primary focus for care when the point of cure has passed.

Each step of the Noble Eight-Fold Path guides the practitioner to ease suffer-ing. My descriptions of the steps are adapted from an earlier interpretation (Johns 2005) to make them more accessible and relevant to clinical practice

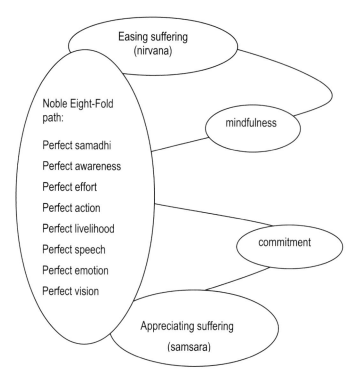

Figure 3.2   The Noble Eight-Fold Path.

(Figure 3.3). Whilst offered as a series of steps, in reality they are woven into a pattern that gathers momentum along the path, commencing with vision and intentionality to realise the vision. Each step, with the exception of perfect action, relates to attributes of the individual practitioner, acknowledging that it is 'who I am' as a person, as a practitioner, that has the greatest impact on my ability to ease suffering within my caring relationships. In practical terms the heart of the Noble Eight-Fold Path is perfect action – it represents what practitioners actually do. The way they do it is influenced by the other steps.

The Noble Eight-Fold Path is a reflective model that guides me toward easing suffering. In doing so it is also my path of spiritual growth. By spiritual, I refer to the idea of cultivating self-awareness so that we become more mindful of our choices to act for the good. Again Nagapriya (2004:47) says:

> The spiritual life involves becoming more and more aware of the choices we make, how we make those choices, *moment by moment*, and changing them in the light of our best values. (my italics)

Whilst the Noble Eight-Fold Path offers me a path to ease suffering, I am mindful not to impose Buddhism on the other person. I assume this is no different for other practitioners who have a strong faith or no faith. The early hospice movement in the UK was driven by a strong Christian ethos that has, in my view, become diminished with the growth of palliative medicine as a

Perfect samadhi	Where both self and the other person transcend suffering to experience higher levels of consciousness and spiritual realisation.
Perfect awareness	I interpret awareness as being mindful. Being mindful percolates through each of the steps besides being acknowledged as a step in its own right, when being mindful is fully realised. It is knowing self within each unfolding moment whilst keeping one's vision of easing suffering in sharp focus.
Perfect effort	Being mindful that my practice requires effort, patience, commitment and diligence despite any difficulty; there can be no scope for complacency.
Perfect livelihood	I like to interpret this step as virtue; being a good person, committed to peace and harmony in the world. In the narrative, I often refer to this step as 'riding the windhorse'.
Perfect action	The wisdom to make good judgements and respond with appropriate and skilful action to ease suffering.
Perfect speech	Being mindful of speaking in ways that are truthful, affectionate, nurturing and which promote harmony within the world.
Perfect emotion	Being mindful of how I am feeling, and to cultivate positive emotions and overcome negative emotions and attitudes. It is fundamental to the ideal of caring, such qualities as giving, compassion, joy in the other's success, equanimity, and faith – perhaps interpreted as a feeling of something sacred.
Perfect vision	Being mindful of the intention to understand and ease suffering and guide the person to transcend suffering towards enlightenment.

Figure 3.3   The steps of the Noble Eight-Fold Path.

specialisation. The triumph of science over religion. Indeed, any 'faith' might now be considered an imposition.

Compassion

Compassion is an elusive concept to grasp. It is a state of being beyond the mind, something felt rather than thought. It is healing energy and possibly my most vital attribute as a practitioner. It vibrates through the narrative with a fervent intensity. Compassion is unconditional love towards easing the suffering of the other. Such compassion is healing energy.

'Learn to look at other beings with the eyes of compassion' is a quote from the Lotus Sutra chapter on Avalokiteshvara. You might like to write this down and put it in your sitting room.

(Thich Nhat Hanh 1987:94)

Well, I accept Thich's invitation to write these words in this book because I can't begin to ease suffering if I am not a genuinely compassionate person. To say I am compassionate is an easy thing to say. Yet in practice it is more difficult when the precious ego and craving for attachment are lurking to distract me.

Sister M Simone Roach (1992:58) describes compassion as:

A way of living born out of an awareness of one's relationship to all living creatures; engendering a response of participation in the experience of the other; a sensitivity to the pain and brokenness of the other; a quality of presence which allows one to share with and make room for the other.

The brokenness of the other – such a poetic description of suffering. And it does seem to me that cancer does break people. Yet somehow words and theories seem inadequate to express the nature of love or compassion. It is not a technique to apply or a concept to grasp, but something from deep within the practitioner, a potential within each of us waiting like the sun behind a dark cloud to shine and radiate its beauty and warmth and fuel our caring quest. Yet it may be difficult to act with compassion in an uncaring world.

Without love the world is a wilderness and caring desolate. Genuine compassion is unconditional in that it has no boundaries. It is always open and generous, a gift to the one suffering that asks for nothing in return. How difficult that can be! How can love or compassion be revealed and nurtured as caring energy? Such questions must be at the heart of caring practice. Certainly it requires equanimity so I am in harmony with myself, others and the cosmos, and my vigilance for any resistance to the other person for whatever reason.

In writing myself as compassionate, factors that enhance or blunt my compassion are revealed. To be compassionate is to be mindful. Compassion has a natural flow yet is not something that can be taken for granted for it always has a shadow side of hatred. Compassion is also a collective energy. Being with compassionate people nurtures my compassion. Just spending a few moments at the shift report reading a poem or remembering a patient who has died are powerful reminders of the compassionate and spiritual nature of palliative care. I needn't say palliative – compassion is vital for all practitioners no matter where they practise. Yet, strangely, the word compassion is missing from the Nursing and Midwifery Council: Code of Professional Conduct (2002:3). The code states:

> You have a duty of care to your patients and clients, who are entitled to receive safe and competent care.

What difference would it make to state *receive safe, competent and* **compassionate** *care*? Would such an expectation lead to a romanticism of nursing that is striving to be more objective? Would explicitly stating compassion within the Code lead to inevitable failure and create a collective guilt? Yet, compassion is the natural response to the vulnerability of the other person. It *is* caring. It is an ethical demand (Hem & Heggen 2003). Do I *really* care for this person, warts and all?

Compassion and concern are interchangeable. Simply put, the more concerned I am for you, the more available I am to you. I pay attention to you because you matter to me. The Danish philosopher Knud Ejler Logstrup captures this attitude profoundly (1997:18):

> By our very attitude to one another we help to shape one another's world. By our attitude to the other person we help to determine the scope and hue of his or her world; we make it large and small, bright or drab, rich or dull, threatening or secure. We help to shape his or her world not by theories and views but by our very attitude toward him or her. Herein lies the unarticulated and one might say anonymous demand that we take care of the life which trust has placed in our hands.

However, no one has the right to make him or herself the master of another person's individuality or will. Neither good intentions, insight into what is best for him or her, nor even the possibility of saving him or her from great calamities which would otherwise strike him or her can justify intrusion upon his or her individuality and will.

Pause and dwell in the stillness of Logstrup's words. Do these words inspire? Does your practice reflect these beliefs? The idea that compassion is not possessive is profound. To be compassionate is to be non-attached to the other person. This may seem a paradox because logic suggests that the more compassionate I am the more attached I am likely to be.

In Buddhism a *Bodhisattva* is someone who is committed to helping others ease suffering and learn through the illness experience. Of the many qualities attributed to being a Bodhisattva, it is the balance of compassion and wisdom. Compassion sets the ground for wisdom. The wise person is mindful in approaching every situation from a perspective of not knowing so as to be open to the possibility of the moment. In a world of science governed by the need to know and control, this can be difficult. However, the wise person is in no doubt as to their vision of practice, and responds with purpose, generosity, patience, certainty and joyous energy to guide people to overcome suffering These attributes of the Bodhisattva are called the *paramitas* (Trungpa 2002, Sangahrakshita 1979).

The wise person sets aside their own concerns in order to see and connect with the experience of the other, rather than see the person through a lens of self-interest. I am very conscious of projecting my presence into the situation, so the other person can feel my compassion and feel cared for. In other words I intend to touch the person with my caring presence.

The greatest gift we can offer anyone is our true presence.

(Thich Nhat Hanh 2005)

As I go about my practice I touch people in different ways. I assume that touch is a vital part of healing, not just physical touch but also the sense of touching someone in an emotional or spiritual way. As a complementary therapist I use my hands in a very deliberative way. As a nurse I also use my hands but less deliberatively. In Paramananda's words (2001:37):

My hands are invoked as a symbol of connectedness, a reaching out to others.

Paramananda continues:

The importance of coming into full relationship with ourselves is that it is through being fully aware of ourselves that we begin to have a real sense of our relationship with others and with life in general.

Knowing the person

The stories in the narrative reveal how I get to know someone and develop relationship. To know someone is a mystery waiting to unfold. The key to knowing the person is to *listen* to the person's story. Coles (1989, cited by Bochner 2001:132) says:

> The people who come to us bring us their stories. They hope they tell them well enough so that we understand the truth of their lives. They hope we know how to interpret their stories correctly. We have to remember that what we hear is their story.

In knowing the person, I have to know myself. I bring to the encounter my own background; the meanings, experiences, expectations, and uncertainties. To listen well I must set my stuff aside in order to hear the patient's perspectives and meanings.

Listening, I ask myself – Who is this person? What meanings does this person give to their experience of dying? What does this person's family feel and think? The reflective cues (page 14) guide me to tune into the person's wavelength and flow with them on their dying journey. Without doubt, appreciating the meaning people give to their health–illness experience is the most vital aspect of knowing a person simply because it provides the foundation for care. In response to my concern, the person reveals who they are, not just to me, but to themselves. As the practitioner listens, she or he picks up and probes signs that lead to deeper revelation. Such revelation is often cathartic. It requires great sensitivity, for delving into the mysterious void is unpredictable and may bring to the surface untapped emotions. This has been most powerful with spouses of men who are dying. This emerges as such a vital aspect of care; supporting someone as they face up to who they are right now, as death begins to unwrap her tentacles. It is to touch their spirit.

Sometimes the people I meet are close to death and unable to talk to me about their lives and their thoughts about dying. Relatives or other practitioners will tell me bits about the person. Sometimes I have no words and so I must sense who the person is by reading non-verbal signs and by moving my hands over the person's energy field to scan the signs that tune me into the person's wavelength and to read the unspoken pattern.

Knowing a person is empathic and imaginative . . . what must it be like for that person? What must it be like to die? It is an astonishing question to consider. I often imagined dying as I sought to get alongside the person, to feel their wavelength, but it is never easy. I sense death is momentous and would want my carers to acknowledge this momentousness. Without doubt, I have learnt that caring for people who are dying demands utter reverence.

Getting to know the person is caring. It is not a prelude, like assessment, before caring. It is not a task to be done. Rather, it is a continuous, unfolding, spiritual process of finding and flowing with the other's wavelength and provides the basis for appropriate response to help the person and their family know and meet their health-illness needs.

The medical model approach is focused to know the person from the perspective of recognising and investigating the 'symptoms', diagnosis and curative treatment. The person is reduced into systems and the status of a patient, an object to be manipulated. The risk is to lose sight of the whole person. Recently Susan, my partner, had an ear operation. The nurse 'admitting' her asked her a number of questions written on the assessment form. The nurse actually had her back to Susan as she asked and wrote the answers down. We were amazed at such practice. The questions were perfunctory as if Susan was merely some object being processed. But does it matter? Do people want to feel cared for? Ask yourself these questions.

The holistic approach is very different from expecting the person to fit into a normative and authoritative wavelength characteristic of the medical model. Indeed patients are often concerned to 'learn the ropes' and 'fit-in' in order to be accepted as 'good 'patients (Stockwell 1972, Johnson and Webb 1995). Hence, a distinction can be made between a holistic model whereby the practitioner seeks to tune into the patient's wavelength and a medical model system whereby the patient is expected to fit into healthcare norms. The medical model wavelength can be represented by a straight line to symbolise how the person's individuality and the uniqueness of situation is *ironed* to fit within the norms of the medical model with its emphasis on reduction of the person into symptom management.

The blankness, anonymity, conformity of a straight line. A risk is that the practitioner's own individuality is also ironed out to ensure conformity with little scope for autonomy, creativity and holistic practice. Such contradiction is demoralising for both the patient and the practitioner. Wilber (1998) describes this is as 'flatland' – whereby the human element of I and WE is subtly reduced into the IT of scientific gaze. Welcome to the matrix!

The aesthetic response

Aesthetic Gk. Aisthetikos – things perceptible by the senses
Anaesthetic Gk. Anaisthetikos – numb, without feeling

(Tufnell & Crickmay 2004:41)

My aesthetic response; feeling, interpreting, and responding to the situation reflected in my movement, my performance. Caring practice is a dance, a performance, movement of purpose and grace. My quest is to learn to dance expertly in helping the patient find rhythm and purpose in their step.

Patricia Benner et al. (1996) throw light on the nature of expertise:

The non-conscious holistic discrimination of the patient's state and fluid, skilful response, with little evidence of rational calculation, is characteristic of expert clinical judgement.

Knowing how to respond within the complex and indeterminate situations of clinical practice always requires intuitive interpretation. There are no universal solutions that can be applied. To imagine such solutions did exist would be an anaesthetic response. There can be no prescription without reducing the human encounter into a mechanical problem to be solved. I would become a technician and the patient an object to be manipulated towards specific outcomes. The risk is that an emphasis on 'the problem' diminishes the personhood of the patient and may increase rather than ease suffering, what Frank (2002) describes as de-moralisation in contrast with re-moralisation that ensues through caring presence (Johns 2004a:131).

We might hold a tentative local theory of a situation based on knowing the person, past experiences and theoretical ideas of issues within the situation, yet even such local theory would need to be interpreted for its significance to inform the particular situation. Note – to inform not to prescribe!

The work of Benner, Tanner and Chesla (1996) is, in my view, a benchmark for knowing and developing expert practice along a continuum from novice to expert based on the Dreyfus and Dreyfus (1996) model of skill acquisition. In this model, six interwoven aspects of expert clinical judgement can be discerned which offer a model for reflecting on my expertise within any clinical situation:

I can ask myself to what extent:

- Did I approach the situation to ease suffering?
- Had I tuned into the patient's wavelength and appreciated their story?
- Did I appreciate the unfolding pattern of their situation linked to past experiences?
- Was I mindful of my emotional involvement?
- In what way did I respond intuitively?
- Have I checked out the whole situation and my effectiveness within it?

Each aspect is vital within the whole pattern of clinical judgement, especially in complex and indeterminate situations that characterise Schön's (1987) metaphor of the *swampy lowlands* of everyday clinical practice. Every situation is a mystery when seen as a unique human encounter. The idea of mystery reflects the significance of intuition, that somehow I do know how to respond. If uncertain, I can experiment drawing on my tacit knowing. As Delmar comments (2004:9):

> When experiences are to placed at risk, the nurse must develop a special kind of attentiveness. The nurse must be open in order to sense the patient and to obtain a sense of what the situation requires. This demands a clarification of what a situation really is. Is the situation always unique or will there also be something typical about it? After all, there is always something unique and some typical feature of the patients who enter into situations.

The typical features are known through experience of many previous experiences. Yet experience can lull the mind into complacency, thinking it knows that can lead practitioners into repetitive and habitual patterns of response. Being mindful, I am conscious I have a certain style but that I can never predict, at least for certain, the way I might respond. Reflection as a learning process is both conscious and subliminal, sharpening my perception, honing my aesthetic response.

Knowing and managing self within relationship

The narrative is my journey of coming to know self within relationship with patients, families and with colleagues. Only in relationship can I know myself. In my experience, 'knowing self' is neglected work. For example, no emphasis was given to the development and sustaining of self during my complementary therapy training. The emphasis was on technique within a stance of professionalism. The word *professional* is often used as a barrier to retreat behind to keep distance from or detachment from the patient. Menzies-Lyth (1988:51/54) commented (in context of her work on defence mechanisms against anxiety within institutions):

> The core of the anxiety situation for the nurse lies in her relationship with the patient. The closer and more concentrated this relationship, the more the nurse is likely to experience this anxiety . . . a necessary psychological task for the entrant into any profession is *the development of adequate professional detachment*. (my italics)

From a holistic perspective, *detachment* is an inadequate response to the person's suffering. Indeed such indifference would heighten rather than ease the patient's suffering. It follows that if healthcare practitioners want to be holistic then they need to learn to embrace and survive intimacy rather than resist it because it is painful at times. Perhaps Menzies-Lyth should say *the development of an intimate personal involvement*?

In easing the suffering of the other do I also suffer? Perhaps I do, yet suffering tells me I am human. The narrative throws light on the nature of the human-human encounter. Nåden and Eriksson (2002:35) identified encounter as a fundamental category of nursing as an art. They describe encounter as:

> 'Nakedness', deep solidarity and closeness, being on the same wavelength, and giving oneself over.

I prefer *vulnerability* to nakedness. The patient is vulnerable in revealing self, and gives self over in trust. In response, I too must make myself vulnerable and give myself over in the demand to care. Deep solidarity is intimacy that brings comfort for our anxiety. Even though I am vulnerable to such suffering I know it is not my suffering. I suspect the natural instinct is to protect self from one's vulnerability. Noddings (1984) noted practitioners' sense of being overwhelmed, resulting in feelings of guilt and conflict that were 'the inescapable risks of caring'.

Benner and Wrubel (1989) claim it is the *loss of caring* that causes burn-out, not caring itself. Through reflection, I am reconnected to caring. My anxieties are expressed and worked out. My resistance to relationship is confronted. The joy of realising caring melts anxiety. Rather than defend against such anxiety, I am mindful to recognise the pattern of anxiety and learn to manage the anxiety and any resultant resistance to the person, i.e. not to project my suffering onto others. Mindfulness is a protective bubble without diminishing intimacy. Being mindful enables me to see things for what they are before they penetrate and overwhelm.

Creating and sustaining an environment where it is possible to be available

My relationship with patients, with families and with colleagues exists within an organisational context that can be symbolised as a circle inside a square:

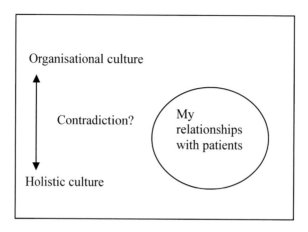

I shall (not unreasonably) assume the organisational culture is primarily concerned with ensuring that practitioners like myself can realise desirable practice. However, this is not a passive relationship. My responsibility is to actively work toward creating an organisational culture that fully supports my practice. To do so I must appreciate the organisational culture and work towards resolving any organisational contradiction that constrains the realisation of holistic practice. From the perspective of *team learning* practitioners across practice disciplines would work in harmony and collaboration toward realising their *mutual* vision of holistic practice. Conflict would be dealt with assertively with respect. Leadership would be transformational to realise the optimal caring environment based on the power of collaborative relationship and expertise in contrast with power based on position and the threats of sanction and promise of reward.

So why is it rarely like that? Why is it practitioners get embroiled in unresolved conflict, harbour anger, guilt and frustration? In the face of a growing medical dominance the nursing voice at the hospice has become increasingly disempowered. Fifteen years ago, when the hospice was opened, it had strong nursing leadership that valued holistic practice . . .

> But now medical directors walk the floor
> The nursing voice no more
> than a faint whisper
> pleading cause
> that caring is something beyond the 'symptom',
> Something less easily known,
> A mystery even,
> Where suffering tolls the bell
> A place where we need to dwell
> and hold the other's hand
> as they stumble around the crater's edge.

My poem reflects the passivity of the nursing voice to assert holistic *practice*. The growth of specialist palliative care has eroded nurses' autonomy as doctors at the hospice claim authority for decision making. Psychologists compete for psychological care, chaplains for spiritual care. Whose responsibility is it to give a hand massage? As symptom management fragments the person, so specialists emerge in response to fragment the delivery of care. It is all very well having the knowledge to make effective judgements and respond appropriately with skilful action, yet do I have the autonomy and authority to act?

Summary

I have set out my holistic vision structured through Buddhist beliefs on suffering and the Being Available Template that offers the reader a framework to reflect on the reflexive development of my holistic practice through *The heron & the tree* narrative.

Chapter 4

Exploring narrative dialogue

In chapters 1–3 I set out my background of reflective and holistic practice. In chapters 4 and 5, I set out my narrative approach to *The heron & the tree*.

Guided reflection is a journey of self-inquiry and transformation for practitioners like myself, to realise desirable practice as a lived reality. The journey is written as a narrative that reveals the transformative drama unfolding. Along the journey, the vision of desirable practice is constantly explored and shifting as new understandings emerge. Barriers to realisation along the journey's path are confronted and action taken towards overcoming them.

At the core of narrative is dialogue:

> Dialogue requires careful listening . . . it requires people to be critically conscious of their own thinking so this does not corrupt the effort to find true meaning. Bohm (1996) calls this proprioception of thought in much the same way that the body is aware of itself in space.

(Johns 2002:33)

Constructing narrative can be viewed as six layers of dialogue that are being constantly woven into the coherent narrative pattern:

(1) Dialogue with self (written in a journal or spoken) as a 'naïve' or spontaneous *story* (that reflects dialogue with persons and self within the story itself)
(2) Dialogue with the story (written in a reflective journal) as an objective and disciplined process (using a model of reflection) to produce a *text*
(3) Dialogue between the *text* with other sources of knowing in order to frame understandings emerging from the text within the wider community of knowing (theoretical framing)
(4) Dialogue between the text's author and a guide(s) to develop and deepen insights
(5) Dialogue within the emerging text to deepen insights and weave the narrative into a coherent and reflexive pattern of form that adequately plots the unfolding journey
(6) Dialogue between the narrative and the curious narrative reader responding to the invitation to dialogue

The first four levels of dialogue are dynamic movements towards patterning the narrative. Each idea within the whole pattern slowly emerges and ripens until it is transformed through the weaving dialogue into its potential narrative form rather like pieces of a complex jigsaw. The narrative is then presented to the reader where a further level of dialogue is invited to challenge and deepen insights. Hence narrative is never completely formed. It is always evolving through dialogue.

But first, I must bring myself into a suitable frame of mind to reflect.

Dialogue with self

Bringing the mind home

> We are fragmented into so many different aspects. We don't know who we really are, or what aspects of ourselves we should identify with or believe in. So many contradictory voices, dictates, and feelings fight for control over our inner lives that we find ourselves scattered everywhere, in all directions, leaving nobody at home. Meditation then helps to bring the mind home.
>
> (Rinpoche 1992:59)

The truth of these words hits people after they have spent just a few minutes relaxation through breath work. It takes practice first and then reflection to realise this simply because we are so used to being fragmented. Through my own meditation practice I came to directly experience the value of bringing the distracted mind home. Senge (1990) recognises the value of meditative practices in developing personal mastery to deepening the rapport between normal awareness and the subconscious.

Reflection is about creating a still point within self and yet a prerequisite of reflection might be creating a still point in order to reflect. Easy? In theory yes, but in practice no, despite the apparent simplicity of breath work. That who we truly are is a mystery and potentially terrifying feels astonishing. People may actually seek distraction simply because they don't have to look in. I know that silence in particular can feel very uncomfortable and make people feel very self-conscious. Rinpoche (1992:74) guides me:

> So, have a spacious, open and compassionate attitude towards your thoughts and emotions. When we do not intrinsically understand what they are then your thoughts become the seeds of confusion. Before them be like a wise old man watching a child play.

Before them be like a wise old man watching a child play dramatically captures the reflective posture. Often people say to me that thoughts rush into the stillness and they can't concentrate on their breath. Rinpoche's words help to alleviate the need to control the breath by seeing it as a process rather than an outcome. So when thoughts come, pay them attention, be tolerant of them like a wise old man, notice their content and they will melt away. Use the line – breathing in, I calm my mind, to return to the breath.

It is as if the body is addicted to its thoughts. It has to learn to be different and this is only possible through discipline. I encourage students to write their reflective journals daily and perhaps spend the first five minutes 'bringing the mind home'. Slowly, we learn to cultivate the sense of stillness and through reflection liberate the habits and open to the possibilities for holistic practice. For, without doubt, it is vital that we know and manage ourselves to practice from a holistic perspective.

I use breath work with students before commencing a reflective practice session in much the same way that I use breath work with patients prior to therapy to bring people into a place of stillness where they can let go of the attachment to the body, the mind, to anything. In doing so, I open a space where learning and healing can take place; a sacred space both inside self and in physical space; to create a sense of reverence for the sharing of stories that I feel is significant given the profound nature of their stories. Bringing the mind home is finding the still point within as the essential ground for reflection.

Finding the still point

I wrote the following poem for the annual reflective practice conference held in Amsterdam in 2001.

Finding the stillness within

There is a point of stillness
beyond the grasping ache of everyday
that I can rest within.

A point of stillness
where the layers of concern can fall away
to reveal the clarity of heart and mind.

A point of stillness
from the rushing river that sweeps me
headlong in chaotic frenzy.

A point of stillness
between the pulse of each heart beat
between each aching thought.

A point of stillness deep within me
where I can reflect and see things for
    what they are;
to see myself for who I am.

A point of stillness
beyond the rational demand
and the ego's clinging pull.

A point of stillness
where I am free to reveal my authentic self;
to shed the cloaks that mask.

A point of stillness
where I make sense of the chaotic frenzy
and surf the stormy waves.

A point of stillness
where I nurture my compassion from the
    flames of guilt, anger, despair
that distort my mind and darken my spirit.

A point of stillness
where I can honour my experience
where I can honour myself as caring.

A point of stillness
where the mysteries of my practice
    are revealed,
my limitations no longer concealed.

A point of stillness
where I nurture my resolve to
    move beyond
to realise my caring self.

A point of stillness
within each unfolding moment
where 'who I am' is present for all
    to see.

Beyond the point of stillness is
    a white light
reflected through a prism of
    dazzling colours
revealing my beauty deep within.

And if I close my eyes
and let go of attachment to my
    thoughts
and release my compassionate self
I hurtle towards this light
and dissolve in its radiance.

A point of stillness lies within each of you
within reach of you;
It is the essential ground of reflection.

Doodles in my journal: revealing the storied self

The first layer of dialogue is a dialogue with self to write or tell the story.

As I sit at the computer I wonder: How do I write this part of the text? How I do write my stories? Remembering a moment . . . the look on her face, a word said, a tear, the feeling I feel inside, a sad smile, the smell of curry, a picture on the wall, the dance of the trees outside the window . . . so many signs to trigger my story. Reflection is awakening to self . . .

Knowing I am going to write a story prompts me to be mindful, pay more attention to what is unfolding moment to moment within practice. It always seems remarkable how much detail the body absorbs. To write I find a quiet eddy out of the fast current of life, to pause, muse, to clear and let go of the mind and open the body to pay attention to the experience, to create a space where I can get back into the experience with all my senses.

One evening after a shift at the hospice I wrote in my journal:

> *Entering the four-bedded ward I notice that Veronica had no visitors again this afternoon. I sit with her and say 'Hello Veronica, it's Chris the nurse'. Veronica has been blind since September as a consequence of her brain tumour. I wonder what she thinks, lying here alone in the hospice knowing she is dying. I ask if she would like me to massage her hands. She consents but only if I'm not too busy. So typical of her . . . always thinking of others and making no demands for herself. I sense the other women in the ward are watching me . . . I sense they are waiting for their turn for my attention . . . that's always one of the problems of entering the ward not that I had deliberately gone in there to see Veronica . . . Just that she caught my attention being alone . . .*
>
> *I hear one woman say to her relatives 'he's a complementary therapist . . .' As I leave, I smile at the other two women, they both have relatives . . . they all look at me with interest . . .'*

I tend to write my journal in a factual way to recapture the moment, usually straight onto the computer, sometimes referring to notes scribbled earlier in my journal, scribbled words that capture words spoken. I prefer to write in the present tense to better capture the moment. I like the computer because I can move words around as I seek to find the flow between words. But first just let the words come as a spontaneous flow in rich description, paying attention to as much detail as possible, pursuing signs, running off on tangents. At a recent workshop I asked people to write for 10 minutes without taking the pen off the paper . . . The time limit is a good idea because it creates a rush . . . no time to think.

When we conversed about the experience of writing, one person said she had not yet got to the point of the experience. She, like so many other particip-ants, was astonished with the amount she had written. Revealing the storied self. Putting together the pieces of self, of life itself. A creative, restorative act.

> We come to know more of what matters in our lives, less through an in-tuned search for self, than in conversation, in relationship to what is around us. We rarely know what currents flow beneath what we are doing and feeling. The impulses, instincts and intuitions that impel our thoughts and actions are as animals moving in the shadows of our everyday awareness. As we create we discover events, characters, places, sights and sounds, whose significance we cannot quite define, yet whose presence makes more visible what is moving through our lives. Creating is a way of listening and of trying to speak more personally from within the various worlds we

inhabit. It is a way of discovering our own stories, refreshing and reawakening our language and giving form to the way we feel.

(Tufnell & Crickmay 2004:41)

I know practitioners who find journal writing easy and natural, whilst others struggle to express their experience – especially in written form – as if some censor is at work in their minds limiting their potential. If you have never written about self before it may feel strange, even threatening. The mirror is not always kind, especially if we create false impressions of ourselves. Hence writing requires effort, honesty, and perseverance. It also requires meaning, that writing is a movement towards something worthwhile.

> Reflective practice is part of the way I work with others in my nursing practice. Journaling is both a professional and personal way of making sense of everyday living. It may be called a journey to wholeness and well-being. It is the process of journaling that is by far the most significant act in my practice, for it records the process of my evolving as a human being and connects me with the other in my nursing relationship; it is a journey from the 'I' to the 'we', the consciousness of the collective soul journey of each human being. The journey begins with the self, *the awakening to the self*, in relation to the spiritual path each of us is destined to follow.

(Gully 2005:151, my italics)

Resistance to writing about self is resistance to self. Writing is confrontational and begins to loosen the self from its ego bondage. It is much more than a cognitive exercise of recall. It is as if I seek to dwell within the situation as a witness. In this way I tap into the right side of my brain and stir the centres for imagination, creativity, perception, intuition. These qualities of self are not just useful for reflection but are also pivotal in developing clinical expertise.

Reflections can be expressed as painting, poems, dance and movement, photographs. . . . I rarely use painting in my own reflections except in art workshops, although I do find myself writing more poetry, as if poetry enables me to touch the essence of the experience in few words.

At the workshop I asked people to use art-form as a reflective medium. One woman said she couldn't paint and had never written a poem. Earlier she had written a reflective account, so I suggested she broke her description into lines as a sort of prose poem. I did this with Veronica's description.

Veronica tucked away in the corner,
no visitors again this afternoon
blind, yet what does she sense
as she approaches death?
What does she see in the darkness?
Perhaps childhood memories?
Or bright lights of spent romance?
Or perhaps regret?
Perhaps I should ask or would I intrude?
I sit with her.
A touch of sadness stirs within
Yet smiled away in the moment.
'Shall I massage your hands,
Play you some music?'

She turns her head towards me
A faint smile
As she fold her hand over mine
'Only if you aren't too busy'.
Her spirit glows
And lifts me beyond the throws
    of sadness
As my hands respond to ease
    her.
Even as she dies
she turns her thoughts to others
makes no demand for herself,
So easy to pass by.
She takes me to my still point.

Rewriting my experience with Veronica as a poem is a creative and imaginative response to my experience. Words seem to emerge and flow from a spiritual source of creation that opens up the words, moving me into a more reflective mode than description. New images emerge as the imagination is stirred. In particular, I pay attention to how I was feeling, reflecting the way writing poems stirs the senses. Lei, one of my students, reflected on the way his painting had revealed so much about himself that normally he wouldn't reveal. He felt both vulnerable and elated at his revelation, surprised that his painting could be so revealing and cathartic. It seems as if our bodies hold dark secrets that can only find expression through the imagination, bypassing the censoring ego. Perhaps artists and art therapists know this well. The work of Michele Angelo Petrone, who painted his own *Emotional Cancer Journey* (2003) and worked with others to express their cancer stories through art in *Touching the Rainbow* (1999), inspires me to develop reflective practice through art, just as Miranda Tufnell's work *The Widening Field* (2004) inspires me to explore movement as an expression of reflection.

The poem captures something of the beauty, mystery and tragedy of caring, its light and its shadow. I wrote the poem *The heron & the tree* (page 86) one evening to honour my relationship with Jackie after she died in the hospice. We had often gazed out of the window of her hospice bedroom at the bronze metal heron and the small Japanese maple tree in the garden. They seemed to accompany us on our journey as Jackie slowly descended into death.

I am sometimes challenged – 'isn't it "soft" to write poems?' but such prejudice reflects ignorance grounded in left brain dominance that rejects the professional's expression of poetry. Writing narrative naturally challenges accepted ways of writing 'professional text'. I want to begin using paintings and photographs, perhaps collages in my narratives, even dance, to capture more exquisitely the passion, the beauty, the horror of my experience. What I write is a *text* for a deeper, more objective and critical dialogue with self.

Dialogue with the story text

I pause from my writing. Description is exhausted. I can say no more, at least for the moment. In front of me is my 'story text'. I step back from the text in order to see it more clearly, to bring it into a more objective focus. Curious, I can now ask questions of my text, to pull it open for its significance and meaning, to expose contradiction between my practice and my vision of desirable practice and open up the learning space. More words from Tufnell and Crickmay (2004:41) – these authors nurture me, encouraging me to find expression for my own language.

> Creating becomes a conversation when we enter into a dialogue with whatever we are doing. In this conversation we are drawn along in the moment by moment flow of sensation, interchange and choice, rather than following a predetermined intention or idea. Conversations grow as we listen and explore – a constantly shifting process of discovery that changes in momentum, rhythm, clarity or chaos as we work.

Reflective cue	MSR map*
Bring the mind home	
Focus on a description of an experience that seems significant in some way	Aesthetics
What particular issues seem significant to pay attention to?	Aesthetics
How were others feeling and why did they feel that way?	Aesthetics*
How was I feeling and why did I feel that way?	Personal
What was I trying to achieve and did I respond effectively?	Aesthetics
What were the consequences of my actions on the patient, others and myself?	Aesthetics
What factors influence the way I was/am feeling, thinking and responding to this situation?	Personal*
(personal, organisational, professional, cultural)	
What knowledge did or might have informed me?	Empirics
To what extent did I act for the best and in tune with my values?	Ethics
How does this situation connect with previous experiences?	Personal/ Reflexivity*
Given the situation again, how might I respond differently?	Reflexivity*
What would be the consequences of responding in new ways for the patient, others and myself?	Reflexivity*
What factors might constrain me from responding in new ways?*	Personal *
How do I NOW feel about this experience?	Personal *
Am I able to support myself and others better as a consequence?	Reflexivity
What insights have I gained? *(framing perspectives)*	Reflexivity
Am I more able to realise desirable practice? *(Being Available Template)**	
What have I learnt through reflecting?	

* changes from the 14th edition

Figure 4.1   Model for Structured Reflection (15th edition).

Model for Structured Reflection (MSR)

To guide my questions, I can use a model for reflection of which I can find many 'on the market' that offer practitioners a systematic mode of reflective inquiry located in the reflective practice manuals. I use the cues set out in the Model for Structured Reflection (MSR). These cues are internalised and used naturally over time. The MSR was first constructed in 1991 through analysing the pattern of dialogue between practitioners and guides in guided reflection (Johns 1998). The 15th edition (Figure 4.1) reflects my constant effort over the years to refine it as a more adequate guide to reflect on practice.

Drawing out significance

Bringing the mind home, I can better pay attention to the text and pull out from the text those issues that seem significant. Whilst I pay attention to all experience, what is significant in my encounter with Veronica? Initially I sense that my encounter with Veronica was spiritual – that easing suffering is fundamentally a spiritual encounter for both of us – that giving therapy is always spiritual, reflected in such words as *she brought me to my still point*.

Yet, what else is significant? I am caught by the idea of Veronica being alone.

In *The Powerbook*, Jeannette Winterson (2001:103) captures the intention to pull out from the big screen (the story text) meaning:

There are so many lives packed into one. The one life we think we know is only the window that is open on the screen. The big window full of detail, where the meaning is often lost among the facts.

   If we can close that window, on purpose or by chance, what we find is another view.

   This window is emptier. The cross-references are cryptic. As we scroll down it, looking for something familiar, we seem to be scrolling into another self – one we recognise but cannot place. The co-ordinates are missing, or the co-ordinates pinpoint us outside the limits of our existence.

   If we move further back, through a smaller window that is really a gateway, there is less and less to measure ourselves by. We are coming into a dark region. A single word might appear. An icon.

If we can close that window . . . for me this involves seeing with soft eyes rather than hard eyes tuned to search for what I expect to find, to the meanings that I might project into the text, trying out the familiar, the world I already know and feel at home in.

We find another view . . . that what the text alludes to, signs between the lines (cryptic) what is not said. These signs are not read on the surface but at a higher level of consciousness. Gadamer (1975) challenges me to read the text being open to its possibilities, to the unexpected, to soften my eyes.

Ones we recognise but cannot place . . . I have a sense about this meaning, something intangible, something read perhaps? I have met so many people like Veronica – old, cancer, dying, hospice, alone . . .

A single word might appear that bursts onto a smaller screen, a gateway to an unknown path.

alone

   Are patients like Veronica, alone, who make no demand, so easily passed by? If so, it is a shocking recognition that deeply confronts me. I do not witness staff sitting with her, especially in the quiet of the afternoon. Where are they? What are they doing?

   At different times different issues emerge as significant, yet as you will see, I did pick up the significance of being alone within the narrative, albeit with a twist (see page 224).

Paying attention to feelings

Often strong, usually negative feelings such as anger, guilt, frustration, sadness, draw our attention to the experience. Feelings are gateways into our stories because they ripple and disturb our habitual and taken-for-granted consciousness.

   In my description of Veronica, I do not say how Veronica was feeling or why she felt as she did although I ask myself what is she thinking as she approaches her death. However, this is not the same as appreciating her feelings within that moment. So I might have asked her: 'How are you feeling, Veronica?' Perhaps I didn't because I knew the answer – that she would smile and say she's fine. She did not want to burden me or anyone with her deeper feelings. Perhaps I might have written that in my journal and edited it from the narrative as not being an issue that needed highlighting. The cue is vital for the development of empathy – how can I know how Veronica is feeling or what meanings she gives to her experience? My own feeling of sadness is interesting to explore deeper. Perhaps my sadness is tinged with pity; pity that she is alone, even anger – anger that she is alone, that no-one is with her, anger at her family for not visiting and at my colleagues for passing her by. Indeed as I write I feel a residual anger even now, two years later, as if unresolved feelings reside in the crevices of the unconscious. Yet I never acknowledged this anger in my reflection.

What was I trying to achieve?

I have suggested that I was trying to respond to Veronica on a spiritual level, to ease her suffering through touch. This care was not acknowledged or negotiated with Veronica. It simply emerged in the flow of the day, as part of the holistic background of what I do in the hospice. I felt I responded appropriately and effectively. Veronica appreciated my attention, yet whether I 'eased her suffering' is difficult to judge. I really appreciated sitting with her, to give her my time, my attention, my skill. As I write I wonder if the whole experience was self-indulgent . . . perhaps sparking a deep quandary that care should be for the benefit of patients not staff. Do I really believe that? Certainly, at the time I felt no such thing. Perhaps at the time I was drawn into intimacy with Veronica and now, in the cold light of day, I put another spin on things.

Influencing factors

The cue 'What factors influence the way I was/am feeling, thinking and responding to this situation?' is a most difficult cue to respond to without a guide, simply because people are normative and take themselves for granted, and defensive to ego threat. Influencing factors are embodied as part of 'who we are' that reflect the impact of social, cultural, organisational, and professional socialisation.

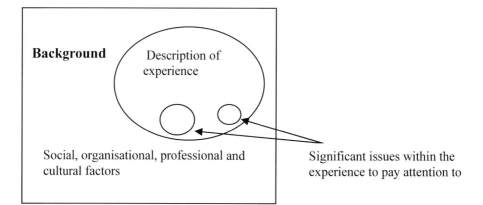

Conforming to 'normal practice/habit'? The weight of tradition	Negative attitudes and prejudice? Racism?	Expectations from others? Need to be valued?
Limited skills/discomfort/confidence to act in new ways?	What factors influenced my decision-making and actions?	Fear of sanction? The weight of authority
Emotional entanglement/ over-identification?		Misplaced concern – loyalty to colleagues versus loyalty to patient? Anxious about ensuing conflict?
Personal stuff/ baggage? Deeper psyche factors?		Knowledge to act in specific ways? The weight of theory
Wrapped up in self-concern? Pity? Stressed? Guilt? Frustration? Other feelings?	Time/priorities?	Expectations from self about 'how I should act' Doing what was felt to be right?

Figure 4.2   Influences grid.

Influencing factors may be deeply embodied in our psyche and not easily accessed for scrutiny. Nagapriya (2004:58) eloquently captures this sense of self-revelation:

> Fundamentally, we create our own world and don't realise how much our own prejudices, desires and habits distort our experience of it; we see the world in terms of ourselves.

My description of being with Veronica gives no indication of response to this cue, yet begs a multitude of questions for the discerning reader. The 'influences grid' offers a useful template to systematically explore potential influences (Figure 4.2). I adapted the grid to make 'racism' a more explicit focus for reflection, inspired by the work of Puzan (2003) and Blackford (2003). As Puzan (2003:194) notes:

> There is so much familiarity in talking about the alleged racial differences of non-white people in public discourse and so little familiarity in talking about those racial properties attached to being white, that the concept of whiteness (or a recognition of racial formation) has little resonance within nursing (Jacobson 1998). While issues related to cultural difference are not ignored, they rarely include the difference specifically engendered by 'whiteness', which is structured to avoid and deflect interrogation or critical reflection.

Reflection then opens a space for such discourse: I was certainly doing what I expected from myself. I didn't sense any issues of loyalty or expectation from other staff. I had time as no other patients had a demand on my time. And yet, I must confess that Veronica would not have been an obvious priority. As I say in the 'text' she taught me well not to pass people by. My feelings of sadness tinged with pity may have slightly entangled me. As I worked with her I pulled myself free from this entanglement by converting these emotions into healing energy and felt a strong connection and intimacy with her.

Dialogue between the text and other sources of knowing

Theoretical framing

The cue *'What knowledge did or should have informed me?'* prompts me to reflect on whether I responded within the experience in the most effective way as indicated by theory, research findings, protocols and suchlike. I describe this as theoretical framing – my ability to access and critique 'information' for its relevance to inform my actions and, as appropriate, to assimilate within my clinical practice.

From a reflective perspective, evidence is never accepted on face value. The reflective practitioner views all knowledge through a sceptical eye (Dewey 1933) for its validity and relevance to inform practice. Knowledge can only inform; it can never be predictive. It always needs to be interpreted for its relevance within the specific situation rather than applied as a prescription.

As Dewey (1933:215) notes:

> Reflective action entails active and persistent consideration of any belief or supposed form of knowledge in the light of the grounds that support it and the consequences to which it leads.

Through reflection I synthesise theory with practice in constructing personal knowing or *praxis* – the knowing I use in my everyday practice.

So I ask:

- What evidence is there to support the therapeutic value of a hand massage?
- Would a particular hand massage technique be more beneficial than others?
- Are dying patients lonely?
- What is the best approach to help a lonely dying woman?
- How best to respond 'spiritually'?

Libraries are lined with row upon row of books. Journal shelves are bulging. Healthcare is obsessed with 'evidence-based practice' – which puts a great strain on me and my colleagues to apply such knowledge to our everyday practice. Making links between practice and theory is a daunting task for practitioners like myself who lead busy lives and simply cannot find the time – even if I had the motivation to explore the vast realm of journals and books. I might easily become overwhelmed. I am reminded of the proverb 'the thin end of the wedge' – once you start that journey of exploration within the literature where do you stop? Perhaps better not to start at all?

Ethical action

The cue *'Did I act for the best'* opens a Pandora's box of ethical principles and conflicting perspectives as I grapple within the ethical maze of knowing how to respond for the best. Would my idea of what's best be in tune with my medical colleague? Ethics offers us a way to mediate our differences with a claim to ethical principles. From a holistic vision, respecting and creating the conditions for Veronica to be self-determining would be the highest principle

(Seedhouse 1988). So, I would always ask Veronica whether she would like a massage rather than impose a massage because I felt it would benefit her alongside other aspects of her care.

Previous experiences

The cue *'How does this situation connect with previous experiences?'* acknowledges that reflection is never an isolated event but a moment of paying attention within the endless flow of experiences. Every experience is informed by previous experiences. Are there patterns of behaviour evident? Do I keep falling into the stream? If I am looking back at the past (with regret, resentment, disappointment, longing, fond memory) then I am not looking forward to new possibilities.

I know from past experience with Veronica and other patients that she likes company and a hand massage but neither can I take it for granted that at this particular moment she would like me to give her a massage or even sit with her.

Looking forward

The cue *'Given the situation again how might I respond differently?'* guides me to move from looking back at a situation to moving forward and anticipating the possibilities for responding differently, more effectively – to be creative and imagine new ways of responding within situations. A challenge to pull open the mind's shutters. This cue is complemented by the cue *'What would be the consequences of responding in new ways for the patient, others and myself?'* This cue challenges me to generate multiple options for responding and then to choose the most favourable in light of its potential consequences. Imagining new ways of responding, of being, is like planting seeds in the body to germinate under the right conditions (Margolis 1993). It prepares insights for action.

Imagining potential consequences for responding differently helps prepare me for responding to those consequences and to consider whether I have the personal resources to respond in desirable ways. So I ask myself the cue *'What factors might constrain me acting in new ways?'* The cue is vital for preparing me for the real world of practice rather than my indulgence in imagination and idealism. I call this 'the reality wall' – the point where I must face reality because of factors embodied within me and reinforced within normal patterns of relating, that are likely to constrain me from responding in new, more desirable ways. It is vital to acknowledge that it is not easy to shift the reality wall, but that's OK – it is a real world and it's tough sometimes. However, I can understand the reality wall in the broad terms of tradition, authority and embodiment, whilst helping me to become empowered to act in more congruent ways. Just because I can understand something doesn't mean I can change it. But understanding it *is* the first step towards changing it. I learn to plot, become strategic, devise tactics. I am resolute, committed and patient.

This cue was not explicit within previous editions of the MSR although implicit within the idea of reviewing the consequences of alternative actions for the patient, others and myself. I felt it required more overt recognition, for many 'ideal' responses may prove beyond my available resources for reasons which can be surfaced, explored and worked towards overcoming. In situations of individual and group guided reflection, scenarios can be rehearsed for taking action.

Would I have responded differently given the situation again with Veronica? Certainly I would give her more attention prior to that situation. I would like to have shared my story at a shift report, to help others see her as beautiful, to challenge if we do pass people by. I can't imagine any constraining factors unless the consultant is present who wants to use this time to focus on symptom management issues. Would I be quietened?

In my experience, these 'looking forward' cues are neglected. Practitioners become adept at looking backwards but not looking forward and anticipating future situations. Yet these cues are vital for making the 'reflexive link' between experiences within the unfolding narrative.

The two cues *'What insights have I gained?'* (framing perspectives) and *'Am I more able to realise desirable practice?'* guide the practitioner to summarise the insights gained, to plant them deeper in the mind.

Framing perspectives

The last cue of the MSR asks *'What have I learnt through reflecting?'* The framing perspectives offer a systematic approach to frame learning through reflections. I can ask myself questions based on each framing (Box 4.1).

Box 4.1   Framing perspectives.

Perspective	How has this experience enabled me to . . .
Philosophical	Confront and clarify my beliefs and values that constitute desirable practice?
Role	Clarify my role boundaries and authority within my role, and my power relationships with others?
Theoretical	Draw on extant theory and research in order to help me make sense of my knowing in practice, and to juxtapose and assimilate theory/research findings with personal knowing?
Reality	Understand those forces embodied within me and embedded within the environment that constrain my realisation of desirable practice (the barrier of reality) whilst helping me to become empowered to act in more congruent ways?
Problem	Shift my pattern of mental models and appreciation of systems to focus problem identification and resolution within the experience?
Temporal	Draw patterns with past experiences whilst anticipating how I might respond in similar situations in new ways?
Parallel process	Make connections between learning processes within my supervision process and my clinical practice?
Developmental	Frame becoming an effective practitioner within relevant theoretical frameworks? (for example, using the Being Available Template, see Figure 3.1, page 22)

Developmental framing seeks to answer the question: *'How might the realisation of effective practice be known?'* It is a challenging question. The framing perspectives tell me something about what I have learned through reflection but they don't inform me whether I have become a more effective holistic practitioner. Developmental framing turns relevant theories into reflective frameworks for framing learning – either specific aspects of practice such as conflict management or developing assertiveness ability, or more global theories for knowing holistic practice such as the Being Available Template that I set out in Chapter 2.

The Model for Structured Reflection (MSR) map

I configured the MSR map (Figure 4.3) to guide practitioners to reflect on clinical reasoning and action. At the core of the map is the aesthetic response influenced by the ethical, empirical and the personal – the four fundamental ways of knowing in nursing explicated by the work of Barbara Carper (1978). I had previously utilised Carper's work within the MSR as a systematic approach to frame learning through reflection (Johns 1995).

The aesthetic response comprises four key processes:

(1)   The way the practitioner appreciated the pattern of the particular situation
(2)   The way the practitioner made clinical judgements in terms of care needs
(3)   The way the practitioner responded within the situation
(4)   Judgement about the efficacy of response in meeting care needs

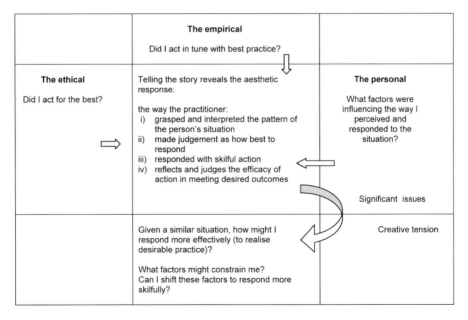

Figure 4.3   Model for Structured Reflection Map.

The practitioner must then ask three questions:

- Did I act for the best? (the ethical)
- What knowledge did or should have informed my practice? (the empirical)
- What factors were influencing me? (the personal)

From the ensuing description, the practitioner can draw out significance and creative tension, and then to anticipate how they might respond differently if given the situation again and what factors might constrain them. I know many practitioners who prefer the MSR map to the MSR because its primary gaze is looking-out at the situation in concrete clinical terms rather than a primary gaze of looking-in at self. However, when the MSR map is skilfully facilitated, it leads practitioners to look at self in relation to the particular experience being reflected on.

Dialogue between the text with other sources of knowledge

Having gained some tentative insights, I return to the literature with the intent to dialogue in order to frame my emerging insights within the wider community of knowledge. I might revisit literature explored earlier under theoretical framing but take it to a deeper level of understanding.

So I ask:

- Does my understanding of spirituality stand up with current theories?
- Are current theories flawed in light of my own understandings?
- Do people facing death feel lonely?
- Is there a difference between being alone and being lonely?
- Does such distinction reflect a difference between solitude and loneliness?

I find Wilber's Four Quadrant model (Wilber 1998) offers a useful framework to dialogue with diverse extant sources of knowing within (Figure 4.4). Wilber was concerned that sources of knowledge offer valid yet partial aspects of the whole. He was keen to integrate these partial views and to discriminate between various truth claims. In Figure 4.4, the left hand path is the subjective path characterised by I and WE type knowing. The right hand path is the objective path characterised by IT type knowing. Each quadrant is termed a paradigm governed by its own rules and injunctions as to what constitutes valid knowledge. As in the nature of paradigms (Kuhn 1970) these rules and injunctions become normative or taken-for-granted. As such, they are imposed on other paradigms. Hence the rules for judging the truth claims within IT worlds are imposed on the subjective paths leading to a denigration of subjective truth claims, given the dominance of IT type knowledge within healthcare. As a consequence, the significance and legitimacy of subjective knowing has been oppressed. 'I' knowing is accessed through reflection and provides the only basis for dialogue with the other paradigms. Through dialogue, other forms of knowing can be integrated into personal knowing.

Framing knowing can be seen at various discrete levels within narrative. On one level I am concerned to inform, frame and develop my understanding of

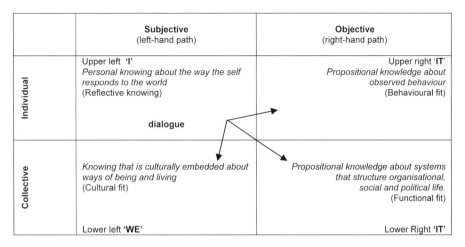

Figure 4.4   The Four Quadrant Model to integrate partial views of knowing (Wilber 1998).

desirable practice. With each reflection I can reflect on the meaning of my beliefs and values, and frame within a relevant philosophical and theoretical literature. Concepts such as holism, suffering, touch, agitation and spirituality can be explored to inform my understanding of these concepts in relation to my practice.

So I might claim that Veronica has a greater sense of well-being as a result of my hand massage. My insight is based on my empirical observation supported by the patient's feedback. Yet what do I mean by relaxation? Can it be adequately measured? Is there any evidence to support my claim, or indeed claims made within the literature? Is a hand massage relaxing? Do my understandings of spirituality stand up with current theories? Are current theories flawed in light of my own understandings? Reading literature sparks ideas, for example reading the words of Jeanette Winterson (page 42) inspired me to break her prose into a poetic form which then triggered a deeper reflection on the word *alone* (see page 43).

Another level of dialogue with the literature is concerned with the narrative process. Do my ideas of narrative find acceptance within a wider literature on narrative inquiry? What makes a valid narrative? For me, this has been a journey of discovery and revelation exploring Buddhist, Native American and ethnographic literature, and writers such as Ben Okri and Jeannette Winterson, who profoundly influence the way I write and view narrative. And so dialogue continues as the river widens and deepens towards the vast ocean.

Summary

The practitioner dialogues with a relevant literature to inform and frame ideas and insights emerging from reflecting on the story text. In doing so, theories and research are critiqued and assimilated within personal knowing to inform future practice and are woven into the pattern of the narrative pattern.

Chapter 5

Weaving the narrative

I construct narrative through six layers of dialogue commencing with my rich description of experience. The result is a 'story text' that I subsequently reflect on by using a model for reflection to reveal significance and gain some tentative insights. These insights are then framed or grounded in dialogue with a wider relevant community of knowledge.

I shall now explore the three further levels of narrative dialogue:

(4)   Dialogue between the text and a guide(s) to develop and deepen insights
(5)   Dialogue to weave the narrative into a coherent and reflexive form that adequately plots the unfolding journey
(6)   Dialogue between the narrative and its audience.

Dialogue between the text and a guide

Firstly, I must emphasise that dialogue with guides or peers takes place constantly. It isn't a neat step-by-step process that follows dialogue with the literature. Secondly, I must confess that my guidance has been both casual and infrequent. As I allude to in the narrative, I received guidance through supervising hospice nurses in clinical supervision, in general conversations, and at shift reports. I have received most feedback (as opposed to guidance) from sharing parts of the emerging narrative at workshops and conferences. As a result I develop the narrative.

Effective guidance is the balance of high challenge with high support underlined by *thick* trust. Only then can dialogue flourish. Cope (2001:152) notes that 'Trust is the oil that lubricates relationships'. Cope identifies five attributes of trust (Box 5.1) to distinguish the quality of trust within a relationship. This is a useful model to reflect on the quality of trust and its significance in creating and sustaining any therapeutic relationship – either with colleagues in guidance-type relationships or within clinical relationships with patients and families.

Why guidance?

Guides are necessary to help would-be narrative writers along the journey for several reasons. Perhaps the first reason is to prod practitioners to wake up to and shake up their inner world. So many practitioners are asleep, complacent,

Box 5.1   Five attributes of trust.

Truthful	The extent to which integrity, honesty and truthfulness are developed and maintained
Responsive	The openness, mental accessibility or willingness to share ideas and information freely
Uniform	The degree of consistency, reliability and predictability contained within the relationship
Safe	The loyalty, benevolence or willingness to protect, support and encourage each other (and here I might add mutual concern or love)
Trained	The competence, technical knowledge and capabilities of both parties

pursuing practice in habitual ways, or lack commitment and interest in what they do.

> People have difficulty awakening to their inner world, especially when their lives have become familiar to them. They find it hard to discover something new, interesting or adventurous in their numbed lives.

(O'Donohue 1997:122–123)

Perhaps left to my own devices I wouldn't bother to keep a journal because it takes effort and discipline. I was motivated because of my passion for palliative care and complementary therapies, my quest for spiritual awakening, and because I wanted to write a narrative for academic reasons.

However, I need guidance to kindle my motivation, or rekindle my commitment to practice, which sometimes get numbed through the pressures of everyday stuff. I meet many practitioners who are tired and turn away from the mirror of reflection because the image of themselves is difficult to face. Yet I also know how guided reflection has turned so many practitioners back on when their caring light had become dimmed. Many of my experiences are tinged with anxiety, when perhaps my natural inclination is to defend against anxiety. Anxiety triggers defence mechanisms that prompt me to protect myself, notably rationalisation and projection. People often say to me 'Don't we all reflect?' I usually say 'Yes, but to defend against anxiety rather than face up to and learn through it.' As such, guidance supports me to face up to and harness anxiety as positive energy to take action.

I also need to be challenged to unearth contradiction between my actual practice and desirable practice. I know that just talking through a reflection with another person really helps me to explore ideas. Just listening to myself helps to reveal contradiction. Eureka moments! The guide is like a listening board reflecting back my ideas and cuing me to explore issues more laterally, more deeply, as I work towards resolving contradiction. It isn't easy for me to see and understand those forces that seem to constrain my realisation of vision as a lived reality; forces of authority, tradition and embodiment. It is difficult work without guidance simply because it is so difficult to see things that are embodied as normative, things about ourselves and the world that are generally taken for granted, even with the help of aides such as the 'Influences grid' (Figure 4.2).

Referring again to that often-asked question 'Aren't we all reflective?' I might say 'Yes, but only to a certain depth.' My answer is based on Jack Mezirow's work on levels of reflectivity (1981). Mezirow distinguished between reflection at consciousness and critical consciousness levels. At critical consciousness level, I am able to reflect on my pattern of thinking and mental models, vital for learning if thinking governs my responses to situations. As I became more reflective, so my natural ability to reflect at deeper levels developed, although I – like everyone – have blind spots! The guide is a facilitator not an authority. They are not there to judge on my practice or impose favoured solutions. As I share my understandings so my guide responds, leading to a fusing of horizons that transcends our previous separate understandings. In this way meaning is co-created between us. It is a dynamic creative process. Based on my new insights, my guide challenges me to identify and consider the consequences of responding in new ways to practice situations.

> Opening shutters
> Pulling me out of my complacency and blindness
> Revealing new vistas of possibility
>
> (adapted from O'Donohue 1997)

Trapped within my habitual patterns and comfort zone I may resist new ideas. A guide offers a challenging yet supportive hand across the messy and indeterminate swampy lowlands of practice (Schön 1987) for without doubt, my stories reflect situations of considerable complexity. Each situation is unique, a mystery unfolding. There is no formulaic response. I need to be challenged to see beyond my normal patterns. It is so easy to get stuck in a rut and not even realise it! Guidance urges me to act on my insights, to act with integrity, infusing me with courage when the will weakens or the threat of potential consequence freezes me. Yet guidance also supports me when I stumble and fall against the hard face of reality, for without doubt, change is painful, like the small child learning to walk falls and bruises her knee yet she perseveres because she knows the gain is worth the pain (Rogers 1969). The guide can seem parental at times – 'this is good medicine.'

I know in guiding others that I can be like that. And most significantly, I need someone to listen to my stories with genuine interest. No longer is my cry unheard across a wasteland where caring has perished. Being heard I am remoralised (Frank 2002).

Clinical supervision

In the narrative, I refer to clinical supervision as a space within practice where practitioners are guided by a clinical supervisor to learn through reflection on their experiences towards enabling them to gain and sustain competence, to take responsibility for their own learning, and to monitor their performance against some idea of standards (Johns 2004a).

The emergence of clinical supervision stems from the *Vision for the Future* document (NHSME 1993). It recognises that practitioners would benefit from ongoing professional development and validates the value of reflective practice to achieve this.

At the hospice during the time of constructing my narrative, I was employed as a clinical supervisor to a number of nursing practitioners. My approach to supervisory relationships is collaborative rather then hierarchical. I recognised that these practitioners were more experienced palliative care practitioners than myself. I was also conscious that the supervision space was essentially their learning space, not mine, hence they should set the agenda for learning. The basic rules were establishing trust, confidentiality and reflective practice. I was a learning resource.

One useful approach was for me to share my own stories and seek their guidance – a type of peer supervision. In this way I would trigger their own reflections and help them to develop their supervision skills to use with other staff. In this way I could test my tentative insights with more experienced practitioners. Whilst such peer supervision was useful, I would have benefited from my own bespoke supervision, ideally with someone with a deep knowledge of complementary therapy working in palliative care and spiritually well developed.

At the core of any guidance relationship is the contracting process whereby both practitioner and guide can decide whether to work together. Is my prospective guide knowledgeable, wise, skilled and committed enough to be my guide? Such questions are vital.

Dialogue to weave the narrative

The narrative is constructed by weaving the first four levels of dialogue into a coherent and reflexive pattern that adequately plots the unfolding journey in such a way that is open to further level of dialogue between the narrative and the narrative reader.

Forming the narrative can be viewed as a hermeneutic circle that represents the 'whole' of the narrative at any one time. The narrative gradually evolves its pattern through dialogue between itself and the various parts that are part of it until it becomes an adequate representation of the journey. What started as 'doodles in a journal' has been transformed into the narrative text.

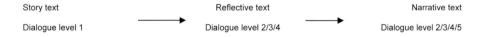

Story text		Reflective text		Narrative text
Dialogue level 1	→	Dialogue level 2/3/4	→	Dialogue level 2/3/4/5

Story text transforms into reflective text that transforms into narrative text.

How do I weave? Initially the narrative contained all the experiences I had reflected on over the two-year period as 'reflective text' in a chronological order. The more significant experiences in terms of revealing my learning or aspects of holistic practice were marked *. I could then link the emerging threads of holistic practice with my insights through the various experiences into a reflexive movement. More than half of my reflected experiences were then discarded. That was very difficult to do because every reflected experience is meaningful but a very necessary cull in terms of the final narrative. How long should a narrative be? When does it become boring?

I had to decide whether to present the narrative in a truly chronological form (as in *Being Mindful, easing Suffering*) or as a series of 'case studies'. Both approaches fragment the narrative in different ways. Using a case study approach breaks up the continuity of time whereas continuity of time breaks up the case studies into bits although each 'bit' is whole in itself. Either approach is adequate. I chose the case study approach because I felt it gave greater coherence to the narrative although perhaps, as a result it is more static and less dramatic. Take your pick. At all times I held onto the plot – what am I trying to achieve and am I portraying this adequately?

The narrative is never complete, hence I prefer to use words like 'adequate' and 'coherence'. What makes a narrative adequate and coherent? The written narrative is a snapshot, a moment in time, for experience continues and narrative insights are constantly being tested and developed. My formulation of guided reflection as a process of self-inquiry and transformation is also ever changing as I explore new avenues of inquiry that reveal methodological inspiration and challenges, reshaping the pattern of methodological influences I first set out in *Guided Reflection: advancing practice* (Johns 2002:6) (see Figures 5.1 and 5.2) As such, the narrative is also a journey of its own forming.

I am not going to explore the journey of travelling from the old to the new template. That is another text to be written. However, I will make some observations about writing the narrative. In doing so, some of the methodological influences will become apparent.

Critical social theory	Hermeneutics	Phenomenology
Evolutionary consciousness	Guided reflection:	Literature
Dialogue	a co-developmental and collaborative research process	Ancient and spiritual wisdom
Empowerment theory	Reflective and supervision theory	Feminism

Figure 5.1   Methodological influences grid (Johns 2002).

Critical social science and Empowerment	Hermeneutics and dialogue	Narrative inquiry
The feminist slant	Guided reflection as a journey of self-inquiry and transformation	Ancient and spiritual wisdom
Auto-ethnography (autobiography)	Reflective theory	Chaos theory

Figure 5.2   Methodological influences grid (December 2005).

Self-inquiry

Narrative is writing self-inquiry. I am at the very core of the narrative. Bochner and Ellis (2002) might describe this research as autoethnography – where self becomes a participant observer of self. Pinar (1981) would call it autobiographical. Pinar (1981:184) captures its essence as movement:

> We write autobiography for ourselves, in order to cultivate our capacity to see through the outer forms, the habitual explanations of things, the stories we tell in order to keep others at a distance. It is against the taken-for-granted, against routine and ritual we work, for it is the regularized and habitual which arrest movement. In this sense we seek a dialectical self-self relation, which then permits a dialectical relationship between self and work, self and others.

Dialectical relationships resonate with dialogue, commencing with self and then, like a pebble tossed into the still water, rippling out to embrace all situations and relationships, peeling away the surface layers to reveal the concealed taken-for-granted that construct unwitting lives, enabling the practitioner to come to a reflexive awareness of self. From this awareness comes movement to move beyond existing understandings.

Plot

The plot guides the narrative form. The plot is unfolding my reflexive journey of realising desirable practice as a lived reality. However, the plot is not deterministic in the sense of achieving some ultimate idea of desirable practice even if that could be known. The plot is merely a guiding light, like enlightenment is for Buddhists.

Reflexivity

Reflexive: a looking back to discern the unfolding pattern as one part flows into another, just as one experience inevitably leads to the next in an unbroken series of experience that makes up human life. Over a two-year period, certain experiences are selected as being of significance to illuminate the realisation of desirable practice. In the narrative I use The Being Available Template to *loosely* mark my reflexive journey on the basis that it offers an adequate representation of desirable practice. I have not revised the template since I first constructed its pattern in 1990 suggesting its adequacy. I say *loosely* because I do not want to reduce or fragment the narrative into a scheme. Rather, the reader can use the Being Available Template over the narrative, as a viewing lens.

Narrative form does not demand allegiance to any specific form beyond the reflexive demand. Indeed it is a demand for a liberation of self from oppressive forms of censorship and expression (Cixous 1996). As I construct the narrative I am conscious of tensions playing themselves out within me, the tensions between finding an adequate expression for my voice in relationship with those I work with and finding an adequate expression to engage readers in ways that might be meaningful. Narrative resonates with chaos theory in the sense that clinical practice is deeply complex in its wholeness and yet within that apparent chaos there is order or pattern recognition. Narrative is *movement*; like a stream gathering pace, rhythm, deepening, widening, being shaped by the landscape as it flows towards the sea. I can tune into and flow with the inherent order rather than resist the flow of energy by forcing ideas into boxes. This was a vital understanding in constructing narrative.

I must also resist an urge to make sense of my narrative by resorting to generalisations and reduction into some explanatory scheme, what Clandinin and Connelly (2000) describe as the formulaic and reductionist boundaries with narrative inquiry. In a world largely governed by professional texts in a formulaic and reductionist vein it is a difficult pull to resist. Elaborate concept identification and analysis obscures rather than illuminates possible meanings when the narrative needs to be open for the reader for potential dialogue.

> And I think that this is better. When words are born of love, it is better to leave them open, so that each person can benefit from them in their own way and at their own spiritual level – this, rather than tying the verses down to a meaning that not everyone could relish.
>
> (St John of the Cross, cited in Matthew, 1995:15)

A feminist slant

In the narrative I pay descriptive attention to detail to give the reader a strong sense of experience. The real drama lies not in heroic acts but in the fabric of relationship. Virginia Woolf in her 1945 essay *A Room of One's Own* influenced me to explore the idea of a feminine narrative that pays attention to and honours caring in contrast with the grand heroics that characterise masculine narrative. Perhaps in an ironic way, such small moments of caring are the understated heroics. Living with and dying of cancer *are* heroic. My narrative simply tries to illuminate that. In my experience these moments of caring are often invisible yet make a profound difference to the experience of being cared for and for practitioners who care. Narrative endeavours to capture caring in its wholeness characterised by discrete caring events, each caring moment unfolding into the next. Writing makes such moments visible and reveals their significance.

To give an example:

Rachel visibly relaxes seeing Callum so still. She says 'It's like magic.' I take her hand and say 'it must seem like that.'

We pause and still holding her hand I say 'your hands are dry.'

She says 'they are always like that.'

'Let me massage them for you.'

Her subdued smile radiates through the gloom. Holding her hand is an invitation to intimacy, a gateway to opening a healing space. Like a prop to ease the burden of her suffering. Like an olive branch of peace.

Such moments often pass unnoticed in the heroic din. Words come alive in ways that the reader can relate to; feel, engage with, engendering personal reflection and imagination in ways that theory or conventional texts fail to open up the mystery of human existence. Jeannette Winterson in her book *The Passion* (2004:155) eloquently expresses this mystery:

> Words like passion and extasy, we learn them but they stay flat on the page. Sometimes we try and turn them over, find out what's on the other side, and everyone has a story to tell . . . We fear it. We fear passion and laugh at too much love and those we love too much. And still we long to feel. (her spelling of extasy)

Passion words to inspire passion: passion for my practice, passion for my writing, (com)passion for others. Can you love enough? Has the world become so sterile that we fear passion? If so, my narrative is a public exclamation that passion is vital that I want the reader to feel and *flow* with. The rewards are vast for those who come to live their passion.

Being playful, being disciplined

Writing narrative must be an imaginative, playful and joyful effort to release the creative spirit. Indeed, so must clinical practice. Both require hard work and discipline. Okri (1997) challenges me to write playfully to free the spirit and as an act of transgression; to challenge the taken-for-granted as a creative act of realisation whereby I seek to both enchant and confront the reader with the beauty and horror of caring in a broken world.

Perhaps many health care workers are broken, resentful and feel they fail to ease suffering of their patients and families. Perhaps they fail to see the beauty of their practice too tightly wrapped up in their own suffering. Perhaps they cope by becoming complacent and thick-skinned. Perhaps 'caring' has become diminished in healthcare. If so, then practitioners need reminders to confront the loss of caring in their lives and to help reconnect to the beauty of caring as vital to their practice. I know that my caring is both beautiful and horrific as I dwell within suffering. People are fearful, people die and loved ones look on helplessly. Yet within suffering is a great humanity, full of warmth and joy. I know the reader will relate to the caring enfolded within the narrative and deepen their own humanity. It is offered as a gift for the reader's reflection and interpretation.

Between the lines of my narrative description I plant signs that point direction to the significance and meaning of my practice; in a touch, a glance, a pause, a plaintiff smile, a simple action of holding someone's hand. As I wrote elsewhere 'the profound buried in the mundane yet when watched, lifts it into immense significance, valued in its unfolding moment, a light across the reader's soul' (Johns 2002:42). Planting seeds to explode in the reader's mind over time (Ben Okri 1997). The narrative is written to unfold like a serial drama holding the reader in suspense. Due to its reflexive nature, the narrative might seem repetitive; yet a new twist is always present for the discerning reader. Reflection helps me to reveal the complexity and uncertainty of easing suffering for people who are dying and their families, pulling out for deeper reflection on significant issues such as:

- What is a 'good death'?
- What is spiritual care?
- What is suffering?
- What is compassion?
- What is the therapeutic team?

Narrative holds these ideas together as a 'whole' in ways that communicate meaning within the particular situation, revealing the common patterns and uniqueness within each situation. It reveals the subtlety and depth of nursing knowledge (Boykin & Schoenhofer 1991) lifting apparently mundane acts into significance.

Hence narrative illuminates the complexity of practice as a 'whole' and, as such, is the natural expression for holistic theory and practice.

Coherence

Narrative is my journey of realising my vision of easing suffering as a lived reality but whether you the reader agree is another thing. Perhaps to really know if I practise as I write you would need to be observing me from the shadows, assuming you were sensitive enough to the subtlety of my practice. Holism does not exist in any abstract way – it can only known as lived within the particular situation.

Given that the truth criteria for reflection is authenticity you may ask 'Is the narrative authentic?'

The pathway to authenticity is through *genuine* dialogue to reveal the true self and pull away the masks of illusions. By genuine I mean a commitment to the truth. It is astonishing how reflection quickly confronts people with such commitment. Those without commitment to the truth fall quickly by the wayside.

Reflection is an interpretation of what happened given credence through dialogue with self as a form of systematic reflective inquiry and within a wider community of knowing as depicted within Wilber's other quadrants of knowledge (see page 51).

The criteria for judging the worthiness of the narrative are open to interpretation. There are no fixed rules to be rigidly applied, but they must be worked out and judged in response to the particular research project or, in the words of Smith and Deemer (2000:889), 'actual inquiries'. Interpretation is deeply subjective. Others present would probably give different accounts. In my narrative I have my blind spots. I just haven't seen them. Maybe you will tell me? Without doubt, I foreground aspects of experience that seem to me the most meaningful for me at the particular time. But many more aspects of the experience lay like ripe plums waiting to be picked and eaten. Readers will pick them based on what is most meaningful for them.

In this spirit the narrative opens a space for dialogue between the reader and the narrative, a space open to the reader's perspectives in terms of their own diverse experiences and interpretations.

I know that some readers will dismiss the narrative as narcissistic, self-gratifying nonsense. It may give offence to those hardened to caring and love in the seemingly harsh world of everyday practice.

Perhaps the stories will destabilise your taken-for-granted perspectives and create small explosions in the mind. Arthur Frank (2000) makes the distinction between disruptive and destabilisation narratives. Disruption narratives make you pause before continuing in your normal way, perhaps making slight adjustments along the way. Destabilisation narratives are transforming. They turn the world upside down. Reflection is always disruptive in that it cuts across the taken-for-granted and thus always has the potential to destabilise, which I suspect is subtly reflexive. I know through experience that the stories trigger the reader's or listener's own stories and facilitate the sharing of stories and the development of communities of learning, what I call 'camp-fire teaching' (Johns 2004a:256). I know from performing many of the stories in the narrative at conferences and from reader response to 'Being mindful, easing suffering' (Johns 2004b), that my narrative resonates deeply with the audience. When I shared my reflection on being with Carol and her family (page 108) at a recent critical care conference, I was approached by a nurse who said she had never thought of asking relatives to bring in photographs of the dying person. It seemed a revelation to her that photographs could open a way for her to dwell with the relatives around the dying person and to humanise the dying patient in the stark surrounds of the intensive care unit. So simple, and yet so profound.

As such, the stories change lives as they have changed my own life. They are a mandate for social action towards a greater humanity.

> I would argue very strongly that the self that is writing the story
> is changed by the process of writing it.

(Laurel Richardson, cited by Flemons & Green 2002a:91)

Part 2

Chapter 6   The heron & the tree and other stories   65

Chapter 6

The heron & the tree and other stories

The fact that I meant well will not absolve me from the consequences of my lack of forethought. It is our responsibility to think through the consequences of what we do.

(Nagapriya 2004:44)

It is October 2002. The morning is very still. The first leaves of Autumn washed along the side of a road in the early light. I drive up the narrow lane to the hospice set back approximately 400 yards from the main road. Built around 1987 as a charity, the hospice has 10 beds, now comprising six single rooms and a four-bedded ward. The original matron was passionate about hospice care, yet like many passionate people, she was also controlling, anxious to ensure effective care amongst a newly-recruited group of nurses who lacked formal palliative care training. After 10 years she departed under an acrimonious cloud that coincided with the rise of medical leadership, marking a shift of emphasis from hospice to specialised palliative care.

I commenced working at the hospice in September 2000. My role at the hospice has always been opportunistic, first as somewhere I could develop my clinical skills to teach palliative care at the University, and secondly as a formal volunteer complementary therapist working within the inpatient unit on average eight hours weekly. The hospice has a day care unit, where therapists also work as volunteers co-ordinated by the day care sister. For a short period of time, the hospice employed a therapist as a co-ordinator, but she left and was not replaced. Within the inpatient unit I claim autonomy to respond as appropriate in consultation with the nursing staff although with little contact with medical staff. I deeply appreciate the opportunity to practice with people and families experiencing terminal care. I know I make a positive difference to these peoples' lives, as my stories will testify.

Edward

At the hospice I am working with Carol (care assistant). We call ourselves the 'P team' because whenever we work together we are always up to our arms in pooh and piss. We have Edward to look after, a 70-year-old man who has a rectal colon and liver metastases reflected in his jaundice. He was transferred to the hospice from the general hospital following investigations for grand mal fits. He is quite alert and accepts our offer of a jacuzzi bath. As we turn him before his bath, he is incontinent of faeces. Knowing looks between Carol and myself, the inevitability makes us smile. He likes the jacuzzi bath and hair wash and scalp massage. He has such a small head and I think how frail and vulnerable he is.

He is going home on Wednesday. Glenda, his wife, has been persuaded to accept him despite her fears he will be abusive to her as in the past. Can a leopard change its spots? Will his frustration at being so dependent on her spill over the edge and pierce her? Yet, he is so jaundiced and close to death I wonder why we talk of discharge and create this family conflict. It is as if we get locked into a pattern of thinking that limits our ability to flow with people on their wavelength. It is easy to see Glenda as a solution to our problem of discharging Edward just as it is easy to not see Glenda's perspective as a suffering and abused wife as if she is peripheral to our caring gaze. A dent in our holistic vision. As a result, Glenda resists us as we resist her. A breakdown of dialogue resulting in staccato rhythm, where we dance awkwardly at a time when we need to flow together within the apparent chaos.

The caring dance. We move together along an unfolding but also familiar trajectory, seeking rhythm, harmony, as if dancing. Gabrielle Roth, in her book *Sweat your Prayers; movement as spiritual practice* (1997) identified five rhythms of dance (Box 6.1) that offer an intriguing reflection on the caring relationship.[1]

Two days later

Agnes (care assistant) sits with Edward. He had been fine this morning, 'his usual self' but then something snapped inside him and now he is close to

Box 6.1   Five rhythms of dance.

Flowing	Being able to tune into natural rhythms and flow with them with least resistance. It reflects my intention to tune into the other's wavelength and flow with them in relationship
Staccato	Gives the dance its creative form. As I flow with the other's wavelength I try and shift it toward a more therapeutic trajectory, aligning my own wavelength. It is easy to step on toes or lose my stepping for the dance is unique and never been danced before. It may seem awkward at times, frustrating even as we try to find the flow. Of course one of us may not want to dance!
Chaos	Going with the flow as the music takes us. It is resisting imposing pattern, yielding to the intuitive. As such chaos is unpredictable and yet chaos is the creative edge; the artist rather than the technician at work
Lyrical	Emerging through the chaos to realise the deep trust and spiritual nature of the caring relationship – just as the surrender to the dance can lead to ecstasy so the caring dance leads to a spiritual uplifting, a sense of something special
Stillness	The profound sense of connection with the other person within relationship, of being one with the other. It is experienced as a sense of lightness, even spiritual awakening

---

[1] I have previously explored Roth's work (Johns 2004b:125–131).

death. He is unresponsive, his mouth gapes open, his breathing laboured. Glenda cannot be contacted. I stay with Agnes and Edward, feeling the poignancy of the moment. As Edward dies, I sit with him for about 10 minutes and practise the *essential phowa*, a Buddhist practice to guide Edward's spirit to merge with the divine light and ease his journey into another dimension (Longaker 1997:124–125). I am now more confident in openly practicing the *essential phowa*, a reflection of my own spiritual confidence yet mindful of imposing my spiritual trip. I have not always been so confident (Johns 2004b). Perhaps I do impose it but in good faith. It does not matter that Edward is not a Buddhist. The divine light is a reflection of any religious affiliation, and for those without affiliation the phowa is simply a gift, an honouring of a life passed beyond the mortal coil.

A few minutes later, Glenda arrives. She doesn't want to see Edward. It's tough to observe unresolved or unforgiving conflict within families as death looms. Although we cannot fix things and make them perfect, we can flow with compassion to nurture forgiveness.

Reflection

> The finest achievement for men of thought is to have fathomed the fathomable, and quietly to revere the unfathomable.
>
> (Goethe cited by Sangharakshita (1997:31)[2]

Edward's story reveals the frailty of human existence exposed along a fine edge. We can see the practitioner's art of acceptance without judgement, dwelling within the family, encouraging reconciliation yet without enforcing it; connecting people with a soft touch, a smile, simply being present in the moment.

In the dimmed glow of someone's death there is always poignancy. Poignancy is an expression of the soft lens of the spiritual. Something that touches the meaning of existence, that binds together the human predicament into a meaningful whole. Not something grasped. Such assertion sits uneasily with efforts to know spirituality as a phenomenon, assessed and competently met as a 'patient need' – an attitude that dominates contemporary spiritual palliative care literature. For example, Wright (2002:125), a hospital chaplain, notes in his abstract:

> This study used a phenomenological approach founded on the Husserlian tradition to discover the spiritual essence of palliative care in the lived experience of (16) stakeholders who held a variety of roles linked to palliative care.

A futile search for the holy grail? Leeuwen and Cusveller (2004) state:

> In order for nurses to provide holistic care, nurses must be competent to intervene on a physical, mental, social and spiritual level.

---

[2] Goethe: *Maxims and Reflections (Penguin 1999).*

These authors undertook a literature review to distil a complex set of com-petencies as a framework for training people to be spiritual. My counter claim is that I can only respond to the other's spirituality as a reflection of my own spirituality. As a Buddhist, I strive to be mindful of my spiritual presence within each unfolding moment, i.e. that is part of who I am, and naturally reflected in the way I am with people like Edward and with the other patients I reveal through my reflections. At its essence spirituality, like life itself, is a mystery. It can never be a technique to apply. The scientific quest by its very nature strives to know this mystery as if it is something concrete out there to be discovered and known. The science approach to spirituality will turn it into something mechanical and stifle the imagination. The spiritual life is an ima-ginative life. The liberation of the senses to touch and connect with self.

> For our lives to have meaning we have to be in relationship with them. Meaning comes through a depth of connection to ourselves and the world. For many of us there is little room for the imagination, rather we are full of information and ideas.
>
> (Paramananda 2001:76)

As I held Edward's hand before he died, I asked him how he felt about what was happening to him. I wrote:

> He understands and says he knows he is going to die and that's OK. He is ready. He has been a staunch catholic, he believes in God and an afterlife but he is in no hurry to go. He has no fear about dying.
>
> (Johns 2004b:249)

I was deeply humbled by his revelation. It was a deeply spiritual encounter, as if our spirits touched. It was not just the words spoken but the ambience of my (spiritual) presence liberating his own spirit to express itself. It was as if we had emerged through the chaos into a place of stillness.

No distinction need be made between the religious or spiritual; people are as they present themselves, with or without religion. It makes not a scrap of difference to my spiritual response. Wright (2002) notes that spirituality is a deeper current than religion, fundamental to the human condition, whereas religion might be viewed as partial and divisive. I take Walter's (2002) argu-ment that spirituality is an idea to replace secularised religion. Bereft of reli-gion, people seek something that is labelled spirituality, something that gives meaning to life. As Bradshaw (1996) notes (cited in Walter 2002), traditional orthodox spirituality, the human being in relationship with God, has been replaced by a conception of spirituality as a personal and psychological search for meaning. Perbedy (2000), in her attempt to differentiate spirituality from religion, concurs. Yet it is not the search that is spiritual but the meaning itself – whatever that might be. Edward was quite serene about his predicament, yet often people are not at ease with themselves and experience what might be described as an existential or spiritual fear, as if in a blind panic they come to realise they lack meaning. Heyse-Moore (1996) describes this as spiritual pain and Kearney (1997) describes it as soul pain.

From a Buddhist perspective, spirituality might be used to describe the noble path from samsara to nirvana, the pathway toward enlightenment (Figure 3.2, page 26) that suggests an instinctive energy of the human condition to realise and transcend its human potential. But what is enlightenment? Cohen (2002:77) says it:

> is the liberating discovery of the profound mystery of our own self, a mystery that we will never be able to understand with the mind.

We must loosen our attachment to our partial and often dogmatic views in order to be open to the possibilities that the mystery holds. Sahajananda (2003:148) notes:

> A wise person is not one who accumulates knowledge and knows all the scriptures, but one who has realised the limitation of all knowledge and all scriptures and who looks into the sky of eternity for the appearance of wisdom.

Knowledge only gives us an idea. Wisdom is beyond knowledge, letting go of attachment to knowing to be open to the possibilities of the moment. Knowledge belongs to the past, whereas wisdom is the flow of the present, having faith at ease dwelling in the mystery. Sahajananda (2003:165) summarises poetically:

> Life can either be creative or it can be mechanical. Mechanical life is a life of repetition, fixed and inflexible, in which there is only imitation, the past entering into the present and the present projecting itself into the future . . . creative life cannot be defined, for the moment we define life it becomes mechanical.

When the situation is approached from a situation of 'knowing', then the practitioner becomes concerned to apply that knowing and narrows the viewing lens to see it that way. Paradoxically it is ignorance. Yet that is the dominant message of science – to know the world so it can be predicted and controlled where the subtlety and intimacy of the human–human encounter becomes a dim memory.

Learn from eagle:

> Look up! See how eagle rides the invisible. Up and down, coasting, then back up and down again. With deliberate intent, she manoeuvres her wings in order to catch the next current, rising to a new height. Levelling and riding a straight course, she gains new sights. Then, accepting the inevitable downward drift, she surrenders to each experience. Invisibly changing and unpredictable, the air currents carry eagle to the places she must go. Eagle understands the dance of life and accepts the downward as naturally as she accepts the upward.

> (Blackwolf & Gina Jones 1996:185)

Perhaps the air currents are the breath of life, a description of spirit derived from the Latin word *spiritus* (Hoad 1986). Like eagle, we who care must learn to ride the air currents and tune into the rhythm of the caring dance in order to journey with our patients. Perhaps that is the essence of spiritual practice – to offer patients a ride to go to the places they need to go.

Jim

Jim is an Irishman in his early 40s with terminal lung cancer. He wants to take his eight-year-old son to Ireland to see his relatives before he dies. Sharron (staff nurse) feels he may struggle to survive the plane journey although it's only one hour. Of course he must go and we must smooth the journey as best we can. He greets me warmly, having just returned from the smoking room. His body is emaciated yet I am struck by his neat thick hair. Very dapper. George Best's autobiography lies on the windowsill. He reads my mind.

'I've smoked and drank all my life.'

The rooster coming home to rest – but I have no need to judge him in a negative way. On the contrary, I admire his determination to reconnect with his roots and be with his son at this time. It is his spiritual quest. His breathing is difficult and the room has a dank smell of bad breath. I suggest an aroma-stone with eucalyptus and lavender essential oils might help to ease his breathing and sweeten the air. Jim agrees.

Two days later

The aroma-stone is switched on but dry. I frown and replenish the stone, informing the nurse caring for Jim of my action and reminding her to ensure it doesn't run dry again. Yet, in reminding her, I am anxious. I try to be mindful not to project my frustration and evoke a defensive response. She thanks me for my action but says she has been busy and wasn't even aware that Jim had a stone in operation.
  I say:

'It's in the notes . . .'

but without response. I want to shout:

'Why haven't you read the notes?'

but I am silenced. 'Being busy' – the ubiquitous avoidance scam that nurses have learnt as the universal excuse for non-engagement.
  The maintenance of aroma-stones is a recurring problem as if their use is peripheral to the scope of normal practice. Clearly my 'aromatherapy prescription' lacked authority in comparison with pharmacological approaches to Jim's symptom management, despite the widespread rhetoric of embracing complementary therapies. I must confront it if I am to make the use of aroma-stones visible within everyday practice. Even signs stuck on the front of notes 'aroma-stone in use' have failed to ease the problem. People only seem to see what they are looking for.
  I ask myself 'Why do I struggle to communicate my concern?' I sense I tread on eggshells wrapped up in the culture of niceness that pervades the hospice,

as if myself and the nurse collude to avoid transgressing an unspoken rule. To be overtly critical might break open the containment and cause an emotional mess. Have we learnt to contain our frustration perhaps because of the anxieties that working with people who are dying evoke? I can position my conflict managing style within Thomas and Kilmann's (1974) styles of managing conflict grid:

Competitive

Pursues his/her own needs at the exclusion of others – usually through open confrontation (win–lose situations).

Collaboration

Involves an effort to effectively problem-solve the issue towards mutually satisfying conclusion – a win–win situation; i.e. concerned with needs of self and others. Openly discuss issues surrounding conflict and attempt to find suitable means to resolve the conflict.

Compromising

Realising that in conflict situations, every party cannot be satisfied – accepting, at times, to set aside personal needs in preference to others to resolve conflict.

Avoidance

Characterised by a negation of the issues and a rationalisation that attempts to challenge the behaviour of another is futile.

Accommodating

Essentially a co-operative interaction but one in which the practitioner is not assertive – prepared to give up give up their own needs for the sake of maintaining harmonious relationships and need to be accepted by others. 'Apologetic'.

I sense I am a conflict avoider yet keen to collaborate. I am not alone. Cavanagh (1991) notes that avoidance is the dominant style of nurses and nurse managers. Can I be collaborative, a win–win situation where the patient's best interests would govern the dialogue between myself and the nurse without either of us taking issues personally, and where I can assert my perspective without the fear of ensuing conflict? Not acting collaboratively injures my integrity, weakens my spirit and depletes my energy. I must act toward creating an environment whereby I can be fully available to patients like Jim. Or, put another way, to work toward collaborative relationships in common purpose to ease suffering.

Outside Jim's room I bump into Sister Mary, a Roman Catholic nun who is a 'spiritual visitor'. She comments positively on the aroma and her interest in the spiritual dimension of essential oils. We discuss the prayer group at the Convent and the impact of prayer on healing – thinking of a recent paper *Prayer in your Practice* by Rossiter-Thornton (2002). I always tingle when I'm with Sister Mary. It is the love she radiates. I am certain that people's suffering is eased simply by her presence. Suffering is the other side of spirituality. People suffer because their spirit is not at ease. Perhaps *easing suffering* is a better expression of practice *than meeting spiritual need*.

Jackie

Jackie was admitted to the hospice on October 7 from her home. She requested admission because she feared dying at home. She had recently been discharged from the general hospital, where she had had a pleural tap. Her chemotherapy was stopped after an adverse cardiac reaction. Her pulse had shot to over 200 beats per minute on exertion. She was very breathless due to her lung cancer and extremely anxious. It was thought she would deteriorate and die quickly.

However, she did not die.

A week later, I first meet her, no more than in passing. I introduce myself as a nurse and complementary therapist, rather like a tradesman setting out his wares. In response to the idea of reflexology or a foot massage she says her daughter Nikki massages her legs with some moisturising cream when she visits in the afternoon. Jackie senses how important it is for her daughter to do this act of caring. Nikki needs to do something useful and touch is such a physical connection, such an act of love that brings comfort to both daughter and mother. I understand this intuitively. However, Jackie succumbs to the temptation of a 'pukka' reflexology treatment on Wednesday.

A moment's pause . . . I stand by her side and smile. Hovering-in-the-moment. She invites me to sit down. She talks about her struggle at home because her family is very distressed and how she feels burdened by their feelings. At home she was still mum. Coming to the hospice is a sanctuary from this responsibility. She is very open with her feelings and talks easily about her death, which she accepts, at least on the surface, with grace.

I enjoy the experience of being with her; she is full of warmth and laughs easily. I marvel at her ease in the shadow of her imminent death. I feel a strong connection with this woman, a synchronicity or what Newman (1999) describes as a rhythm of relating. Newman poses the question: *How do we know when we are really connecting with another person?* It is a vital question because it is at the core of any relationship. Newman argues that we need to listen to the silence between our words to feel the rhythm and its emerging pattern. Listening to the silence is listening to the other's spirit. When we tap into each other's rhythm we can begin the caring dance. Newman notes (1999:227):

> Moving in synchrony with someone else . . . brings with it a feeling of closeness and unity with a greater whole.

These words are vital. I quickly felt close to Jackie. The idea of unity with a greater whole seems to me another way of expressing spirituality – a realisation that we are all connected together. Spirit is then this unity of wholeness that Jackie and I could connect with through our (spiritual) connection with each other; tuning into and flowing with each other's wavelength as a process of synchronicity, shaping a wavelength most suited for caring and healing. The patient's wavelength may be in crisis and needs re-patterning. Yet to re-pattern we must first appreciate the old pattern for all shifts in pattern must evolve from it.

Reflection

I am intrigued by the idea of *hovering-in-the-moment* to open a space where Jackie invited me to listen to her story rather than me inviting her to tell it. In hovering I communicate *I have time*. By smiling I communicate care. The art of creating therapeutic space. I might even radiate love, but I suspect that comes from somewhere deeper, somewhere I have yet to reach.

Perhaps when Agnes spoke of *being busy* it is the effort to retain control of time, yet it reflects an attitude of doing things to people rather than being with people. 'Having time' is a quality of holistic practice.

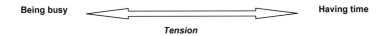

Being busy ← → Having time

Tension

Two days later

I pop my head round her door to say hello. Jackie is propped up in bed, her oxygen mask covering her face as clouds of nebulised air cascade about her. She is very breathless. Two friends flank her, as if guards to mark her dying journey. She reminds me she is looking forward to her reflexology later. We negotiate a time of 3 pm.

I am 10 minutes late returning. Brian, her husband, exclaims:

'Here he is! I told you he wouldn't have forgotten.'

Gavin, her son sits in the corner, everyone seems so at home at the hospice and I feel welcomed into their domain.

Jackie likes the aroma of the patchouli and frankincense essential oils that I have added to the reflexology cream but she can't place the smell. Frankincense is a new smell for her. She asks about the oils. I say the patchouli is to help her positively contemplate her life or, in Worwood's words, to 'bring a sense of the sacredness of life' (1999:240). Frankincense is to protect her spirit until she is ready to move beyond the earthly realm. It will also help ease her constricted breathing and feel calmer. I like the idea of oils touching the other's spirit, especially when the person is dying and contemplating what that means. Talking to Jackie about the spiritual characteristics of these oils helps open a sacred space where we can dwell and dance.

I apply the cream to Jackie's feet and guide her through a variation of the relaxation ritual I use with reflexology treatments:

- First, I place my hands along the base of each foot with the intention to centre myself. By this I mean to bring myself fully present free from any distraction and in tune with the universal energies for healing
- At the same time I ask her to concentrate on her breathing . . . to follow her breath in and to follow the breath out . . . slow deep breaths in and slow deep breaths out

- After about six breaths in and out I ask her to imagine that she is surrounded by a warm healing light
- And then, with each in-breath, to breathe this light into her body move this warm healing light to each part of her body, especially any part of her body that has cancer or has pain
- I then ask her to smile at how good that feels, this warm healing light healing her body
- I then suggest that with each out breath she let go of any worries, concerns or fears, to let them drift away on a gentle breeze so she can be fully present in this moment
- I then guide her to relax each part of her body commencing with the scalp . . . down to her toes until her whole body is relaxed, at peace until she feels like a fluffy cloud floating in a clear blue sky
- As she continues to follow her breath in and follow her breath out

And all the while I focus my own breath, harmonising my body with Jackie's body through my hands until we become one. Placing my hands along each of her feet I become one with her so I can read her body more intuitively.

> In order to understand something, you have to be one with that something.

> (Thich Nhat Hanh 1987:38)

The idea of asking Jackie to smile is inspired by William Bloom from his book *The Endorphin Effect* (2001). Bloom suggests that turning on the inner smile releases endorphins in the body that act to ease pain and engender a sense of well-being. The whole ritual creates a sacred ambience of deep healing intent.

Jackie says the treatment was wonderful:

'I had this sensation of green.'

I suggest the green was her heart chakra bursting with love and she says that's exactly how she felt. Balancing the chakras is integral to my reflexology treatments (Johns 2004b:232). She enthuses with Brian and Gavin. Gavin says he almost went to sleep himself as if the smells and sense of occasion had drugged him!

I feel strange leaving the room, leaving behind this family I have dwelt with as if I have become one with them. I know it is unlikely that I will see her alive again. It feels a strange way to say goodbye . . . just a gesture when I want to embrace her and wish her a good journey. And yet I am constrained, not wishing to draw the family's attention to this inevitability even though they dwell within it. Simply saying goodbye feels an ironic lack of intimacy, an affront to our spiritual connection. I imagine if I felt this so must Jackie. I must not be hard on myself. I must rest easily in the belief that I have helped Jackie and her family find some stillness amidst the stormy sea. Stories do not always have perfect endings. Yet I have another sense that I have again avoided something that constrains my caring.

I ask myself:

'What can I learn from this if faced with a similar situation'?
'Maybe you could have been more authentic and acted on your instincts.'
'How?'
'Maybe you could have said something like – *it has been a privilege being with you today* and then be silent and let her respond.'

That sounds good.

Reflection

I am intrigued by Brian's reaction to my being 10 minutes later than planned. Setting a time created a sense of expectation. Brian's relief reflects his anxiety, a reflection of the family's helplessness as they wait for the inevitable. I can contrast waiting anxiously – as a projection of the future, and waiting quietly – as dwelling in the present.

My intent is to help the family dwell in the present to find that place of stillness within their suffering. Therapy helps to create this sense of stillness or waiting quietly free from the future's incessant fearful chatter. Perhaps they felt they could not do much themselves to ease Jack's suffering so they put greater reliance on other's doing. It may have been better if I had said *this afternoon* rather than *3 pm* so as to ease the burden of expectation? If appointments are made then they need to be met, to guard against increasing anxiety that puts trust at risk. Without doubt trust is vital if I am to be available to work with this family, especially within the palliative care setting where these people have had long and traumatic illness journeys and are vulnerable to being let down by careless action.[3]

Nine days later, October 25

Rain lashes down in the early morning. As I drive to the hospice, I am mindful of my breath as I had no time to meditate before leaving home. When I am going to the hospice I like to meditate using the *metta bhavana* or loving kindness meditation to nurture my compassion for what lies ahead.

In the car I use a guided meditation by Thich Nhat Hanh (1993:15):

> Breathing in, I calm my body,
> Breathing out, I smile,
> Breathing in, I dwell in the present moment,
> Breathing out, I know it is a wonderful moment.

My body is transformed with a sense of pleasure. How is it that something seemingly so simple can transform me? Another of life's mysteries, but one

---

[3] On page 53 I set out the TRUST model (Cope 2001) that sets out the dimensions of a trusting therapeutic relationship and offers a model to reflect on the extent to which thick or thin trust has been achieved within the relationship.

that might help all people prepare positively for the day ahead no matter what work they do. I often use this guided meditation with patients who need help to relax and develop a more positive mind-set:

- The first line – breathing in, I calm my body, helps the person to focus on quietening the body
- The second line – breathing out I smile, helps the person focus on and release any negative emotions and engender prostaglandins
- The third line – breathing in, I dwell in the present moment, encourages the person to let go of fear (associated with the future), and such feelings as guilt, regret, anger, hatred (associated with the past)
- The fourth line – breathing out, I know it is a wonderful moment, encourages the person to honour and value each moment as precious despite suffering. It helps to orientate people to a healing presence

Driving in the early morning, the sky and land have a surreal presence. It is a good time for mindful breathing. It brings me fully present within the new day. Henry Miller (1963:26) captures perfectly this sense of being present:

> To image a new world is to live it daily, each thought, each glance, each step, each gesture killing and recreating, death always a step in advance. To spit on the past is not enough. To proclaim the future is not enough. One must act as if the past were dead and the future unrealizable. One must act as if the next step were the last, which is it. Each step forward is the last, and with it a world dies, one's self included.

Not just good Buddhist philosophy, but words of action, for myself and for the patients who face death and yet are wrapped up in regrets of the past, or fears for the future. By being present myself, I can better help others be present. It is refusing to avoid reality so the spirit can flourish. Just like being with Jackie.

At the hospice Jackie did not die. She has deteriorated yet holds her own. I negotiate being her carer this morning. Gladys (staff nurse) and Rita (care assistant) are helping her with her medication as I slip into the room. She greets me warmly. I take her hand and say how good it is to see her. I sit with her as she inhales her nebulisers. We are like old friends. She is happy for me to care for her this morning. We negotiate her wash around 10 am and then I will give her some reflexology. She says how much she benefited from the last session. She likes music and would like to listen to some relaxation music. I find an Enya CD.

Just before 10 o'clock, Jackie asks for the bedpan to pass urine. Gladys helps me hoist her onto the bedpan and then we wash and change her nightdress and bedding. Her hair is thin and greasy but she declines my invitation to wash it.

As I help her wash I ask:

'Do you dream?'

She is uncertain if she has dreams but she has visitors during the night. Her mother and twin sister, who both died in their 50s, come to see her. I ask how that feels, this gathering of family women?

'Very comforting . . . as if I am not alone and will soon join them.'

I imagine the women gathering to comfort Jackie as she approaches her mortal death in preparation to guide her into another dimension of being. Other people have told me about visits during the night from loved ones who have died. Patricia's son came to visit her after he died to tell her he was OK (Johns 2004b:147). A mystical experience beyond rational explanation. I have a deep sense of awe.

We finish the wash. I tidy up her room and mix the vanilla Complan she loves. She says:

'Yesterday I had some fruit . . . the first thing I have eaten in six weeks.'

Such small things seem important.

Her three grandchildren gaze at us from the photograph that sits on the bedside table. I suggest losing our relationship with grandchildren is particularly hard. My empathy is speculative but comes from previous experience. For example, Tony was tormented with losing his relationship with his four-year-old grand-daughter. Her painting on the wall was a constant reminder of his pain (Johns 2004a:101). Losing this type of relationship seems most poignant. The things we care about are the things that make us vulnerable. Jackie says the children know she is dying.

'Children are so resilient.'

I know this to be generally true. They bounce easily. She continues:

'One of the children has asked if she can go to heaven with Grandma.'

We both smile. Half an hour later she is comfortable, recovered from the exertion of being hoisted and washed, ready for her reflexology. I play Enya's *Watermark* album as she surrenders to my attention. I recently read a paper by Prashant (2002) – *The Art of Holding Space* – about using breath to create and hold a healing space. Now, as I practise, I am more mindful of using my breath to create a healing space where I can dwell with Jackie. I surprise myself with the difference. Being more mindful of staying with my breath I am more present. I must confess that sometimes I lose concentration in giving reflexology and find myself unwittingly surfing mind waves as I often do in meditation.

Jackie's feet are pale and crinkled. I sense her body has little energy. As I work her feet, her colour returns. I finish with therapeutic touch (TT). So much heat from her chest area that I sweep away. Sensing the shift in therapy she opens one eye. A thin smile. She is deeply relaxed. Eventually she says:

'That was absolutely wonderful.'

Jackie has tightness of breathing that makes her anxious, which in turn affects her breathing and increases the tightness in a vicious cycle. She feels the reflexology beaks the anxiety cycle *and* eases her breathing.

Later, in the afternoon Jackie is surrounded by her best girl friend, Brian her husband, and another woman I do not know. Jackie is slowly peeling grapes. I have come to say goodbye at the end of my shift. This time I sit with her and hold her hand to say goodbye. A knowing smile and wave. I inform her that I am at the hospice again next Wednesday and express my hope that I will see her.

Outside the room I hear Brian say to the nurses congregated at the nurses' station:

'She has picked up today.'

They say it's because she's had reflexology. Smiles all round. Perhaps it is – if love could heal she would walk out the door. Reflexology, when approached from a spiritual perspective in contrast with a functional approach, has this impact of inducing a deep relaxation that is also energising. It literally drains stress. It is such a spiritual attunement with the other person.

As I say goodbye to Brian I hold his shoulder. Unspoken words reflect the uncertainty. Brian suffers waiting for Jackie to die. Her admission notes read:

Jackie feels she is dying now and her wish is for it to peaceful and dignified with sedation there for her is she requires it. She fears fighting for her breath.

It is now 18 days since her admission and Jackie has, in everyone's opinion, deteriorated. Her wish to die peacefully and with dignity is holding. She does this by negotiating increasing doses of midazolam to combat her creeping fear of suffocation in response to the sensation of increasing breathlessness. It is a waiting game, a temporal vacuum in the passing of time in which we all dwell and wait; Jackie waits, the carers wait, the family waits. Brian bears it with equanimity as Jackie is in no apparent distress.

Reflection

I am intrigued by my earlier reflection about the 'art of creating space' and Prashant's 2002 paper *The Art of Holding Space* – space, a place continually being recreated moment to moment yet also being held as a continuous movement through caring. I want to be flippant and say 'space the final frontier' and perhaps that is what it is.

Past experiences inform my practice creating a sense of familiarity that is reassuring although I must be mindful not to impose my previous understandings into the present. The reflective practitioner learns from the past but is always open to the possibilities of the present moment.

Five days later

A still, wet morning. I arrive at the hospice at 7.20 am. Jackie has not died. I feel a thrill at the thought of being with her again. Tentatively I ask how she is? Melanie (staff nurse) says her condition seems stable, no obvious deterioration of her breathing. After the shift report I tiptoe into her room. Her eyes are closed. I pull her curtain a little open and sit on the edge of her bed. She opens her eyes and slowly greets me. I am *so* pleased to see her; so pleased to have this new opportunity to dwell in our relationship.

Jackie peers out of the window. Our friend the ornamental heron has a dripping nose from the rain. The small tree has lost more of its leaves. We have watched the leaves change colour and now fall over the past three weeks. She says she is OK, as Melanie said 'she is holding her own'. The tightness around her chest borders on pain but that is the only sign of deterioration.

Boldly I ask:

'Are you surprised not to have died?'

Holding my hand, she takes this in her stride.

'Each night I wonder . . . my grandson visited me yesterday and I did wonder if I would see him again. I don't want to die but I know I am dying . . . we must all die sometime.'

I interject:

'But most of us don't have to face it up.'
'No but I am content . . . this is my home now. This fear persists that I may get thrown out.'

I reassure her that would not happen. She knows this but the fear lurks in her mind.

'It is a comfort for me to be here. I don't miss the home or the garden. I know that if I was at home I would not still be here, if that's not a contradiction! It's been comforting watching the family change and lose their fear.'

I say:

'It's amazing we can have this conversation talking about your death.'

She smiles:

'It feels important to talk about my dying isn't it? One thing though, if I need sedation . . .'

Again I reassure her that we would increase her analgesia and sedation as necessary to ensure her comfort. These insights into her fear are profound. She can relax knowing and trusting us to do this for her, feeling that she can control and negotiate her treatment regimen. Her recurrent fear is that, in handing over her body to us, we will fail her and do what we think is best. If anything we err on the side of over sedating the patient rather than under sedating in the quest for the 'good death' where the patient drifts off peacefully on time with no apparent pain or distress. For Jackie it is about finding a fine line between managing her anxiety and clouding her consciousness.

I ask her about the effect of the reflexology last Friday. She said it was deeply relaxing.

> 'Did it give you more energy?'
> 'When I came in here I felt I couldn't move my legs. My arms felt strong but then I was using them to move myself up the bed but now I find I am wriggling in bed at night moving my legs again.'
> 'Would you like reflexology today?'
> 'Please!'

We arrange an appointment for two o'clock. In the meantime, I set up an aroma-stone with lavender, frankincense and bergamot essential oils to ease her breathing and anxiety. She finds the odour very agreeable. I fetch her favourite vanilla build-up drink and leave her.

Later in the afternoon I give Jackie reflexology. Her feet have more colour although her heels are purple and congested. As before I finish with TT to take the heat from her chest area although less hot than last Friday. Afterwards she is again deeply relaxed. She asks if she can listen to the music again – *Serpent's mound* by Rusty Crutcher.

Later, Brian and Gavin are with her. Jackie enthuses with them that the music was incredible. She tries to explain to Brian what she means, that the music took her to another place. Once she opened her eyes and Sister Mary was sitting in the chair. She could only smile. Rusty Crutcher's music resonates with the soul and helps the body to vibrate on a different transcendental frequency, what Gerber (1988) describes as vibrational healing. Music seems to heighten the healing potential of reflexology, aromatherapy and TT to bring the self into harmony. Gavin will borrow the CD and copy it for her.

Leaving the room I linger and chat with Brian. He is at peace visiting Jackie. He could visit like this for the next six months without feeling anxious about whether Jackie will die. He wonders about my question. 'How do you feel?' Not an easy question because Brian has no yardstick for feeling in such a situation.

> 'Everyone thought Jackie would die within 48 hours of admission but she hasn't. Life is a mystery, even my feelings.'

Reflection

I am struck by Jackie's comments about being at the hospice so her family didn't suffer. They had suffered watching her at home where she still tried to be a mother and wife. The hospice was not a place she would have chosen to die, but it is a sanctuary for her family. She had absorbed their suffering and being here she can release it and as she says, she sees it released within them. Suffering has this interpersonal dimension that floats on the surface of any deeper existential crisis of facing one's own extinction.

Jackie gives me a sense of the *good death* as a spiritual encounter where she can accept her destiny with grace. This insight reinforces my view that my own spirituality is my most potent caring attribute within the holistic approach and it is incumbent on us who work with the dying to nurture our spirituality. The caring space contains the whole family. I dwell with Brian and Gavin, helping them to find meaning and responding to their suffering. Different wavelengths, yet moving in the same direction, like interconnected rivers moving inexorably towards the vast ocean.

Five days later

Silently I stand at the end of Jackie's bed and watch her resting with her eyes closed. She must sense me for she opens her eyes. Her smile is beautiful. She is pleased to see me. A mutual feeling. Her aroma-stone is caught under a bed wheel. It is dry so I replenish it knowing how much she enjoys the aroma. Sitting on the bed we gaze again out of the window. The small tree outside has just a few leaves left clinging. Heron is inscrutable. After her reflexology she is deeply relaxed. Gavin has arrived but remained outside rather than disturb us. I feel very close to him now as with all this family. He holds her right hand when I say goodbye. I hold her left hand and arrange to see her on Friday all being well. I feel confident that I will see her but also know her future is unpredictable.

Three days later

Early November. A wind swept and rainy autumn day. Leaves line the road verge in sodden heaps. The trees are alive with remnants of vibrant colours. As I enter the hospice, Brian is sitting alone in the corridor. Immediately I think the worse! I am not used to seeing him in the mornings. He says:

'They are just washing Jackie.'

He explains that Jackie had called him on Wednesday to come to the hospice because, in her words, *the time had come*. Brian had been in hospital himself on Tuesday night because of atrial fibrillation. At 8 am Wednesday morning in A&E he flipped back into normal rhythm yet was surprised when the cardiology team discharged him – they knew something he didn't know – that

Jackie had called him. He has an old history with his 'ticker' and wonders if the stress of Jackie's illness has caused this.

> 'I've always got stressed easily with small things like DIY . . . obviously there has been a change in Jack's condition although she's still here . . . she's brighter today though. Wednesday night they put a bed alongside her. I got about four hours' sleep . . . we've always liked our sleep but it was better last night. I went straight to sleep around 11 pm when my head touched the pillow and I didn't wake until 6 am. I went to sleep holding her hand and was still holding it when I woke up. Jackie doesn't want to see people so much now, she became quite agitated when her best friend wanted to visit . . . just the family now.'
> 'After Jackie dies will you continue to live in your house?'

A tough even confrontational question, yet Brian takes it in his stride.

> 'We've been married 42 years and lived virtually in the same house. I will stay on. I have some close friends. One couple we met married the same year, same date and even the same time. His wife died quickly of pancreatic cancer two years ago. He has met someone new and is planning a future. I've brought Jackie in some Neil Diamond music – she was tapping her finger with the music . . . she then asked for Louis Armstrong, so we've been alternating the music.'

I listen as Brian fills me in with the detail. Brian's comment that Jackie didn't want to see her 'best friend', that it was 'too much effort' intrigues me. I sense Jackie's need to withdraw from the world, that she has said her goodbyes. It must be an effort to maintain relationships, reminding me of what Toombs (1995) described as 'existential fatigue' as an 'impetus to withdraw' from the world (cited in Lawton 2000:89). However, I do not perceive any associated loss of self despite the physical effort to do things and the loss of mental will to maintain relationships.

I dwell with Brian for about 20 minutes as he talks, listening as he reminisces on his life with Jackie and enabling him to find meaning in the present and envisaging a future without Jackie. I know from experience that such talk is vital grief work. His tears are close to the surface and as he talks he cries and laughs, apologising. It is sacred work. The hospice as a sanctuary, a place of refuge.

Linda (care assistant) finds us.

> 'She's ready for you now.'

Brian goes ahead. I hold back to give them some time together.

Jackie looks glazed, as if a degree of consciousness has been stripped from her. Brian tells me the midazolam had been increased on Wednesday to compensate for her increased anxiety. As usual, she is attached to the oxygen. Sitting on the bed I smile and hold her fragile hand. From the window I gaze again upon the ornamental heron and small tree outside the window. I say:

'The tree has lost more leaves since we last sat here.'

I explain to Brian that Jackie and I have watched the tree over the past weeks change its colours and lose its leaves. A marker over time. The dropping of leaves seems symbolic, that the tree is nearly bare and will mark Jackie's death when the last leaf falls.

Just sitting with Jackie fills me with compassion. She squeezes my hand.

'Just a short reflexology today I think.'

I smile because it is no exertion at all for her to melt into the treatment. Perhaps she has been pulled about being hoisted onto the bedpan and washed. Perhaps even contemplating being 'treated' conjures more work. It is a pattern I know well.

She closes her eyes with Brian holding her hand. I have never been so present giving a treatment. It is simply a beautiful experience to be with these people in this room at this time, with this music, pure *dana* yet in giving I receive so much. Afterwards I ask if she sensed any colours?

She smiles.

'Pinky colours.'

As I move to leave the room Jackie gestures me to hug her. It has been a very emotional treatment, I feel slightly overwhelmed yet with no sense of distress . . . love spilling out mixed with sadness knowing that she has deteriorated and her death climax is approaching. It is as if I am saying goodbye.

Reflecting on her increasing sedation, I sense Jackie is dying the 'good death' as well as she is able. To begin with she determined her need for midazolam, but now we have taken over this role, in response to her signs of distress. Parentally we act in tune with her anticipated wishes, fulfilling the ethical principle of respecting patient autonomy (Radbruch 2002). Maybe it is natural to experience a certain panic as death unfolds its tendrils around the dying person. It is a momentous moment in one's life. How can one not face death with trepidation as a step into the utter unknown? I wonder if fear is better remedied by dwelling with the person rather than sedating? The answer is indeterminate because it depends on the individual, but it does require the nurse to be mindful and read the signs well, and challenge her own need to experience the 'good death'. Radbruch (2002:239) notes:

> Sedation does not offer an easy way out of all the problems of palliative care. It is an ethical decision . . . the palliative care team should reflect on our own attitudes towards sedation in the dying.

As Lawler (1991) suggests, Jackie is relinquishing her dying body to the nurses to be cared for. Or perhaps as Lawton (2000) suggests, that it is not so much that Jackie relinquishes her body but we take it over. It is a subtle yet crucial distinction to understand. Are we, as Lawton suggests, concerned primarily to ensure a 'good death' by increasing the midazolam. In doing so, we render the body docile toward ensuring a public demonstration of a 'good death'. It is as if the person crosses a line where the loss of agency to be self-determining melts into the dying role. Perhaps it is the line that makes the terminal phase.

After lunch I meet Nikki, Jackie's daughter, for the first time. She sees me in the corridor and asks 'Chris?'

I joke that I had usurped her foot massage role. She laughs. She is open and warm. Jackie's feet are our reference point for connection. Gavin sits with his mum holding her right hand. She has a flannel on the top of her head feeling very hot. Is this heat a 'crisis' from her reflexology this morning or a marker of general deterioration? In a sense it does not matter. Can I help? Indeed I can try to take the heat away with TT. Gavin and his sister move into the rest room although I would be happy for them to stay.

I hold Jackie's brow with my left hand and my right hand on the back of her head at the base of the skull. Words are difficult to describe the immensity of holding Jackie in this way. Her head feels so small and vulnerable and I feel so powerful. It feels as if I hold the Universe. I close my eyes and focus my breathing – drawing in universal love and breathing out compassion through my hands until Jackie's body is flooded with love. How does she feel? Does she sense this enormity? I have become one with this woman on her journey. Working the TT my hands are cold and tingly, her energy field is not as hot as I expected. Initially I asked Jackie to visualise a cool waterfall cascading over her yet now I am uncertain. It is as if her energy is so deleted that I must draw energy into her yet after twenty minutes I feel the energy field has changed little. As I work small gasps emanate from Jackie, as if her suffering is torn. Afterwards she says it was beautiful. I have brought her into a clearing of stillness when the heat of the jungle had been stifling her. She feels more comfortable in body and mind. We exchange few words yet our eyes speak volumes to each other. She knows I care for her deeply and she reciprocates. I listen to her body and respond with my own. Being silent opens up this new clearing where we can dwell in stillness. I sense we both feel joy.

> Silence is important for listening and hearing the message. You must be silent if you wish to listen to another, to listen with openness. This involves silencing not only your mouth but also your mind.

> (Perry 1996:9)

As I write I wonder about my dark humour on meeting Nikki? Was it appropriate considering how she must be feeling as she waits for her mother to die? Is my effort of humour a means of coping with some anticipated anxiety? I am conscious of Jourard's (1971:181) words that:

> Joking behaviour tends to evoke joking behaviour in return from the other.

If so, does humour close down a space to express sadness? *She laughs. She is open and warm* – perhaps she is thankful for the light touch to lift the gloom? Intuitively it felt right.

Tolle, in his book *The Power of NOW* (2001:41) says:

> The whole essence of Zen consists of walking along the razor's edge of Now – to be so utterly, so completely present that no problem, no suffering, nothing that is not who you are in your essence, can survive in you. In the Now, in the absence of time, all your problems dissolve. Suffering needs time, it cannot survive in the Now.

This is true for both the carer and those being cared for. My effort is to focus my being in the Now. Then suffering cannot leave its mark. When this happens joy can burst forth, a state of being beyond the ego where I can dwell with compassion and equanimity. It is to such places I work to move Jackie and all other patients; a place beyond fear and pain; a place of unfolding stillness and love.

Four days later

Message on my mobile phone from the hospice – Jackie died at 5.04 pm yesterday with her family around her. How do I feel? Perhaps wistful is the closest word to describe the feeling. I sit and practise the *essential phowa* for Jackie, helping her spirit merge with the divine light. But I wonder if I am too late – has the moment of fusing with the light passed her by? Does her spirit float anxiously in cosmic space? But I do not think 'futile' – I focus my energy and visualise her spirit taking courage and move into the divine light. Perhaps it is more a form of closure for me, a final act of dwelling with her. I am comforted through this act. Tolle (2001:18) writes:

> When you become conscious of Being, what is really happening is that being becomes conscious of itself. When Being becomes conscious of itself – that's presence.

To dwell with the other I need to have presence, i.e. to be self-conscious in a non-egoic way – a witness to self within the unfolding moment, with mind clear of chatter in order to be present. When the mind is chattering it is simply not possible to be present. The conscious use of breath stills the mind and helps me become more present. *Dwelling with* is a sacred space amidst the chaos of the unfolding illness drama, where we can be ourselves in peace and love. In *dwelling with*, I appreciate the pattern of the whole and respond to guide the patient and family to find meaning and harmony. Richard Cowling (2000:18) asserts that wholeness is irreducible into parts yet the (whole) person can be appreciated as a merging and unfolding pattern in context of his or her environment. He writes:

> My own view is that the nature of nursing is one of responding (with reverence) to the wholeness of human experience . . . In human terms, the pattern gives identity to and distinguishes one person from another. It is the essence of being who you are; thus, pattern appreciation is reaching for this essence in each individual and seeing the wholeness within pattern.

I resonate with the idea of reverence, that what I do as a nurse and therapist is sacred work. It is vital not to fragment wholeness, for then we lose sight of the person. So appreciating someone's life pattern is a distant cry from assessing their problems. From the perspective of *dwelling with*, I become a part of the pattern itself, appreciating it from within. As Jackie withdrew then I flowed with her on her journey, hopefully reading the signs and responding appropriately, embracing her suffering, finding meaning, experiencing a paradoxical sense of joy. There was no withdrawal on my part.

I have dwelt with Jackie and her family these past 27 days. We have waited patiently for that inevitable moment of her death. Being with her has been moments of profound beauty stretched along the dying trajectory, and yet, can dwelling with someone who is slowly but inexorably suffocating be described as beauty? It is as Okri says (1997), a place where beauty and horror lie side by side, as if beauty is itself an act of transgression.

I write Jackie a poem to honour our time together and work through my sense of loss and to let her be free of my attachment. Writing the poem is a creative act revealing the artist within, an artist often submerged in the torrent of rational thought. Writing the poem connects me with my spirituality, as if opening a valve to reveal the mystery and majesty of suffering and caring, lifting and transforming the mundane into its spiritual significance; a hermeneutic interpretation in its portrayal of meaning.

The heron & the tree
Each day we dwelt beneath the small tree
That stood outside your window
to witness the change of colour
From green to yellows and reds
And then brown to mark the leaf's
descent into the earth.

Each day fewer leaves
were attached to the tree's life
Reflecting Autumn's time for death
Within the cycle of life

In the shade of the tree sat heron
as if a guide who waited patiently
To guide your journey
From this dimension of life to the next.

I know heron brought you comfort
Even a sense of stillness
In those poignant moments
When fear gripped the raw edge of emotion

Some days heron would catch a leaf
Or two as it fell from the tired tree
Damp with rain the leaf held fast
As if reluctant to let go.

The leaves are a symbol of life
Each day a few less leaves
Until the last time I sat with you
just one or two clung tenaciously
    to life

Reluctant to let go.
As if each leaf falling was a
    countdown
To that inevitable moment
when your breath would cease.

Yet you did let go
In peace
Surrounded by your family
To melt into the divine light.

Eight days later, November 19

Yesterday I felt certain about going to Jackie's funeral but this morning I am less sure. What is my purpose? Do I seek closure? Am I simply paying my respects? Do I really want to go? I have never been to a hospice patient's funeral even though it is common practice for nurses to attend funerals.

I drive past the church about 20 minutes before the service. People enter dressed in black. By the time I find a place to park and enter the church it is nearly full. I love the old church despite the coldness. I feel its presence. Four of my colleagues from the hospice are already seated and shift up to accommodate me. The undertakers place the coffin before us. Jackie's family follow the coffin and take their pews. I feel the utter sacredness and silence of this moment.

After the service Jackie's favourite music fills the air – Neil Diamond and Louis Armstrong play us out of the church. Brian's face erupts into a smile of surprise and delight as I offer my condolences. Now I know why I have come. Glenda, one of my hospice colleagues, says later that she sensed in Brian's greeting how much I meant to the family. I give him the poem *The heron & the tree*. I met Nikki only once but in the emotional moment, the hug feels natural. Afterwards I tread lightly to my car and return to the hospice. I am fulfilled.

Reflection

I had always considered funerals a closure ritual. Now I sense the funeral creates a space to honour my relationship with Jackie. Perhaps it is less a closure ritual and more about moving my relationship with Jackie into a new space deep within my being, not as a memory but as a convergence of spirit. Brian's response to me at Jackie's funeral reflects that funerals are a ritual to affirm living relationships. My attendance says I remain available to you. I am reminded of Logstrup's ethical demand (1997) *that we take care of the life which trust has placed in our hands* (see page 28). I sense that if I had not attended the funeral Brian would have looked for me but not demanded I be there. In other words, the ethical demand is unspoken. It is simply implicit within the human relationship.

My narrative of being with Jackie and her family hints at the complexity of caring, one question like 'Should I attend Jackie's funeral?' set against multiple backgrounds.

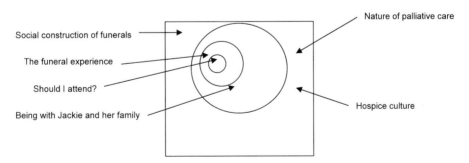

Brian

Three months later

I meet Brian in the hospice corridor. He has been fundraising for the hospice and has popped in to to see the nurses. He says the poem *The heron & the tree* is being calligraphied and framed as a tribute to Jackie and the care she received at the hospice. He spills his plans, and between the plans he spills his sadness. I feel his loss and his need to be with us at the hospice as a sanctuary; a loving place to dwell for a while. I sense the poignancy of maintaining the connection between Jackie's death and the present. We are that connective thread to pull him through, a lifeline. The image of a sanctuary as spiritual; a place where Brian and other families whose loved ones have died can remember and be held. Perhaps in this sense the hospice becomes a secular church. Such moments make hospice work joyful and nurture my spiritual growth.

Gerard

Wednesday October 16

It is a cold damp autumn morning. The leaves are beautiful in their changing autumn colours. Esme, a Macmillan nurse, has asked me to visit Gerard, a 38-year-old man who had a primary cancer of the tip of his penis that was excised about a year ago. The cancer has now spread to a lymph node in his left groin. This was also excised but has grown back and failed to respond to chemotherapy. He now has a large fungating wound spreading rapidly down his left thigh and across his abdomen. Gerard has rejected further chemotherapy, preferring, at least for the time being, to explore alternative therapies to conventional medicine. Esme had asked him whether he might like to meet me to discuss some complementary therapy. She mentioned I worked in the local hospice. Gerard agreed although remained adamant he did not want to be a hospice patient. When I rang Ginnie, his district nurse, to say I would be visiting today, she felt that Gerard wouldn't be unwrapping his Christmas presents. She has a way of putting things. Yet I am confident of being able to help Gerard and Lisa, his wife, whom I am informed is very stressed. They have two children aged five and eight. So young to watch their parents suffer.

I arrive at 9.30 am. I warmly shake Gerard's hand, with strong eye contact. His grip is strong. In contrast, Lisa's hand is limp. Ginnie sits on the edge of the sofa discussing with Gerard and Lisa wound self-management as Gerard and Lisa are going to the New Forest next week for a half-term break. An urgency to make the most of life as the dark clouds gather menacingly? Pictures of the children line the windowsill and I sense the huge loss Gerard's death will create. The wound stench drifts in the room. It is not pleasant, a constant reminder of the cancer's increasing presence. I ask about the wound dressing. Gerard is using charcoal dressings to counter the stench. He changes the gauze pad every two hours because of the heavy exudate. I suggest a drop of lavender on the gauze pad each time it's changed to help counter the smell. The wound is very painful, and the lavender may have a local anaesthetic effect. I also suggest using bergamot in an aroma-stone for the room odour. I could lend them a stone from the hospice? They respond enthusiastically and Lisa writes these things down to purchase. These offerings are like crumbs of hope eagerly grasped.

Being forewarned of Gerard's antipathy to the idea of the hospice, I emphasise I am *not* the hospice invading their home, conscious of Gerard's fear that hospice is a euphemism for death. His gaze is firmly toward cure so I must help him focus yet without offering false hope, even as he seeks hope to counter his fear. They tell me about their decision to reject chemotherapy and pursue an alternative approach. He talks about 'quality of life' and does not want to be ill with the side-effects of chemotherapy. If things don't do well with the alternative approach he can fall back on the chemotherapy. Gerard has started a particular diet involving bark from an exotic tree. They found the diet via the Internet. He is also being treated by a spiritual healer. Warning bells ring inside. The alternative approach will not stem the tide of the cancer's advance. Perhaps he should be blazing away with every gun of conventional medicine, especially as the cancer is rampant. But I do not surface my doubts. He is confident in his approach and it is not my place to contradict him, at least not today. But I do make a mental note to explore my warning bell with Esme.

Gerard says he doesn't feel particularly stressed, and it's true that he does have a calm demeanour that perhaps masks a deeper fear. On this first visit, I very much move along the surface of things tuning into and appreciating the pattern of their lives. I read the signs along the surface that lead to deeper and possibly darker aspects of Gerard and Lisa's lives – yet it is not the time to venture too deep. I am mindful of the impact of my presence on them, careful not to overwhelm or beguile them.

I suggest to Lisa that she might also benefit from some complementary therapy? Gerard chips in saying how much harder it is for Lisa; at least he has the cancer and knows he must deal with it. For the looker-on it can be so much harder. Gerard's equanimity surprises me. I was informed that he was very anxious, as I might expect him to be. Is he the 'strong' husband, stoic for Lisa's benefit? In response, Lisa smiles but is silent. She masks her suffering but nevertheless it is palpable.

I suggest reflexology and therapeutic touch (TT) may be beneficial. I say these therapies would help to bring his body into balance to fight the cancer. He feels this is in tune with his alternative medicine approach. Ginnie takes this as her cue to leave, wishing them a good holiday.

I ask what type of music helps him to relax. He laughs, confessing a preference for heavy rock. I suggest a CD I have brought along – *Chaco Canyon* by Rusty Crutcher. Gerard laughs at the name 'Crutcher' – genital humour. He rises and puts the CD on, enthusing about a Pink Floyd tribute band he had tickets for tomorrow night. His type of music. He cancelled them because of his deterioration. These small losses accumulate . . . nibbling way the quality of their life.

I tell him I have added patchouli and frankincense to the base reflexology cream.

'The patchouli is for positive thinking and the frankincense is to help you feel calm.'

Gerard laughs.

'I need plenty of that then!'

Such a throwaway comment reveals a deeper fear beneath the positive mask. The mask is his coping front to the world. We all must cope with our predicaments in the best way we know how. He needs to keep it together or otherwise he will crack open and be lost on an ocean of despair.

During the reflexology, Gerard drifts on the edge of sleep. Afterwards he is enthusiastic, exclaiming how relaxing it was! He asks me to visit again. He loves the music and Lisa asks where she can get it. I give them Emerald Sound's website.[4] I get sucked into Gerard's enthusiasm and offer to teach Lisa TT when I next visit so she can use it with Gerard. I am mindful that she feels helpless and would like to do something positive to help. Of course, she does help but I sense her desperation to do more. TT offers a tangible opportunity to do something specific to help Gerard and help dissipate her despair into positive energy for helping Gerard. However, I do not say as much to her.

Outside the house, I breathe in the cool air. Meeting Gerard and Lisa has been intense. Their suffering lies thick on the surface. They are full of hope yet the signs are deeply ominous. I sense dark clouds looming and wonder just how much I can help them. They clutch at straws and I am OK about being another straw. That may sound trite but it does reflect how I read the situation.

Two weeks later, October 30

Ginnie is leaving as I arrive. Brief words on the doorstep – Gerard's wound has worsened. The outlook is gloomy. Jessie, their eight-year-old daughter, answers the door in front of Lisa. She has a lovely open face. Lisa explains:

'She's off school as she has a cold.'

I shake Gerard's hand but not Lisa's. I sense her distance both physically and emotionally, as if she is in a bubble as protection for her fear and vulnerability. Gerard is cheerful; he says the New Forest break had been good if windswept! He feels the wound is stable. The odour from the wound is not so penetrating although he says he can still smell it.
Lisa says:

'I think I've become acclimatised to it . . . he's not using the charcoal dressings because their hard edges digs into his wound.'
'Did the lavender and bergamot help at all?'

Lisa replies:

'We haven't used the oils because the smell was too strong . . . I have asthma and need to be cautious . . . I feared they might trigger an asthma attack.'

---

4 www.emeraldgreensound.com

'That's OK . . . it was only an idea. You know your body and you must take care and stay in good shape.'

I wonder why I reassure them. Do I think they feel they have failed in some way? I can see the way health professionals prescribe treatments that create an expectation of compliance. At the core of *being available* is dialogue . . . of working with the family, exploring ideas and negotiating the best way forward as we read it.

Gerard's left leg has become swollen. He says it just happened. I suspect the damage to his lymph nodes has blocked the lymph flow. Local pressure may also compromise the venous return. However, I am happy to continue the reflexology. I am cautious of mixing patchouli and frankincense essential oils into the reflexology base cream because of the threat to Lisa. I mix a little for her to smell. It has a subtle non-intrusive yet enticing aroma that she senses offers no threat and gives her consent.

I commence the reflexology with my relaxation ritual by placing my hands along the base of each foot (see page 73). I stay in this position until I am *centred.* By this I mean until I have tuned into myself and centred my healing energy free from distraction, until I have tuned into Gerard and become one with him so the healing energy can flow between us without resistance, and tuned into Avalokiteshvara, the Bodhisattva of compassion, for Gerard and myself to bathe in his infinite love. Then, and only then, are the conditions right for healing.

As I finish the treatment, Gerard is asleep. He looks so peaceful, a respite from the insidious progression of the cancer devouring him. After a few moments I wake him. He says:

'That was fantastic.'

Lisa, on cue, comes down stairs with Jessie – Jessie so full of life, bubbly, interested, chatty; a real joy. Such innocence amidst this unfolding tragedy. Within their own home, I feel the children's presence much more than when children visit at the hospice.

I leave some oil for Lisa to massage Gerard's feet because they are so dry without any essential oil added! I emphasise the importance of keeping the skin hydrated to minimise the risk of infection, especially the leg and foot swollen with lymphoedema. Massaging Gerard's feet will help Lisa feel she is contributing something positive and to some extent compensates for me not teaching her TT today because of pressure of time. A slight wave of guilt makes me feel uncomfortable but she doesn't remind me about the TT. I am reminded of the saying 'Don't make promises you can't keep'. In the pressure of the moment it is easy to promise things especially when people have great suffering.

Guilt immediately creates a barrier and diminishes my ability to be authentic. Perhaps, on reflection I could have said:

'Lisa, I don't have time to teach you therapeutic touch today.'

Tomorrow Gerard and Lisa are going to Lourdes for a couple of days with his parents. Gerard says:

> 'Who knows what might happen. I'm not particularly religious but maybe a miracle?'

Another throwaway comment that reveals his pessimism. I don't verbally pick up the cue. Our eye contact and silence are enough. We make an appointment for next Monday. Lisa will be at work and the children at school creating an opportunity for Gerard to explore his deeper fears with me if he so chooses.

Later I meet with Esme. She doesn't feel Gerard and Lisa are being realistic. They are seeing the consultant tomorrow but Esme doubts whether the consultant will be honest enough with them. She wonders how much the family should be prepared because Gerard's femoral artery could easily rupture resulting in a fatal haemorrhage. I sense the dilemma – would being totally honest crush Gerard and Lisa's need for hope? Should the consultant respect their right for autonomy or act with beneficence to protect then from harm? Positioning self within the ethical tension between patient autonomy and professional autonomy is not easy.

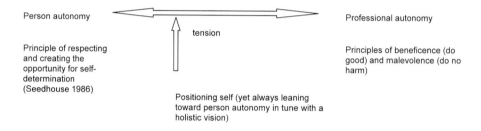

Knowing Lisa and Gerard, my gut instinct is to be honest. Once practitioners distort the truth or collude with what Lisa and Gerard might want to hear then trust becomes a slippery slope. Breaking bad news well is an act of caring – and needs to be given by someone who is available to them. Being honest does not have to be brutal. It may enable them to surface their deeper fears and focus them on making the most of their life together. It may help them make different decisions than the ones they are making now. It gives them control of their destiny yet with professional support as appropriate. Perhaps some professionals instinctively prefer to be in control in order to control their own feelings, their own comfort.

I wonder what Jessie thinks seeing three health practitioners in one day? She must sense that something bad is happening to her daddy. I wonder how perceptive children are? I gaze at her, seeking give-away signs but I cannot tell.

Five days later

The first thing I notice entering the house is the stench. It is not as bad as my first visit but it hangs like an ominous cloud. I shake Gerard's hand.

'How was Lourdes?'
'Now there's a story to tell . . . we discovered the evening before departure that Lisa's passport had expired. It would have been impossible to renew the passport the next day before the flights so we didn't go. My parents went as planned. We are hoping to get the insurance to cover the costs and hopefully go in December before it's too late.'

Gerard fixes me a stare when he says that:

'I mean to get the most benefit . . . Dad brought some holy water back and poured it on my leg . . . it felt warm.'

Gerard is animated. I sense how much this act meant to his healing. I ask:

'Are you Roman Catholic?'
'No . . . I'm not humungously religious . . . it's worth trying.'

I am mindful of the way people turn their gaze towards the spiritual when their taken-for-granted immortality is questioned. However, I sense the significance of a religious connection. I say:

'Sister Mary, a Roman Catholic nun and a volunteer at the hospice says prayers each day for people at the hospice. Would you like me to ask her to say prayers for you? Research[5] indicates this can be healing.'
'Yes please.'

His left leg remains swollen, perhaps a little more than previously, although it's hard to judge. I ask:

'How is the wound?'

Gerard describes the wound. It has a deep core in the lower groin. It spreads up the groin crease although not as deep. It spreads down the groin crease with his inner thigh. It has burst out in several places on his inner and rear thigh. More recently, it has tracked across the top of his pubis. He noticed a series of small lumps that then break down.

'When I get the lumps I know what's coming.'

I think:

'Wow, it's voracious, eating you alive . . .'

but I am silent. Silence between us. An image of cancer on the rampage. Mindful of the moment I ask:

---

[5] For a summary of prayer healing research see Dossey (1993).

'Do you ever contemplate that you won't beat this thing?'
'I'm hopeful it will get better . . . but sometimes it does cross my mind that I won't.'

A dark shadow creeping ever closer.

'You're not considering conventional medicine again yet?'
'No, not yet, although the chemotherapy remains an option if things don't go so well with the alternative approach.'

As Gerard talks, I'm thinking:

'Well things aren't going well so do you need to make that decision? But then I suspect it's too late anyway and why would he want to suffer chemotherapy on top of everything to no avail. Perhaps the doctors would not offer it now anyway'

After the reflexology, Gerard is again asleep, so I work down his body using TT, in particular focusing on his energy flow down his left leg. He opens an eye but says nothing. Just then Lisa arrives, sent home from work to look after Gerard. Her work people had picked up on her distraction. She looks stressed, although her taut smile attempts to mask her despair.
Gerard says:

'I was drifting in and out of sleep, catching up on lost sleep. I didn't get much sleep last night.'

Lisa responds:

'It's been a difficult weekend in the aftermath of the Lourdes fiasco . . . Gerard's been confused and restless.'

She asks if I was doing TT with Gerard. I say:

'Yes . . .'

Lisa responds:

'And did you say you would teach me to do that?'
'Yes . . .'

I feel the guilt twinge in not delivering what I said I would. Careless me.
Lisa says that Gerard's leg has swollen up again – it had gone down after my last treatment. Maybe the reflexology helped to reduce the swelling although I do not reinforce this possible connection.
I offer Lisa reflexology next visit to help relax her. She is uncertain.

'Not if it takes away from Gerard!'

I reassure her that it won't. Gerard urges Lisa to accept my offer, which she eventually does with a flourish. I need only look into her eyes to touch her aching and exhausted spirit. Yet she turns her eyes away as if she cannot bear the pain reflected back.

Four days later

I am at the hospice preparing to visit Gerard. However, after my last visit I decide to discuss Gerard's care with Esme, the Macmillan nurse. Entering her office, she is on the phone speaking with Lisa. I listen to the grim tale. Esme tells Lisa that Gerard will die, and the need to tell the children. I wonder about saying these things on the phone.

The call is finished. Esme looks shattered.

'That was tough . . . I visited them yesterday and could see that Gerard had deteriorated, that he was dying. I told Lisa what I felt about that. The wound was a solid black necrosis, infected and had haemorrhaged . . . Lisa just phoned me, not wanting to believe what was happening.'

'I'm about to visit . . . I'm pleased I popped in to to see you.'

Leaving Esme I drive to the house. I feel I am walking into a cauldron, the door opens, Lisa offers a faint smile through her faint complexion. Both children are around her legs. Blank faces peering out, shocked. Lisa trying to be brave for them. She says:

'Gerard's in bed. Go up . . . he will be pleased to see you.'

Gerard lies on the bed . . . his leg exposed, swollen in its bandages.

'Gerard . . . I've heard the news.'

Gerard is tearful, shocked, devastated by his bad news. I sit with him, helping him talk through his tears and fears. He is waiting for the GP to arrive at any moment so declines any treatment. He would like me to come next week if that's OK. I hold his hand to say goodbye . . . my heart feels very heavy but I put on a brave face.

Downstairs Lisa is waiting for me. I ask her to tell me how things have been and she pours out her heart. Jessie is distant from me, but Greta the youngest daughter asks me what I do with her daddy. I kneel before her and say I touch his feet to help him feel better.

She wraps herself around Lisa's legs and says:

'Can you touch my feet?'

I laugh.

'Of course I can . . .'

Greta throws herself onto the sofa and offers me her foot. I massage it. She giggles and says it tickles but wants me to play with her. After a few minutes

Jessie joins in the fun. Even Lisa relaxes observing the scene. It feels as if we burst the tension . . . allowing expression for the pent up emotion that was suffocating them. Children bounce easily and remind us that life continues. Lisa is grateful.

Five days later

Lisa answers the door.

> 'I tried to contact you. I just missed you at the hospice to stop you wasting your time . . . the district nurse now comes at 11 am so we are less rushed in the morning getting ready for her visit. Gerard is in the bath now . . .'

Lisa shouts up the stairs:

'Gerard, it's Chris!'

Gerard shouts his greeting down the stairs. Lisa says:

> 'The weekend was just turmoil but things have now settled down a bit. The children have gone back to school today, they have both been off sick with colds. I managed to sleep better last night because Gerard's pain control was improved by taking three spoonfuls of oromorph at night. Before that, he was restless with pain throughout the night. Getting up the stairs stirs the pain. Now the movement is still painful but overcome.'

I *gently* listen as Lisa releases her words. By *gently* I mean in a way that reinforces my availability to her. I am mindful of being there to ease her suffering, of easing the stress that has accumulated over the weekend. Her life is a rollercoaster reacting to what unfolds. She feels out of control because Gerard's illness trajectory is so unpredictable and because she resists the inevitability of his death. She seeks out signs of recovery but finds none. Nothing positive to cling to except morsels of comfort in that Gerard's pain control is better. It is as if she has absorbed Gerard's suffering as her own. His pain is her pain. His pain control relieves her.

I want to hold her, to contain her but wrapped up in her suffering she is distant from me, wound up like a *taut spring*. Something inside me wants to fix it for her and makes me feel anxious. I must take refuge in simply being present. It is enough although it seems so little. Sometimes the moment, like a large wave sweeps me away just when I thought I could surf well! I emphasise it is no bother for me to visit. I arrange to visit again on Friday and depart.

Reflection

The comment about three spoonfuls of oromorph is obviously advice in tune with current opioid therapy. Maybe I could have given that advice if I had explored his pain history in more depth using the reflective cue 'How has this health–illness event affected Gerard's normal life pattern and roles?' It is clearly my role to complement conventional allopathic approaches to pain.

Two days later, Friday November 15

Driving to the house, I anticipate that Gerard's condition will have deteriorated and that their suffering will be thick in the air. It has also been a tough morning at the hospice with Saved's death (see page 107). As I drive, I am mindful of my breathing using a variation of Thich Nhat Hanh's meditation taken from his book The Blooming of the Lotus (1993:15) to calm my mind and ride the windhorse. The windhorse is a powerful healing image taken from the Shambhala teachings (Trungpa 1984). The wind is the exuberant and brilliant energy of goodness that exists deep within each of us and which connects us. With true compassion, the wind can be harnessed and ridden to heal others.

> Breathing in, I calm my body
> Breathing out, I smile
> Breathing in, I touch my goodness
> Breathing out, I ride the windhorse

This meditation has such a positive effect on me. It transcends me onto another dimension where I can be fully present beyond my residual suffering of Saved's death this morning, to be available to Gerard and Lisa.

Lisa opens the door. I half expect her to say that she has been trying to contact me not to come. But no, Gerard is sitting in his usual chair with his feet elevated. He has more colour in his face and feels less tired. He is cheerful and looking forward to his reflexology. Despite all that has happened and the 'bad news' of his prognosis, he is continuing with his 'alternative diet' although he confesses that he is struggling to keep up with the prescribed water intake of five litres a day. He is hanging in there.

The reflexology is uneventful. As before Gerard falls asleep. When he wakes he says the therapy was immensely relaxing but more than that, he was transported to a place beyond fear, another level of consciousness. He can't explain it. I say that sounds good. When people tell me this I am very pleased, because I sense this place is beyond fear, a spiritual sanctuary, a cleansing place where Gerard returns refreshed, less fearful, more accepting.

Lisa is impressed listening to Gerard. His positive talk comforts her. I ask her how she feels. Whispered through a sad smile she says:

'I'm very tired.'

When I empathise, she says:

'Does it show?'

I say she hides it well but nevertheless I can feel it. She agrees but she has no choice.

'Would you like some reflexology?'
'Yes please.'

Her acceptance of the reflexology surprises me. I imagine her *taut coil* has been overstretched and buckled. She sits on the sofa next to Gerard's chair. I guide her through the relaxation ritual. She relaxes well despite the phone ringing and Gerard talking to his work boss for about 15 minutes. It interferes with our rhythm yet I must flow with it . . . treating people at home is always subject to such disturbance. Life doesn't stop because we wish to suspend it.

Afterwards, Lisa says:

'At one point I was conscious I didn't have any thoughts in my head.'

Such a perfect statement of relaxation.

Ten days later, November 25

Lisa's mother opens the door. Lisa comes to the door and informs me that Gerard was admitted to the hospice yesterday. Things took a turn for the worse last Wednesday when Gerard became increasingly confused. Her mother is staying at the house as both Jessie and Greta are sick. Lisa says:

'Jessie had been crying all night . . . I would have slept at the hospice but couldn't because of her . . . I didn't get any sleep.'

My heart weeps for Lisa. If I could scoop her in my arms and take the pain away I would. We are back in the cauldron where the threads of her life are hanging loose, torn from their safe hem. I say:

'I am going to the hospice now . . . I will see you there shortly?'

She replies:

'Yes, I'm coming in now.'

At the hospice Gerard's sister Leanne is at the bedside. She looks so much like her brother. Gerard's other sister lives in New Zealand and is flying home on Wednesday. I am mindful of creating a space or clearing amidst the chaos of Gerard's dying where we can dwell together; a place where we can become one in our mutual endeavour to ease Gerard's and each other's suffering, being open to and accepting each other's vulnerability, and where people can be themselves rather than act out any expected role.

Frederiksson (1999:6/16), reviewing the literature on presence, notes that:

> The power of presence as 'being with' lies in making available a space where the patient can be in deep contact with his/her suffering, share it with another, and find his or her own way forward.

Again, the idea of creating and holding a healing space with the intent to move through the staccato rhythm, embracing the chaotic to find meaning until we reach a place of stillness.

Gerard lies in bed, apparently unconscious and unresponsive. I move close to greet him . . . he stirs and Lisa jumps in expectation but the moment has gone. We sit by his side . . . she holds one hand and I hold another as she recounts Gerard's last few days and deterioration. Gerard's erratic breathing bothers Lisa. In response, I suggest giving Gerard TT to ease his breathing pattern. Lisa accepts the offer. His energy field is cold. Over the next 20 minutes I gradually warm the energy field, in fact almost too much! I then had to cool him down again! Yet my efforts have changed his breathing pattern – his laboured breathing has eased. Lisa is grateful. She says that Gerard's hands are warmer.

She accepts my offer for reflexology but only if she can continue to hold Gerard's hand. Not a problem.

I play an Enya CD and for an hour we dwell in the rhythm of the music as I work my reflexology movements. I cannot describe the sense of stillness in the room in the midst of the unfolding tragedy. Lisa says she went to sleep at one point. Now she feels more relaxed and energised. I joke that we weren't disturbed this time by Gerard's mobile phone and his conversation with his boss. It's a kind of black humour that Lisa finds very amusing. It's also poignant because it triggers memories and refocuses the attention on Gerard.

Lisa suddenly exclaims that Gerard's breathing has eased. I say the TT has balanced his energy field and eased his soul pain, helping him to relax in his deeper level of consciousness. Lisa's own spirits lift. It is not easy to watch and listen to the laboured breathing of a loved one. I move to comfort Lisa by putting my arm around her shoulder in a sort of camaraderie way but immediately I sense her tautness and my transgression across an unspoken barrier and quickly withdraw. The gender difference is significant because a few minutes later, Brenda (staff nurse) enters the room and puts her arm around Lisa's waist as they stand facing Gerard. Lisa responds by putting her own arm around Brenda. I feel rejected and isolated especially as I had dwelt with Lisa and Gerard for much of the day and know them from my home visits. I realise the taboo of touch. I also realise my need to touch is beyond an expression of care but a release of my compassion, as if it needed physical expression.

Before I depart, I set up an aroma-stone with neroli to infuse the room with a sense of reverence, ensuring first that Lisa will not be compromised by the aroma. Neroli is an absolute oil I use extensively in such moments. It has a beautiful fragrant aroma. Its spiritual dimension is expressed by Worwood (1999:235):

> Neroli touches the realms of the angels, and anyone who uses it is brushed with the light of angels' wings.

Nothing could be more appropriate as Gerard dies.

Reflection

Later, writing my journal I am plagued by doubts as to my use of touch. Through the text, I describe using different types of touch for different purposes:

- Touch as ritual greeting by shaking hands
- Touch as a technique (e.g. reflexology)
- Touch as play with the children
- Touch as hugs
- Therapeutic touch as a non-touch massage with the intention to nurture relaxation
- Touching the other with presence
- Being touched by events

Shaking hands is a normal social greeting. Playing with the children's feet burst the tension. It was spontaneous and effective. Touch as reflexology involves touching a relatively safe body area, which transcends the social mores on touching because it is an accepted therapeutic approach that Lisa consented to. Touch as therapeutic touch is non-touch, and again an acceptable treatment approach.

It was my use of touch to comfort Lisa at Gerard's bedside that was problematic and unskilful. Clearly, I was not mindful enough of the signs. I had assumed an intimacy and responded to my own need to contain and comfort her. The idea of containment by holding her is a powerful response. Would she want that? She is young and distressed, and my touch may be easily misconstrued, transgressing social mores. Perhaps to be held by another man in front of your dying husband was an affront. Clearly my relationship with Lisa was not safe enough for her to accommodate my use of intimate touch. Davidhizar and Giger (1997) suggest that some patients do not like to be touched, let alone young grieving spouses. I speculate, yet I cannot ask her how she felt at that time.

As I touched her I recoiled, like a reflex action. I knew I was on dangerous ground. My body knew even as my mind was distracted. I had invaded 'her space' even as I am part of her space. It is helpful to consider 'space' in the way I position myself and the way Lisa positions herself within the caring environment. It seems to be a reciprocal positioning, reflecting how touch is always an interaction. In touching I am touched and vice versa. Many patients accept having their space invaded as a consequence of illness and treatment. It is a surrender of autonomy in exchange for care. Edwards (1998:3/17) notes that:

> Touch breaks through the personal space of the individual into their intimate zone and as such will require permission or at least acquiescence if it is to be personally or socially acceptable.

I assume 'socially acceptable' refers to situations when the other is unable to negotiate the use of touch for themselves and hence the use of touch is judged from a more objective social norm.

Carter and Sanderson (1995:4/10) state:

> Autton (1989) believes that nurses must be in tune with themselves if touch is not to prove inappropriate. Autton states 'touching involves risk . . . nurses must also bear in mind that individuals have thresholds of intimacy similar to thresholds of pain.'

Reflecting on the idea of transgression by touching Lisa suggests that I had not gained Lisa's agreement to be touched. Chung Ok Sung (2001:8/15) notes that:

> Physical touch in caring as a behavioural process of skin-to-skin contact between people is based on commitment to humanism, and is oriented to addressing emotional and physical discomfort in humans. It is a process of intervention through which physical and emotional comfort is promoted and spirituality is shared. It is an intentional, shared, and mutually understood process, which has specific social role meanings and is based on a specific framework of the caregiver.

Chung Ok Sung's idea of physical touch being based on a commitment to humanism is flawed. On the contrary, I might argue that it is based on a Buddhist philosophy of wisdom and compassion. I struggle because I was not mindful enough of Lisa's position. I agree that touch should be intentional as with any nursing response yet sometimes events overtake us. I agree my response intended to bring emotional comfort. However, my use of touch with Lisa as she stood by her dying husband was flawed, reflecting a misunderstanding of her needs and/or a misunderstanding of my own motives. For Lisa, my *arm round her shoulder* touch was physically uncomfortable for her at that time and negatively detracted from the more positive messages. Lisa was bewildered and searched for meaning in Gerard's dying. I sensed my use of touch was to communicate more overtly my presence – that she was not alone on this journey and was intended to ease her suffering. Here I sense ambiguity, of Lisa's mixed interpretation. On one level, I feel certain she did recognise and accept this message, but on another, more embodied level, she sensed a threat. Perhaps touch does convey sympathy yet it must be safe and interpreted by the other on an unambiguous level. I should have made myself available and let her initiate any touch outside the safe zones.

Perry (1996:13) noted, within her study of male and female expert nurses' use of touch:

> The men were more inhibited, limited perhaps.

Perry asks the question if this finding is still a reflection of societal norms with which I undoubtedly identify. Evans (2002) researched eight male nurses to explore their experience as nurses and the ways in which gender relations structure different work experiences for men and woman as nurses. Prevailing gender stereotypes are embodied; men as sexual aggressors and men nurses as gay which creates caution in nursing both women and men. I am haunted by the idea that Lisa might perceive me as a sexual predator. Evans (2002:12/15) concludes that:

> The gendered nature of men nurses' caring interactions reveals the ways in which gender stereotypes create contradictory and complex situations of acceptance,

rejection and suspicion of men as nurturers and caregivers. Here the stereotype of men as sexual aggressors creates suspicion that men are at the bedside for reasons other than a genuine desire to help others. When this stereotype is compounded by the stereotype of men as gay, the caring practices of men nurses are viewed with suspicion in situations where there is intimate touching, not only of women patients, but of men and children as well. In each of these patient situations, men nurses are caught up in complex and contradictory gender relations that situate them in stigmatizing roles vulnerable to accusations of inappropriate touch.

Evans suggests that for these reasons men as caregivers goes against the grain. I sense a grain of truth in what she says. When I trained as a nurse issues of sexuality and intimacy were not discussed because patients were depersonalised. Even my training as a complementary therapist barely touched on these issues.

The emergence of holism and its implications in terms of the nurse–patient relationship inevitably creates these concerns for the sensitive practitioner. Previously (Johns 2000:27), I reflected on sexuality and gender when working with a female nurse one morning shift at a hospice:

> We started by helping Alice, a woman who required some assistance to wash. She was happy for me to help her, although I was sensitive to any sense of intrusion and embarrassment on her behalf. Would a woman who was terminally ill like to be helped to wash by a strange man? However, I didn't sense any resistance. Nurses can be insensitive to patients requiring intimate care. They take it for granted that patients will accept being nursed by any nurse, male or female. This seems more taken for granted by female nurses because of the stereotypical societal role of women as carers. In considering the Burford NDU model cues – 'Who is this woman?' and 'What is important to make her stay in hospital comfortable?' the practitioner develops a sensitivity towards the sexuality of the patient.

Perhaps I might be accused of being oversensitive, but my concerns are reinforced by the experience with Lisa. I feel as if I have embodied the stereotype Evans (2002) discusses. Why else would I be so concerned? If I have embodied the stereotype then so have other people, which must make the idea of being nursed intimately by a male nurse disconcerting for many patients. Do they grin and bear it, or suffer the indignity in silence? Perhaps they are silent because they do not want to reveal their prejudice against men, conforming to a competing stereotype of giving up part of one's identity in becoming a good patient.

Evans' observations are supported by Edwards' study of space and touch with patients over 75 years old. Edwards (1998:9/17) cites female patients are ashamed of their old bodies if seen by a man and a male patient who says 'It didn't feel right a man doing such intimate tasks'. In other words, it is not necessarily how I project myself but deeper social norms at work in the way Lisa faced me. The men in Evan's study (2002:6/15) noted they use touch less than their female colleagues and were more sensitive in how they touched:

> Participants voiced concern that women patients might be uncomfortable and/or misinterpret their touch – a situation that in turn might lead to accusations of inappropriate behaviour or sexual molestation . . . to quote one respondent: 'You have to be very careful that you assess the situation and know that this might be an inappropriate place to touch.'

These men talked of a line they did not cross . . . and yet I am conscious of transgression. Again I struggle with my containment, of being contained within a stereotypical box. Mindful of that idea, it is I who contain myself and fret over possible transgression. Evans (2002) draws on studies that reflect the way men have to learn to touch in contrast with women who are credited with natural ability and that men are judged against a feminine norm of what constitutes caring expression through touch.

I know that touch is a significant response to ease the suffering of the other person by communicating compassion and sympathy. Beyond the normal social rituals of touch, it is an intimate expression of care which the health practitioner is given licence to transgress normal social boundaries. However, touch must be mindful, as a response to invitation especially if it involves family members rather than the patient and considering the age and gender of the person receiving touch. I know this intuitively, yet my experience with Lisa suggests that sometimes in our effort to ease suffering we may unwittingly transgress and that such actions may create anxiety and detract from the caring relationship.

As both the literature and my story suggest, touch is complex. The literature on touch reflects an intellectual effort to explain touch as some entity that can be applied, whereas in reality, touch – like caring itself – is a response to a situation that is relational, unique, embodied and contextual. The key to using touch as with all caring practice is mindfulness – the ability to read the signs, interpret both self and others' motives and respond in appropriate ways to ease suffering.

Three days later

Gerard died yesterday in Lisa's arms with Jessie and Greta present. Christine (staff nurse) says it was beautiful. Can death be beautiful? I wonder if Lisa or Jessie would describe it as such. Christine's words reflect both a hospice need to realise the 'good death' and her need to alleviate her personal suffering by romanticising the death. Perhaps her words reflect a sense of relief given the traumatic circumstances of Gerard's condition and his young family. I know that when death is perceived as 'not good' nurses doubt themselves, that somehow they have failed in some way. Such is the emotional tag of death work. The quest for the 'good death' is a social defence mechanism in the effort to normalise and sanitise death.

Mary (staff nurse) says that staff are reeling after six deaths in one week. Why should staff be reeling? Isn't it what we do? Perhaps, but young patients dying, young widows, horrific wounds and the cries of young children cut across normal sensibilities. In the face of such suffering nurses absorb it – it becomes their own suffering. The words of White (2004:440) et al. from their investigation of the impact of unrelieved patient suffering on eight palliative care nurses ring true:

> All the nurses reported that they tried very hard to relieve a patient's suffering and when they were not able to do this there was a feeling of helplessness, distress, vulnerability, frustration, sadness, of being overwhelmed with a sense of failure.

As often happens when staff are deeply affected by a patient's death, a number of reflections have been organised. I facilitated one session attended by Christine. She expressed her suffering and emotional exhaustion.

'I have little left to give.'

Christine has been deeply affected by the shocking nature of Gerard's fungating wound. She showed me an anonymous poem called *Hibiscence* – a nurse's reflection on the shocking horror of a deep fungating wound. The poem had profoundly touched her. I suggest Christine tune into an aspect of Gerard's care and write her own poem as a way of working out her feelings and honouring the caring moment. I share my poem *The heron & the tree* with her. She is touched and inspired. She feels comforted.

Reflection

Christine's words *I have little left to give* highlight what is termed *emotional labour*. Whilst emotional labour is hard work (James 1989) it can also be construed as a 'gift' (Bolton 2000). Emotional labour is regarded as not simply the emotional work of caring but in maintaining a *correct emotional climate* (Bolton 2000:580) whereby the emotional climate is a social norm, a reflection of the way staff are expected to manage their demeanour. In a hospice this may create difficulties where messages are mixed, for example the demand to be both a human being and to be professional creates a tension, *a balancing act between intimacy and distance* (Hem & Heggen 2003:101). The idea of emotional work as a gift is a reflection of compassion and intimacy. This was evident within Jackie's story, where compassion made it possible to be intimate and become one with her. If I become wrapped up in my own concern, then I am likely to get snared in the tension between intimacy and distance and become anxious.

Debriefing events are arranged to enable staff to unload emotional strife. They acknowledge that caring for dying patients and families *is* emotional work. Without release, suffering can accumulate until the person, like Christine, feels she is drowning. Hence the need to create and sustain a caring environment, through normal hospice talk, and through more formal events such as debriefing and clinical supervision (Johns 2004a).

Eleven days later, December 9

A clear blue sky yet a bitter cold wintry day. The dark indigo slowly melts into the dawn as I approach the hospice for the early shift. All the men have urinary tract infections which has me researching which essential oils are best to combat *Escherichia coli* bacteria. Price and Price (1999) advise me to mix lavender, tea tree and marjoram. This mix in an aroma-stone should also help to relieve John's arthritis and ease Brian's anxiety besides masking the unpleasant odour typical of such infections.

Before I leave to attend Gerard's funeral Christine gives me her poem titled *Blue*. She is animated and says that writing the poem helped her to recover her emotional balance.

'I did what you said . . . I just thought of one particular moment – the look in Greta's eyes as she clung to her dying father. I don't know where the words came from . . . they just flowed once I had tuned into the idea.'

Blue . . . for Greta

The moment had come. . . .
But, you were unaware of what was
   unfolding,
The bewilderment in your beautiful
   eyes told me that.
Eyes of the same vivid blue as your dad,
So startling,
So trusting,
So sad.

You could see mummy crying,
You could feel her sadness
As she held you tightly,
Kissing you, stroking your hair,
Softly speaking,
Softly crying,
Softly, softly . . .

She held daddy to her, reluctant to
   let him go
Knowing there were no more options;
She was losing him,
The battle was being lost,
He was going,
He did not want to,
He had no choice . . .

Through my own tears
I was aware of yours
As you looked from mummy to
   daddy;
You had your thumb in your mouth,
You touched your mummy's hand;
She did not notice.
She could not help it,
She was oblivious . . .
For the briefest moment,
She was aware only of him,
She went with him to the brink

But could go no further;
This was now his solo voyage.
Breathing together,
Breathing for him,
Breathing alone.

Then she looked up into big blue
   eyes,
Your blue eyes,
His blue eyes,
His legacy to her
And held you close to her.

Christine's words are beyond cognition; they flow from a deeper consciousness triggered by the horror and poignancy of the moment. Okri (1997) challenges the poet or storyteller that words should be both beautiful and shocking; and in doing so move the writer and the reader into new places, to transgress the line, to transform self. The poem is Christine's closure and yet paradoxically an opening of her heart.

As I drive to the crematorium, I sense the leafless trees are in mourning against the clear blue sky. A bitterly cold breeze penetrates my clothing. The hard edges of the crematorium sharpen the image of coldness. We wait patiently for the funeral cortège to arrive. People wipe away their tears as we wait; so many young people, reflecting Gerard's young age.

As I take my pew with Brenda near the front of the crematorium chapel, I note the familiar pattern of the congregation filling the pews from the back forwards, as if sitting near the front brought them closer to the coffin and death itself. I want to sit as close as possible to the front, perhaps to feel the occasion more keenly. Lisa and the children are just across the aisle. Lisa turns and gazes into my eyes. I feel her sorrow flow from the darkness.

Towards the end of the funeral service, the chaplain pays homage to the hospice for its comfort to Gerard and Lisa. The collection is dedicated to the hospice. Gerard's favourite music plays as the congregation file past to offer condolence to Gerard's family. Brenda hugs Gerard's father, his gratitude is strongly expressed. My turn – I had not met him before and felt his eyes seek me out – as if questioning who I was. As I shake his hand, I respond by saying I am also a hospice nurse and the therapist who visited Gerard at home. His face relaxes in recognition and he expresses his thanks for my care. I had met Lisa's father when he was laying linoleum in the bathroom at Gerard's house to replace the bloodstained carpet after Gerard had haemorr-rhaged. He also looks searchingly at me, seeking out recognition as he shakes my hand, but I do not remind him of who I am. Brenda hugs Lisa intensely. Tears streamed down Lisa's face. I imagine they flowed from a deep well like lava erupting from a blown volcano. Tears that stream endlessly. The hug itself seems endless. Lisa needs Brenda's hug reflecting the profound intimacy of easing the family through dying and death. But then Brenda is very tactile – she once said to me 'You need a hug' after I had returned to the hospice following another patient's funeral; a maternal act that I accepted graciously, yet it was neither invited or welcome. Perhaps it is Brenda who needs the hug as an expression of her own feelings? Perhaps I misread the situation mindful of my *faux pas* of touching Lisa at Gerard's bedside.

It is two weeks since I was last with Lisa. I had considered sending her a card as I had not been present at Gerard's death. Being at the death, sending a card, writing a poem, attending the funeral are all forms of closure. It is why I am at the funeral.

Her eyes are so sad. She moves to grasp my hand and expresses her thanks. I take her hand and move my other hand across her shoulder and pull her gently into a half-hug. There is no resistance, yet I am conscious of transgres-sion even at this poignant moment. The hug is brief. Our eyes connect again and I communicate my compassion. No words, for words could never express the depth of my compassion. Yet I also sense my vulnerability. The key is not to fear vulnerability but to embrace it because its raw edge is healing.

Jessie and Greta gaze at me with eyes wide opened, bewildered. Huge tears distort their faces. Suffer the little children. With each hand I hold their heads, I breathe in their pain and breathe out my compassion. Whew! Some deep breaths to regain my composure. I quickly make my exit rather than linger with the guests.

Reflection

I am confused. On reflection on Jackie's funeral I felt that the funeral ritual was not so much about closing relationships but moving them into a new dimen-sion. Yet with Lisa I sense I am tying up a loose end or making good a frayed edge, because of my residual discomfort. In other words I am not in-place. I am stranded somewhere in no man's land! This feeling interferes with honouring myself and Gerard.

Saved

Friday November 15

Saved is 29 years old and is dying. His Muslim family are about him in the single room that seems too small to hold the swelling family. Their tears and wails fill the air. Saved's father is beside himself. He does not know what to do. In his heart he still hopes that Saved will open his eyes and say something . . . just something to ease the women's suffering; Saved's wife, his mother and his sister. He worries, despite our fervent reassurances, if the diamorphine and midazolam whirring in the syringe drivers have caused his son to be sedated. He is also anxious that his son has passed no urine. Saved's breathing pattern has changed significantly into a cheyne-stoke rhythm. Death is close.

Maud (staff nurse) and I shift Saved's position. His bladder area is distended and tender although Saved expresses no discomfort. Maud cleans his mouth yet Saved's mother must wash him. We move out as yet more family move into the small room. And then the scream pierces the stillness. Saved has died and over the next two hours the family flood in, the women exhausted with their tears. Perhaps 30 or more family spill from Saved's room into the corridor. We nurses can only make ourselves available yet in ways that are respectful to Muslim culture. It is not easy to witness such expressed grief that borders on hysteria. The women throw themselves at Saved's body or cry that he cannot be dead. They collapse exhausted, faint on to the floor. An hour passes and there is no pause in this relentless grief. We have no sense of control, we must simply flow or else we feel helpless. I feel calm and sense the sacredness of death. I find myself doing the essential phowa even from the back of the crowded room. I am conscious of my breathing as I visualise Saved's light lifting and merging with the Allah's divine light. There is no fear – just joy.

Through the grief mist, Ali emerges to discuss arrangements. He asks for two pieces of cloth to bind the feet and head. An old white sheet is found that can be cut up. White seems more appropriate than the pink and blue sheets we use. Ali asks for the death certificate and whether the body can be left here until 2 pm to be collected and taken to the mosque. The idea of 'the body' intrigues me . . . as if Saved's spirit has left leaving behind the shell to be disposed of.

Saved is a young man. He is his father's son. He has a young wife and two small children who were also present. I have experienced other Muslim deaths but nothing so absolutely devastating for the family. Saved's deterioration and death was also quick and caught the family by surprise. They needed more time to dwell with him. Our knowledge of Muslim culture has been tested. For example, someone offered drinks and food yet it is Ramadan where they fast between sunrise and sunset. My lasting thought is admiration that a family can gather and be so linked through strong faith and express their grief so openly. Perhaps other aspects of being a Muslim are constraining, yet I have greater resolve in my own tentative Buddhism. It was important to keep the situation in focus as sacred. Only then can someone sense and flow with the grief rather than feel threatened by the unfolding chaos.

I leave the hospice at 12.30. Before driving away I eat my sandwiches in the car overlooking the fields that unfold across the landscape to eventually merge with the rolling hills silhouetted against the blue sky horizon. I need a moment's stillness after the raw emotions of Saved's death. It is not easy moving from one scene of emotional trauma to another.

Reflection

Whilst death is commonplace, no death has challenged me as much as Saved's death. I felt an outsider touching the edge of this family. But that was OK. Moving closer in, my anxiety to help would have been intrusive. It is a vital skill to read the signs and position self appropriately within the situation yet what did the signs mean? Only by flowing with the unfolding moment could any order emerge from the chaos. Any effort to impose would only have heightened the despair. My ignorance of Muslim grief and ritual was stark and yet by being available it could be worked out with the family. I sense that religion creates a barrier, because it creates uncertainty, anxiety, even fear, that masks the deeper humanness and response to suffering so manifest within the situation. I wanted to reach out and comfort the sufferers yet my hand was tied behind my back by the Muslim labels. I could only look on.

Two days later

I sit with Maud and others touched by this experience and reflect on this extraordinary event, acknowledging the drama, our feelings and helplessness, but most of all our caring. Debriefing restores the blistered spirit rather than dwell on things that might have been better although we all agree we need to better understand Muslim death rituals.

Carol and Amanda

Tuesday December 17

Carol has a brain tumour. She is barely conscious, already heavily sedated. Her mouth moves incessantly, keeping up a barrage of silent conversation. At times I can make out some words. Amanda, her daughter, is better attuned. Carol asks for her two babies; one died after one day and the other after three months. Does she see these babies? Once she cradled the syringe driver thinking it was her baby. The staff gave her a doll to cradle colluding with her needs for comfort. Yet once confronted by Carol, Gladys (staff nurse) had to say her babies were not here. Does Carol hallucinate or does she try to reconcile her torn life? Perhaps as she nears death her babies are there . . . waiting, calling her. Perhaps it comes out wrong, twisted by the cancer and by the large doses of Nozinan, midazolam, diamorphine and ketamine that flood her body. Perhaps, perhaps . . . without doubt dying is a mystery.

Yesterday she walked down the corridor with her arms outstretched, four syringe drivers hanging from her. Now haloperidol has been added to the cocktail to subdue her. She is quietened but is she really relieved of the distress, or delirium if it was that, or does she simmer underneath the subdued consciousness? I wonder – what does she feel? What does she think? Gazing upon her pale face lying there bludgeoned into submission I am uneasy that one drug has been put on top of another until the four drivers purr away with enough sedation to drop an elephant. I feel as if we have been caught in our own trap. No challenge from the family. Do they willingly submit or request it? Perhaps I should ask them – but would I merely open a can of worms?

Yesterday Carol asked Amanda when Christmas was. Amanda told her 'in eight days.' Carol then closed her eyes and has since been unresponsive. Amanda tells me that Carol loved Christmas. I wonder – does she hang on until then? Is she strong enough now? The human spirit is a remarkable thing but does fighting the sedation take her life away? Radbruch (2002:239) challenges:

> Is the primary goal of sedation alleviation of intolerable suffering? If so, what level of consciousness should be achieved? Does the patient have to be unconscious or merely very sleepy but rousable? For longer periods, is sedation designed to be irreversible, or should trials of dose reduction be planned periodically to check the extent of the suffering and whether the patient wants to revise his (or her) decision on sedation? Sedation as a therapeutic option should be the last resort when other options are not available.

I wonder how Carol would be without any sedation. I sense that we have stepped along a certain narrow path and we are unable to turn round. I call it the technology trap, that medications and technology are the solutions to problems. Perhaps they have their use but only to complement the human response to suffering. It seems we often have this relationship the wrong way round. Are we losing our human touch in the urgency to quell the symptom? We did not ask Carol whether she wanted to be sedated but assumed in our parental way that was the way to calm her, or rather subdue her. Were there other options? It is all too easy to reach for the sedation, especially when staff feel helpless. You hear expressions like 'You wouldn't let a dog suffer'. Carol's situation reveals the difficulty of unravelling the complexity of agitation and distress and knowing how best to respond.

Next day

This morning Amanda and Sue, Carol's sister, sit with Josey the night staff nurse by Carol's side. Amanda greets me warmly.

'Hello Christopher.'

Josey expresses her surprise I am called Christopher. I explain that Amanda prefers to be called Amanda rather than 'Mandy' and hence she calls me Christopher. Amanda chips in:

'I don't like shortened names.'

It is an intimate moment, a reconnection that spans the time we last dwelt together. I move close to Carol and greet her. No response. Her small hand feels so fragile in my own. Carol's breathing has a rattle on which a 2.4 mg hyoscine infusion has made little impact. The family are distressed listening. A relentless reminder of her suffering.

The aroma-stone is unplugged, although it is not dry. I replenish the stone with a mixture of lavender and frankincense as before. A strong smell of urine is evident. I suspect her catheter is leaking? The urine is thick and dark leaking from the leg bag lying in the bed. Lorraine (staff nurse) joins us. We decide to give Carol a complete wash now so that we do not have to disturb her more than necessary. As we turn her, thick infected-looking sputum drains from her mouth. After her wash and changing her nightdress, her breathing seems easier. We debate whether to suction her to remove the thick sputum gathered in her mouth and throat. We decide it is better to keep her still rather than encourage the sputum to come up. It would be a never-ending battle that would disturb Carol and her family.

I meet Elsie, Carol's mother and we look through some photographs that Amanda has brought in. The photographs show Carol last Christmas dressed as Santa Claus. They show her with some children of a family she cleaned for. Other photographs show her with her best friend at a party, drunk. She was 'quite a gal', I am told. She has lost so much weight shrivelled in the bed. Other photos show her at home after the chemotherapy. One photograph taken the day before she collapsed when it was felt she would die but she rallied. These photographs really help me see Carol in a new light, as a vibrant attractive woman rather than a dying shell. I can now better tune into her wavelength.

The family ask me when she will die. I cannot say although most likely today, yet her spirit is strong. As the day unfolds, more relatives arrive and gather around the bedside. In the small kitchen Amanda and Elsie prepare a tray of drinks. Jan (care assistant) is with us. Elsie says it's difficult to watch your own daughter die. It seems I have lived these words so often that it is almost legend, as if someone had put these words into Elsie's mouth, and yet I have never heard a mother actually say this before. Once I had said it to a mother as she sat with her daughter but it had felt clumsy, almost banal, almost a cliché. And now Elsie utters these memorable words.

'It is difficult to watch your own daughter die.'

Carol is her youngest daughter. I say:

'Your baby?'
'No. It doesn't feel like that. I had my five children quickly in seven years so they were all babies growing up together.'

Elsie says she hasn't been able to cry. Like the universal mother, she has always been there for her children. Now she tries to be brave, not to show Carol her tears. I suggest I can release her tears by unlocking the tension trapped in her shoulder muscles? She smiles at me as I move my hands across her shoulders and feel the knots each side of her spine close to her neck. She surrenders to my touch as I gently ease this knot . . . and she feels it give way. Her face crumples. I put my arm around her shoulder and she puts her head on my shoulder. Amanda says:

'I love you Nan.'

She kisses and hugs her. Jan in turn holds Amanda:

'A group hug.'

I stand a step back, content that Elsie has released this pent-up energy. In this small space we have touched the universe. I walk back with them to Carol's room. Later I pop in and Elsie turns and looks up at me. I feel her gratitude in her warm, tearstained face.
Carol's best friend is there, her hair spiked with blond streaks.

'I had them done for Carol.'

A young man is also present. I assume it is Carol's son although I do not check it out. He is the only male present. More of Carol's sisters have arrived and now there are six sitting about the bed. I say:

'The family gathers.'

They smile. I have noticed before that when so many members of a family gather it feels more difficult to address them as individuals. I feel more peripheral and feel my way around their collective edge. When just two or three family members are present it is easier to position myself within the family. The young man is inquisitive about the aroma-stone and the oils I am burning. Through his questions he expresses his concern for his mother and his own angst. My role is to be non-intrusive yet be available to guide the family to find meaning and harmony.

Reflection

I ask myself to what extent was I available to this family? This is a difficult question. I might think I was fully available but was I? Could I have been more available? Did I read the pattern of these peoples' lives well enough and appreciate the meanings they gave to Carol's dying? Could I have done things differently? I am intrigued at my response to Elsie in the small kitchen in contrast with my *faux pas* with Lisa (see page 99). Unlike with Lisa, I did seek Elsie's consent to touch her, mindful of touching her and transgressing some unspoken boundary. I interpreted her smile as consent. Perhaps in the privacy of the kitchen and because she is an older woman she saw my touch as caring rather than as a transgression. Perhaps she sensed my unbridled compassion. Intuitively it felt right. It was cathartic and broke open the pent-in emotion.

So many dilemmas reveal the complex ethical nature of everyday practice. Should we suction Carol or not? Should we sedate Carol or not? Perhaps the dilemma of whether to suction was straightforward in the sense we didn't want to disturb her even though the sputum in her throat disturbed her. The use of medication to dry up secretions may be helpful as it is disturbing for the family to listen to the sound of noisy breathing.

The use of sedation is an ongoing saga through my stories. Being a complementary therapist my approach is always conservative with the use of medication. I prefer a non-pharmacological approach although, as with Jackie (page 72) a small negotiated dose of sedation can take the edge off fear. It is too easy, at least on the surface, to reach for the medication rather than invest the time in being with someone. But that is what I thought hospices were good at?

Perhaps for Carol, the sedation created more problems than it solved. Part of the difficulty with responding to someone's agitation is appreciating the cause of the agitation and discriminating between organic and inorganic causes. Yet there seems nothing spiritual in responding to someone's agitation with drugs unless to supplement a more 'spiritual' approach added and abetted as appropriate with psychological techniques – given that agitation is a disruption of the spirit. Perhaps the medical model would put it the other way round, to view a spiritual approach as supplementing the medication.

The increasing medicalisation of palliative care has shifted care towards a more symptom management approach, recognised by Kearney as early as 1992:39:

> It is argued that palliative medicine may be in danger of developing into a speciality of 'symptomatology'. Such a speciality would be confined by the limits of the medical model and its particular view of illness.

Where are we now? Making decisions about care is the core of my, our practice. In doing so I, we are influenced by a notion of what is the right thing to do (the ethical), by a notion of what is best practice (the empirical), and by our own personal perspectives. Perhaps I, we, who dissent from an overly symptom management approach should voice our concerns more clearly. Yet the nursing voice at the hospice has become increasingly mute in decision-making at the hospice with the appointment of a medical director, reflecting a deliberate shift towards specialised palliative care and a narrowing of the gaze towards symptom management. Inevitably, the holistic vision erodes despite its strong rhetoric.

The 'holistic' team is based on collaborative and dedicated effort to realise shared vision as a lived reality in the best way possible through respect for each other – *not* a team dominated by a medical perspective that privileges symptom management under the rubric of *specialised* palliative care practice.

This is not to say that doctors do not profess a holistic approach, just that it is not their primary gaze. The risk is that holism becomes a furtive subculture spoken in whispers.

> The din of symptom management deafens
> Yet, if you listen carefully to the silence
> within the steely din
> You can hear the whispers of holism
> And the muted cries
> that fall on deaf ears.

Tong et al. (2003) in their study to investigate a 'good death' from minority and non-minority perspectives, constructed ten domains that characterised the good death. (Figure 6.1). They note (2003:173/4) that:

> nine of the ten domains pertained to areas often considered outside the traditional realm of clinical medicine

reflecting the broad scope of holistic practice in appreciating and responding to patient and family needs. These ten domains offer a valid framework to reflect on the reality of realising holistic reflective.

Domain	Definition
Physical comfort	Concerns for pain and physical symptoms at the end of life.
Burden on the family	Importance of relieving burdens imposed by end of life individual on caregiver.
Location and environment	Importance of atmosphere during the dying experience.
Presence of others	Importance of having other present during the dying experience.
Concerns regarding prolongation of life	Desire to die naturally and in peace, without the use of machines.
Spiritual care	Importance of spiritual care and support at the end of life.
Communication	Importance of communication between the dying individual, the family members, and health care providers. Adequate and compassionate communication about disease, prognosis, and end of life decisions.
Completion and emotional health	Concept of completing social and emotional tasks before dying. This includes issues like life review, resolving conflicts, spending time with family and friends, and saying goodbye.
Cultural concerns	Importance of respecting cultural and religious differences at the end of life and of not stereotyping minority groups. The important role of the cultural community at the end of life.
Individualisation	Concept of respecting each death as a unique phenomenon without prescribed notions of what a good or bad death is, as well as having the ability to make individual choices concerning death. The importance of being non-judgmental about these choices.

Figure 6.1 Domains of a good death (Tong et al. 2003).

I sensed a tension between imposing a 'good death' and the needs of the suffering patient and family where death and dying is anything but good. The 'good death' mentality emerges as a tyranny to mask suffering and create an illusion of a peaceful death and 'inform' the practitioner that she has done a good job (McNamara, Waddell & Colvin 1994). In other words, the 'good death', as a social norm may impose suffering. It is a distancing technique (Georges 2004) that reflects the medical model whereby death might be a failure. Being *good*, death is then no longer a failure but a success. In distancing self from failure, the practitioner inevitably distances self from the patient and from self.

Ron

Ron is unconscious, slipping towards his final breath. Just 69 years old. When I last met him five days ago he asked to be catheterised because he felt distressed losing his urinary continence. The indignities of dying, as we slowly lose control of body functions. It is no good saying to him 'It doesn't matter' because it does. I hold his hand and sit with him. I sense his sadness but he cannot say anything more. He hands over his physical body trusting us to respect him. Trust is about relationship and a portal into the spiritual realm. I am deeply moved.

Morgan

To be compassionate is to wish that a being or all beings be free from pain.

(Salzberg 1995:109)

January 6 2003

It is a cold clear morning. Morning frost glazes the road and trees. As I drive through the dark deserted lanes to the hospice, I practise the metta bhavana meditation, wishing all beings might be free from suffering.

Morgan suffers from motor neurone disease (MND), a progressive deterioration of her nervous system. Her 'disease' is advanced. She has difficulty speaking and her breathing is compromised. Maud asks if I can ease Morgan's intractable cough. Her sputum gets stuck at the back of her throat because she's unable to use her laryngeal muscles. Next to her bed, besides the oxygen concentrator, is a suction machine used to suck out the sputum when it gets intolerable for her.

Morgan greets me with her thin smile and warm eyes. She is 39 and married to Guy. They have two boys, aged five and eight. The MND was diagnosed five years ago following the birth of the youngest son. Morgan, like other MND sufferers I have met, finds life a great struggle.[6] She says it's difficult to

---

[6] For a deeper understanding of the MND sufferer's despair, see my account with Moira Vass in *Becoming a Reflective Practitioner* (Johns 2004a).

keep positive, especially at home where she is still the mother of two young children. Her struggle is reflected in her words:

'Pleased I am here because I am allowed to be ill.'

Her constant cough tires and distresses her.

Morgan has reduced sensation in her legs and feet and uses supports for her legs to prevent spasticity. She recently had a PEG tube[7] inserted for feeding although this has not been used. She enjoys her food, especially sausages, which she eats by holding in a tissue. She persists with eating despite the risk of choking. Not being able to eat or drink will take away yet another of her life's pleasures. She likes to pass time watching videos and enjoys listening to music. Indeed she has a rainforest CD playing. Its intriguing sounds rise above the drone of the oxygen concentrator. Even so, time weighs heavily. She is constantly tired. Indeed talking to me is tiring for her but she wants to talk. Life is finding balance. She would like some reflexology.

I set up an aroma-stone using benzoin, lavender and frankincense essential oils. I love the thick vanilla smell of benzoin. It will soothe her irritated laryngeal muscle and aid her weak cough as well as easing her stress. I tell her that it was used in former days to help 'cast out devils' (Davis 1999; 55). Morgan is amused by this description; she feels the MND is the devil. I love Worwood's (1999:193) description of benzoin on the spiritual plane:

Helping guide us home to that place within, the inner sanctum of the soul.

It is a message for now and for the future. Morgan knows she will die soon, and these words comfort her, breaking through a silence where issues of the spirit have been avoided. Using such descriptors short-cut conversations into the spirit. All three oils will help with any chest infection. The frankincense will slow and deepen her breathing evoking a sense of calm. The lavender is so versatile and will help her find balance in her body and mind at a time when she is thrown into chaos.

She does not cough during the reflexology, at least for the first 40 minutes.

'Then I became conscious I wasn't coughing and started coughing again.'

Afterwards, she feels relaxed.

'It took me to another place and I can breath more deeply now . . . before my breathing was very shallow.'

So many people say that reflexology 'takes them to another place' – I imagine it is a place beyond suffering, a quiet place where the spirit can fly.

---

[7] A percutaneous endoscopic gastrostomy (PEG) tube is inserted directly into the patient's stomach through the abdominal wall as the means for direct feeding when the person is unable to take food or fluids orally.

I imagine the suffering she endures, yet she never complains. Her life is a time of personal disorganisation and distress, yet it can also be a time of opportunity to find meaning in the experience in the chaos and emerge into a place of stillness. Newman (1994) describes this transformation as expanding consciousness through finding meaning and new ways of living with self if only we can turn our head to face the 'devil' rather than shrink from it. My role is a catalyst to help Morgan dissipate her suffering (negative energy) into positive energy for the journey ahead, so she can smile and be with her young children with joy.

> It's a one time thing
> It just happens a lot
> Walk with me . . .

> (*Cracking*, Suzanne Vega 1985)

Six days later

Morgan has developed a chest infection and become poorly. So much for my prophylactic oils! She greets me with her warm smile. Her irritating cough has gone and now she wants to go home, to get on with her life.

'I can come in here again if I need a rest.'

We sit and talk about living in the 'now' – she feels this is important (the catalyst at work). She says:

'Although I'm not religious I do believe there is a God . . . but not the Jesus thing.'

I didn't prompt this revelation, it simply emerged within the process of making sense, finding meaning and contemplating the future. Morgan radiates serenity yet I sense her underlying sadness. She smiles.

'I am on Prozac but I sometimes wonder about stopping it. I find it dulls me . . . difficult to really laugh . . . takes the edge off things.'

We wonder how she would be without it.

As I give Morgan reflexology we are interrupted first by the physiotherapist, then by the doctor, and finally by her mobile phone leaving a message! Yet as before, she has been somewhere else, somewhere peaceful. A moment of stillness within her chaotic whirlpool. Perhaps the accumulative benefit of reflexology spirals her into higher levels of consciousness where suffering is transcended. Perhaps. Her experience is all that matters.

Two months later

Morgan was readmitted last Friday. It was thought she was dying but she rallied and has had a couple of 'good days'. On her rollercoaster illness–life journey she dips, ravaged by her persistent cough. She coughs for five to six hours each day. It exhausts and panics her. It tears at her weakened spirit. The medical staff have increased the midazolam to stem the sense of panic.

Morgan greets me. Her fragile body propped up in bed amongst her pink bed linen and oceans of flowers. I kneel by her bedside and take her small limp hand. She squeezes mine. A picture of Guy holding their two young sons gazes from the bedside locker. More pink roses arrive. The room is a florist's shop. I wonder if the pollen irritates her throat? She tells me she sometimes dances with the fairies as if the drugs cloud her mind.

Frances and Maud (staff nurses) discuss how best to respond to Morgan's nasal irritation and cough. Can I offer something complementary? Maud says she has used some benzoin in the aroma-stone as it had worked well before. She wonders about using some benzoin in a nebuliser? I pause, uncertain, not wishing to leap to a solution without pondering over the possibilities. I retire to the clinical room and consult my texts.

Walking down the corridor Guy, Morgan's husband, informs Ruth he is going now, and as he talks he falters, words catch in his throat, tears well in his eyes. Maud pulls him into the staff room and closes the door. I glance in and see her hold and comfort him. Maud is so small and he is so large. It feels incongruous. Yet she has such compassion. I would want to be cared for by her.

Using a drop of benzoin in a nebuliser feels risky simply because I have no experience of using oils in this way. Intuitively it feels OK, although benzoin's attribute to ease a cough by relaxing laryngeal muscle is, at least as far as I know, an unsubstantiated claim. Yet it had previously worked for Morgan in the aroma-stone. Morgan is keen to try. So we do it. One drop in 10 ml 0.5% concentration.

Morgan asks me if I can give her a foot massage. However, as I massage her feet she begins to cough, gathering momentum as if each bout of coughing feeds itself. I am uncomfortable, not with her coughing as such, but whether the nebuliser had triggered the cough reflex. I can't escape this thought as I continue to massage her feet. Eventually I stop to wipe away the thick clear mucous along her lips. Her eyes are heavy.

She reassures me that this is her usual pattern, that the nebuliser is not to blame. The coughing has made her hot and sweaty. In response I sweep her with therapeutic touch for about 20 minutes, taking the heat away but not subduing the cough. Eventually it eases somewhat – so I relax and sit with her, holding her hand. I say:

'We didn't stop the cough.'

She gives me one of her plaintive smiles.

'But I felt less panic.'

She absolves me.

Later I discuss with Maud the use of midazolam – how we have reached that point of tension between subduing her consciousness and her desire to live as long as possible to be with her boys; that point where she hands over her body; that point where she struggles to know best; that point where we hold her trajectory in our hands.

I share my attachment to her; how tender and vulnerable I feel because she touches my heart. I feel something wanting to burst forth from inside me. I have given Maud a glimpse of my vulnerability. And in the soft late afternoon sunlight that draws out the colour in Maud's hair, maybe it is enough to dwell in this point of stillness, in a sense of mutual knowing that drifts between us that needs no further delving or understanding. It is the manifestation of the therapeutic team where we can reveal our vulnerability and realise that our vulnerability is a strength, a reflection of our compassion. To be compassionate is to be vulnerable because it is unconditional.

Three days later

Morgan looks exhausted. She seems to be shrinking. Her colour is grey. Partially congealed sputum around her teeth and lips. But, as always, her smile greets me. I hold her hand. It is so small and pale. She says she cannot talk because it exhausts her and her twin boys are coming shortly. Reading the signs, I leave her to rest. Shortly afterwards the two small boys are running about the place in their royal blue school jumpers. Full of life. I wonder – what do they think, what do they feel?

Reflection

Was the decision to use benzoin via the nebuliser a good decision? The 'evidence base' for using benzoin to relax the laryngeal muscles and ease coughing is unproven. But does that really matter? Is it worth the risk in the face of Morgan's suffering and the failure to ease her coughing by more conventional approaches? Morgan is involved in the decision and consents to the treatment. *We* claim autonomy to make this decision and implement the therapy. I ask myself – has my compassion become entanglement in her suffering to the extent it might distort rational thinking? It is the same for my colleagues who suffer in the face of Morgan's intolerable suffering.

Ralph and Maisey

January 20 2003

Ralph is 68. He has a superior vena cava (SVC) obstruction secondary to cancer of his bronchus. His condition is precarious. He quickly goes blue if laid flat. Because of this, a scan to ascertain the extent of the blockage was cancelled. But then I ask myself – why was the scan booked anyway? The medical urge for certainty? Steroids have made no apparent difference to his condition. Ralph wants to go home to die to be amongst the familiar surroundings of his life. Sharron (staff nurse) is arranging his discharge this morning.

After our shift report, I follow Sharron down the corridor towards Ralph's room. Maisey, Ralph's wife, greets us by the door. She has just had a jacuzzi bath after sleeping in the room next to Ralph. She says she is refreshed although sleep was not easy. Ralph is asleep so Sharron leaves the medication on the bedside locker. He struggles with taking the eight small dexamethasone tablets besides the gabapentin and diclofenac tablets. Perhaps the dexamethasone could be give by a syringe driver? Sharron agrees.

Despite everything, Ralph looks comfortable propped in the bed so I sit with Maisey and Sharron at the table outside his door – just social chit-chat about all sorts of things, especially food and cooking. I feel slightly restless, a need to do something rather than just sit here. But the unit is quiet and I must focus on quietening. After about 20 minutes, Sharron excuses herself enabling me to focus the conversation with Maisey towards herself. I need to know this woman. She is 66 and the youngest of 16 children. Her mother first had twins when she was 16 and had Maisey when she was 46, 30 years of constant childbirth. Just six children remain alive, the eldest being 86. Maisey and Ralph live in a large house. Maisey will stay there after Ralph dies, even though the house is so big.

> 'I think out of loyalty to Ralph . . . his presence will be in the house, and also because of my network of friends . . . although a part of me would like a more peaceful place to live away from the traffic.'

I sit with Maisey for over an hour tuning into and flowing along her wavelength, appreciating her thoughts, feelings and fears about what is happening now and about the future. To know someone is to know their suffering. I remind myself that caring *is* patience – one of the qualities of perfect effort steps along the Noble Eight-Fold Path. Effort cannot be rushed, unfolding at its own pace.

> Perfect effort is being mindful that my practice requires effort, patience, commitment and diligence despite any difficulty; there can be no scope for complacency (see page 27).

Tuning into someone is also tuning into self, flowing with someone is also flowing with yourself. It sparks an intimacy, a connection, yet an intimacy never imposed.

Ralph stirs and I help him take his medications. Later I help Sharron freshen him. She asks me to hold him as we roll him so she can do a rectal examination, as she senses that he is constipated, which might further compromise his breathing. It will help him at home if we tackle such problems now. But his rectum is empty. He has sores all over his body. An elbow pressure wound draining copious fluid into a collection bag. He struggles to stand and use a bottle – indeed he is a large man. We feel he should remain in bed so as not to compromise his breathing and provoke the SVC obstruction. We become more conservative but does it really matter? Ralph agrees that standing is difficult although using a urinal in bed isn't easy. A catheter is offered in view of him going home, but he declines.

For Ron (page 114), a catheter gave him dignity when he could no longer control his urine. For Ralph a catheter would strip him of his dignity because he has yet to lose control. Both men could decide what is best for them. Our role is to create the opportunity for these men to decide and to support them in that decision.

We finish Ralph's wash and tidy the room. I note his emaciated legs. Such a contrast from his huge torso. The skin on his legs is rough and dry and must feel uncomfortable. A large pressure sore dressing covers one heel. I offer to moisturise his legs. Maisey says he used aqueous cream but I suggest my reflexology cream with patchouli and frankincense essential oils might be more preferable? Ralph and Maisey appreciate the aroma. And so, for about 15 minutes, I massage his legs and feet, using firm effleurage movements towards the heart, stirring the sluggish circulation. Afterwards Ralph is relaxed and murmurs his approval.

Maisey sits close to Ralph . . . and then she breaks away, tearful and asks me to talk to him – **please**. She gestures through her tears and leaves the room. I know it's about the decision to go home. I sit with him, his lips tremble . . . he is caught in a dilemma. He does not want to be a burden to Maisey but wants to be at home. He doesn't know what to do.

We are silent and then he says he will stay.

Maisey comes back in, more composed. I inform her and she is so relieved because it lifts an enormous pressure from her. She holds him, cradles him and says she will be here every minute with him. He needs this reassurance as I sense the fear rise in him and burst forth . . . his fear of dying, his immense sense of losing Maisey, of being alone.

I touch their love.

It is simply astonishing to be with people at such a moment. Maisey stands up and I sense the emotion flooding through her. I know it's right to offer a hug. She melts into my body and puts her arm around me and for a minute or so I feel the tension ripple through her and then relax.

Ralph has a troublesome cough. In response, I set up an aroma-stone with the same essential oils I had used successfully with Morgan – benzoin, lavender and frankincense. As the beautiful aroma percolates through the room I sense the anxiety dissolve, the stress melt, creating a spiritual space where we can dwell together.

Later Ralph's cough has eased. The family gather like a tribe around the table, six of them. I am reminded of being with Carol's family when I went to say goodbye (page 108).

Maisey says:

'We've been talking about you.'

I know she has been touched by my presence, just as I have been touched by them as the day unfolded. Saying goodbye is never easy. Will I see them again before my next shift on Friday? Nothing can be predicted beyond the certainty of Ralph's imminent death. I bless them with my love.

Four days later

A small candle flickers on the workstation. Ralph died at 6.15 am, not entirely peacefully as the family were disturbed by the 'death rattle' and their huge grief. I cannot find Maisey. Later I see her and instinctively move towards her and hug her, some words uttered that I can't quiet recollect but it is the hug that transmits the depth of our connection.

Two months later, March 21

Walking along the corridor I see Maisey. A wave of emotion washes over me. Open arms. We hug. I ask:

'How are you?'

Her smile breaks into tears. I hold her and stroke her back – it has been very hard for her. She is attending the hospice bereavement group. Memories of Brian's visit after Jackie's death (see page 72). Repeating patterns of care unfolding as if etched in the sand. The hospice a compassionate thread of continuity to help contain grief torn spirits.

Embracing Maisey cherished my own sense of continuity; helping me acknowledge that I too may be fragmented by deaths of patients and the grief of spouses on a deeper subconscious level. My experience in revealing my feelings about Morgan to Maud (page 114) has shown me that I am vulnerable to the suffering of others and that it is OK to be vulnerable. It seems that being vulnerable is a paradoxical honouring of self and other. I have sensed this previously but not brought it into full awareness.

Reflection

Responding to the suffering of others is intimate work. Within the holistic relationship there is always the tension between intimacy and distance in which I position myself (Hem & Heggen 2003). Yet 'distance' is a defensive posture behind a professional barrier to protect self and the person from 'over-involvement', what Morse (1991) suggests leads to an emotional entanglement and a distortion of the therapeutic relationship:

'Over-involvement' reflects the way the practitioner has absorbed the patient's suffering to the extent her therapeutic judgement is blurred. She can no longer see 'the wood for the trees'.

My view is that being professional *is* managing intimacy appropriately by tuning into the person and reading the signs. However, it may not be easy to position self appropriately as my experience with Lisa suggested when I may have assumed an unwarranted intimacy. For whose benefit is intimacy? It is vital that intimacy is not my need whereby failure of intimacy becomes my failure or projected into the other as their failure. Holism has a seductive timbre with an intimacy trap to catch the unwary and romantic practitioner. To be intimate with another I must know myself well. Do I have boundaries to my intimacy to protect myself? The narrative is a quest to embrace my vulnerability so I can dwell easily within intimacy without conditions.

Mona

January 24

I had briefly met Mona as she arrived at the hospice a few days ago. It was an awkward moment because she was clearly distressed being at the hospice and no nurses were available to help her settle in. I had wanted to give some complementary therapies to other patients but had felt obliged to stay and listen to her distressed story.

Today she chooses to have a foot and lower leg massage. During my gentle massage, Mona becomes increasingly relaxed until the pain kicks in. She complains of severe pain in her right calf. It is neuropathic pain shooting from her hip. I know she is diagnosed with spinal cord compression. I give her Palladone as prescribed for breakthrough pain. I rest her knee on a pillow and kneel by her side to wait for the analgesia to kick in. It is an opportunity to explore her story more deeply.

She is a psychiatric nurse. She thought I had known that. I ask:

'How do you feel being here at the hospice?'

It is as if I had pressed a button to release her pent-up feelings. She is overwhelmed with fear for her future:

'Am I dying?'
'What will happen to me?'
'Who will care for me?'
'Where will I live?'

She feels her relationship with her boyfriend is not committed enough. Her ex-husband has offered an annexe at his home but is now backpedalling because of the commitment. She will not be able to do stairs and so her daughter's house would be difficult. What to do! She is waiting for the social worker to speak with her and help her find a good solution. She does not want to be a burden but gets messages that she might be. Now she cannot stand and she feels this pain is yet another marker along a dying trajectory.

A torrent of words

I can only try and listen but have no answers to her predicament. I feel my way along her staccato wavelength, visually smoothing it out with each movement of my hands until she is calm, the crisis worked through. I suggest I give her therapeutic touch to relax her. Afterwards she is relaxed, sleepy even. Between the medication and my treatments her suffering eases.

Later, at shift report, I am mindful of the way the nurses talked about Mona. They struggle to get alongside her. She is demanding yet resists being 'cared-for', not wishing to become a patient, perhaps because she is also a nurse? She is anxious and self-pitying which makes talking with her an emotional demand, especially when there seems to be no resolution to her 'problems' or reward for the carer. A caricature of the unpopular patient (Stockwell 1972). As predicted from this literature, staff tend to avoid her – which paradoxically increases her level of demand. I have often noticed the way staff *react* to more demanding patients when perhaps the answer is to be more *proactive* and take the sting out of the demanding tail. Listening to my colleagues, I felt a tinge of guilt that I too held negative feelings towards Mona. It felt a release to confess that in the shift report. It helped to bring my feelings into consciousness and gave me added resolve to offer Mona further therapy. Perhaps admitting I shared these negative feelings with the staff also helped them to reflect and dissipate their own frustration with Mona. Sometimes the patient's response to their suffering offends and is taken personally. None of us is perfect. We are all vulnerable. The shift report is an opportunity for practitioners to share their feelings and learn together. Such moments are vital to support and challenge practice.

Reflection

It felt like a terrible confession to admit that I too had felt negative about Mona when I first met her. I wonder – could she sense my negative energy? Perhaps that is why I was reluctant to spend time with her on her arrival. The cue intends to help practitioners become mindful of such feelings and deal with them in order to be available to the patient. The reflective effort is to confront and convert negative energy into positive healing energy.

Again the qualities of patience and compassion come to mind. I cannot fix people's problems but I can flow with them. Having advanced cancer and facing death is imponderable. Hence the significance of the reflective cue 'What meaning does this health–illness event have for the person'? Only when I can glimmer the meaning can I begin to flow with the person on their journey as uncomfortable as that may be. I cannot stand in judgement because my own stuff blocks the view. I cannot project my discomfort into the patient and blame her for my feelings. My vision is to ease suffering not increase it through my lack of presence.

Peter and Sam

Monday February 17

Peter is 52 years old and close to death. Someone asks if I can do anything for the odour in his room. I am often asked as an aromatherapist to combat unpleasant odour or what is euphemistically referred to as *perfuming*. However, I must be careful in using essential oils in public spaces as they may irritate people. Sometimes several aroma-stones are in use infusing the air with a heady cocktail that has caused headaches.

Could I also offer Sam, his wife, something? She is very distressed. Walking down the corridor she sits outside his room with her family gathered around her. Her distress is palpable, rippling through her even as she endeavours to contain it. We move into Peter's room and gaze at him. He looks peaceful, his breathing slightly noisy. She holds one hand and I take the other. He is not responsive even though yesterday he took a jacuzzi bath. Today is another story. Yet holding his hand I can begin to tune into him. Meeting a family for the first time under these conditions is never easy.

As I hold his hand I ponder the question – how can I help? Perhaps therapeutic touch? I rest my hand above his chest and abdomen and sense the heat and pressure of the cancer. Sam asks me what I am doing. I suggest that the movement of my hands across Peter's body will help take away the heat and pressure from his body, and ease Peter's suffering. Saying 'ease Peter's suffering' seems to reassure Sam. To treat Peter is to treat Sam especially as she continues to hold his hand. For 20 minutes we dwell in silence as I practice. Afterwards she senses Peter is more peaceful and his breathing is easier. She smiles but I sense the smile is thin.

Sam has been at the hospice at his bedside since his admission. Sam knows Peter is dying and waits anxiously. It is only a week since his diagnosis. For eight months he was treated for stomach reflux whist the cancer ate away his pancreas. He experienced great pain, had lost five stone in weight, then the jaundice appeared and now, just a few days later he is dying. Questions that require answers but not now. Now she must give her attention to Peter. Sam suffers not just Peter's dying but the anguish of his misdiagnosis. Peter is a young man, his life ripped away. I try and empathise with Sam but struggle to connect with the turmoil I sense inside her, inside the container. I ask:

'How are you feeling'?

A sad smile hints at her despair sitting here as her husband deteriorates. She follows me outside his room and says:

'I am bursting inside . . . it is our wedding anniversary today . . . I couldn't sleep last night . . . I kept dreaming I was at home and reaching for him in the empty bed.'

She bursts open. Her tears cascade like a burn in full spring flow. She is tossed on a raging sea of grief. I feel as if I pick my way through the debris, the desolation that cancer leaves in its wake. She has slept at times, and although tired and filled with the stress of being with Peter she wants no distraction from her bedside quest. Like many spouses, she feels that any attention for her would be taking attention away from Peter. She does accept my offer to set up an aroma-stone but does not want a strong heady smell. I choose bergamot, which she likes. Worwood (1999) notes:

> We may cry inside, our hearts aching, but bergamot will lighten the heart and dispel self-criticism and blame.

Perfect words for the occasion. Such is my practice, entering the hospice and finding myself in the midst of such drama. Again I imagine I am the wind-horse, a wind of compassion and wisdom lifting people above their distress into a calmer spiritual place. The caring dance is unpredictable and sometimes breathless as if my wind has been expelled from me, as if in the tension I have forgotten to pay attention to my breath. The extent of the other's suffering can rock my equanimity so I must always be mindful of being in the right place in order to be available to help ease the other's suffering.

Reflection

Uncertain how best to respond, I bought myself time by holding Peter's hand and just sitting silently with him, being mindful of what is happening about me and within me, bringing myself into the right space to give therapy. Yet there seems to be so much pressure from within self and from others to act quickly, grasping at 'solutions' to problems in the face of the other's and one's own anxiety. We need to move away from a *fix-it* mentality to a *being with* mentality.

However, as Schön (1987) noted, there are no easy solutions to the situations that face practitioners in their everyday work. Being with Sam and Peter was a unique human–human encounter under great emotional strain. How best to respond can never be a prescription, even where there is some evidence about the 'best' way of doing something. Such evidence needs always to be interpreted for its value in informing the particular situation. The reflective practitioner never accepts anything on face value but must be able to critique any available 'evidence' for its value to inform practice. Belenky et al. (1986) describe this as the *separate procedural* voice. It is the ability to stand back from something – either self or a research paper – to look at it with the reasoning mind. Belenky et al. contrast the reasoning voice with the *connected procedural voice* – the practitioner's ability to connect with the experience of the other person in terms of the meanings the experience has for that person. The *connected voice* is the feminine yin and the *separate voice* is the masculine yang.

Both voices are significant, yet must be woven together for the practitioner to speak with a *constructed voice* – the voice of the effective practitioner.

Connected procedural voice

Listening to and connecting with
the experience of others within
the particular situation

the voice of **empathy**

YIN

Separate procedural voice

Listening to and critiquing the voices of
authoritative others for their value in
informing the particular situation

the voice of **reason**

YANG

Constructed voice

Speaking with an informed, balanced, passionate and assertive voice

Andrea

February 17

Andrea was admitted this morning. She is 48 years old. She has lung cancer with spread to her mediastinum lymph system. No more treatment is possible. I read her notes and see that she was diagnosed with asthma and that for 15 months her lung cancer was not detected.

She warmly receives my greeting. I perch on the arm of the chair. Her 'cushinoid' face catches my attention and perceptively, she says she has stopped taking steroids but since then her appetite has ceased and she has eaten nothing and drunk very little.

I gently ask:

'Why have you been admitted?'

She says:

'For management of my pain . . . it has got a lot worse recently . . . they are going to commence a syringe driver.'

I note the fentanyl patch on her arm.

'Do you have pain now?'
'No, it's OK at the moment.'

She recounts the story of her diagnosis. I sense the underlying anger at her misdiagnosis but she resists my suggestion of anger. On one level she accepts her fate but on another level she has taken action, asking questions about her negligent treatment. She says:

'I may have a few months, maybe a year . . . I have been deprived of my old age . . . my children will be deprived . . . I feel taking action is not revenge but may stop another woman from having to suffer a similar fate.'

Andrea contains her anger yet it ripples beneath the surface. Unfortunately, such stories are not uncommon. At first Andrea resists any idea of therapy as she is waiting for the syringe driver to be set up. She may also be unsettled, her first admission to the hospice. I notice her feet and jest:

'Seeing your feet makes me want to massage them.'

She laughs and says:

'OK then . . .'

I laugh.

'It sounds as if I want to do your feet for myself!'

She laughs again. The ice is broken.

Her feet are very pale. I suspect her haemoglobin is very low. She says she has no energy. Her feet and lower legs are very dry. She responds by reiterating that she is not drinking much.

'I have dried up.'

Her words a metaphor for the way cancer seems to shrink people.

As I give the reflexology, I gaze at the silver birch trees from the window. The sun is setting through another window. Such beauty surrounds us. Andrea is completely relaxed as if she surrenders to my touch. Words taken from a Rumi poem (translated by Maryam Mafi and Azioma Melita Kolin 2001):

> At last I surrender in the valley of love
> And become free

I imagine how peaceful it must be when someone who suffers so much can surrender into a valley of love. I silently say to Andrea:

'No need to hunt for love anymore.'

Afterwards she smiles.

'I am rekindled.'

Her colon felt stodgy.

'I think you are constipated?'
'I haven't been for two weeks although I don't feel unduly uncomfortable.'

I warn her of the possibility of a healing crisis and how it might present as a sort of hangover and suggest she tries to drink some water to help flush any toxins out of her body.

An hour has passed as we dwelt in the gathering gloom of the fading day.

Two days later, Wednesday February 19 2003

Andrea is on Lindsey's arm by the bathroom door struggling to walk. I greet her and she returns my smile. I ask Miriam (staff nurse) how Andrea has been? Her nausea has stopped and she is eating. Miriam is enthusiastic about the reflexology. She feels the reflexology and cyclizine have done the trick.

Andrea confirms Miriam's report.

'I'm feeling much better. I even slept very well the night after the treatment.'

I note the colour in her face. The soles of her feet are infused with colour.

'I'm even eating!'

Her transformation is striking. I offer another treatment for Friday afternoon and further treatments in day care following her discharge. She accepts this idea with enthusiasm. Andrea's belief that the reflexology can help her is significant. Positive thinking is everything.

Later, I mention Miriam's comment about reflexology to Brenda, another staff nurse. She resists the idea that Andrea's improvement was due to reflexology. She asserts that other staff have been with Andrea, helping her to rest and talk. I acknowledge she is right but I wonder why she is so defensive, as if somehow her own effort with Andrea had been diminished in some way. Of course, it is impossible to *know* the impact the reflexology actually had on Andrea. An audit of reflexology services with hospices demonstrated positive results in terms of patient well-being (Milligan et al. 2002), although the audit could not distinguish whether the reflexology was responsible for the patient's improved sense of well-being. The synergy of caring. Parts come together to weave healing. Neither one thing nor another. All part of the whole.

Two days later

Andrea is being helped back to her bed after visiting the bathroom. Unsteady on her feet she gropes for support. Despite the respite noted above, nausea remains a significant problem for her. She had initially responded well to the cyclizine via the syringe driver, so well that Brenda had discontinued it yesterday and commenced her on oral cyclizine, yet after a sandwich supper she had vomited and continued to vomit so Brenda recommenced the driver.

I ask how she feels.

'Fine.'

Fine – the ubiquitous response. A brave face to the world. Being more focused I continue.

'How is your nausea?'

She recounts the story of last evening. Now, she has a persistent sensation of nausea, so much so that she declines my offer of a reflexology treatment because she feels she could not relax enough. Once again I experience the irony that someone needs to feel relaxed enough to have a treatment when the specific aim of the treatment is relaxation.

However, I do not push the treatment offer. Instead, I ask her if her feet are still dry.

'They are . . . I had a bath yesterday with some oil added (lavender) and it really helped. I loved the jacuzzi.'
'Can I touch your feet?'
'Yes'

Her feet are still dry.

'I can tell you've got more energy?'

She agrees. I offer to moisturise her feet and lower legs. She accepts. I mix peppermint and mandarin to the reflex cream. The peppermint has a strong aroma that Andrea likes. Davis (1999:233) notes that peppermint:

is valuable in vomiting because of its antispasmodic action, which will relieve the smooth muscles of the stomach and gut.

Peppermint may also help Andrea's breathing because it has decongestant properties and will help clear Andrea's head 'leaving the user feeling fresh and bright' (Davis 1999:234). Mandarin also has a calming influence on the digestive tract. Its delicate aroma is dominated by the peppermint, although Andrea can sense it and approves of the mix's aroma.

As before, she surrenders easily to my touch and afterwards says it was immensely relaxing and comforting. Triumph – the nausea has diminished! I'm pleased I persisted. When I know I can help someone it's not easy to simply walk away. I'm intrigued by the way she said *the* nausea rather than *my* nausea, as if it is something, like the cancer itself that has invaded her. Brenda is her usual open and warm self. No obvious hangover from our conversation about the impact of reflexology on Andrea. The conflict has been brushed away but I am mindful to reflect more on the use of complementary therapies with staff alongside medical treatments. I feel outside the decision-making loop, as if complementary therapy is outside the scope of medical management. Perhaps I should assert its value more? Perhaps I would if I had a greater presence at the hospice. As I have indicated in various reflections, I am consulted by nurses but never by a doctor.

Three weeks later, March 14

Arriving at the hospice I am startled to see Andrea's name on the whiteboard against the 'Rose Room' – a euphemism for the room into which we move dead bodies where relatives can view the body before dispatch to the under-takers. In three years at the hospice, I have entered this room just once when Stella was struggling to stem the flow of faecal liquid from a dead person's mouth. A transition room on the edge of the container. A secret place where dark cars arrive with men in dark suits who surreptitiously carry out the dead via a discreet side yard.

I have no desire to see Andrea's dead body but I am slightly shocked at the news. She was discharged home as planned but was then readmitted yesterday, clearly dying. She and her husband had not told their children that she was dying, thinking time was with them. He told them that evening. They came into the hospice to say goodbye. Their mother ripped away from them. What do they feel? Today they chose to go to school. The distraction and comfort of friends.

I sense my loss of the opportunity to treat Andrea and immediately feel shocked at my self-concern and reduction of Andrea into an opportunity. Have I hardened to dying? Hardened isn't a negative word. I am not trying to put myself down, just to say that I do not seem to absorb the other's suffering as mine as easily as I used to. I wonder if I am less compassionate and vulnerable as a consequence. On reflection I do not think so. As if to touch my vulnerability, I write Andrea a poem.

> Today I was expecting to see you in day care,
> To touch your pale feet
> with the poetic rhythm of my hands
> Like gentle waves
> to wash away your suffering
> so you might find stillness within the storm
>
> Instead I find your dead body
> washed up on the shore,
> Torn by the storm,
> Stained with your children's tears;
> Life ripped away,
> No more their mother's tender smile
> To ease life's burden.

Reflection on expertise

How does my reflection on being with Andrea reveal my expertise? Benner's characteristics of expert practice, based on the Dreyfus and Dreyfus (1996) model of skill acquisition, offer a reflective framework:

The practitioner comes to the situation with a fundamental vision and integrity

My vision is to ease Andrea's suffering and to help her find meaning and grow through her experience. It is her life, so I must respect and enable her autonomy to make best decisions about her life and death. All too easily, I can slip into my own perspectives as to what care I think is most appropriate for Andrea. Holism is being collaborative with patients and colleagues and requires an empowered 'voice' to speak out with integrity when I am disregarded or when others' decisions may be inappropriate.

The practitioner knows the patient's story; its meanings, intents and concerns

My intent to know Andrea is the key because it challenges me *to listen and connect* with her story as the basis for her care. Listening, clarifying, interpreting, I tune into her wavelength and flow with her on her unfolding journey ever mindful that my interpretations do not obscure her perspectives.

The practitioner relies on extensive practical knowledge from working with many, many patients that enables her to appreciate the unfolding pattern of the situation and respond appropriately (even when she doesn't know the patient's story well)

Looking back, I can reflect – did I read the pattern well enough? Pattern appreciation is reading the whole situation, mindful of the relationships within it. The whole is always a complex shifting pattern of physical, emotional, psychological, spiritual and cultural factors. Sometimes it is easy to see a physical symptom such as nausea in isolation from the whole. My reflections through the narrative have illustrated that patterns are familiar. The risk is that we don't listen well enough to the particular patient's story because we have heard it before and know it well. It is tailoring reflexology to suit the present situation rather than it being an essentially mindless act of technique. It is understanding her resistance to therapy.

The practitioner's own emotional responses within the context of the particular situation (only emotional involvement makes it possible for her to respond to the family in a sensitive and meaningful way)

At the heart of caring is compassion and being comfortable with the intimacy that flows from compassion. Compassion by definition is unconditional – a giving of the self to the other based on the other's need rather than my own need for comfort. Yet, it is also about accepting my vulnerability. Hence it requires a deep understanding of self so I am able to accept and manage my vulnerability without becoming inappropriately defensive. Of course, situations arise that threaten my personal boundaries but these situations are opportunities for learning rather than flight. I dwell with Andrea and her family, intent on becoming one with her. I use my hands to melt our separateness. Yet to do that, I must also be mindful of not absorbing her suffering as my own and distorting my perspectives as a consequence. *Who I am* is my therapeutic tool. It needs to be in good shape! I could honour Andrea's death and sympathise with her children yet I did not feel sad.

The practitioner's intuition – a direct apprehension and response without
recourse to calculative rationality and reflection whereby expert nurses
use a kind of deliberative rationality to check out their whole intuitions

How I responded to Andrea was intuitive. I picked up cues from appreciating her unfolding pattern and responded. What was the cause of her nausea? The use of cyclizine suggests it was cerebral rather than abdominal but perhaps the nausea had a complex aetiology. Were peppermint and mandarin the most effective essential oils to use? (By no means the oils I generally use in practice). Should I have persisted with the foot massage after she had declined the reflexology? Of course, we can never be certain, so the expert reflects on her actions for their efficacy. So I check my encyclopaedias of essential oils – an example of informing my intuition where previous experience may be lacking.

Being mindful; the art of paying attention to self within the unfolding
moment, conscious of how self is thinking, feeling and responding yet
focused on realising a particular vision of practice

Being with Andrea I am mindful of the situation as it unfolds with the intent to be available to ease her suffering – the hallmark of expert practice and the plot of this narrative. Am I an expert? Maybe not, but I move closer. There is so much to learn that can only be learned through experience and reflection.

Linda

February 17

Linda is 38 years old and has multiple sclerosis. She has pain in her right hip and has a urinary tract infection. Lying on her bed in the four-bedded ward, she catches my eye and smiles. I kneel beside her bed and introduce myself and say I was wondering if she might benefit from any complementary therapy? She says she has reflexology at home with a friend; they do each other's feet.

'It helps to keep my hands active.'

She says it is very beneficial. She asks:

'What treatments do you offer?'

I talk through my repertoire. She declines reflexology and feels she's not comfortable enough to have a massage. She says:

'I used to massage with aromatherapy but it is too difficult now. I would like something different, maybe therapeutic touch?'

Mindful of creating a relaxing environment, I comment:

'It's noisy in here.'

She says:

'When I was here two years ago for respite care I had a single room . . . I had hoped I would be offered that again.'

I suggest she asks the staff but sense her reluctance to assert herself.

'I don't like to make a fuss.'

She likes the idea of an aroma-stone.

'What oils would you like?'

She suggests clary sage and lavender. I suggest adding sandalwood or perhaps bergamot, as both are renowned for combating urinary tract infection and easing stress. She thinks sandalwood is a good idea but is less keen on the bergamot.

As I go to fetch my essential oils, I inquire about the possibility of a single room to Kirsty (staff nurse). She says she will see what she can do. Two vacant single rooms are booked for men. On my return, I inform Linda of my action.

The oils smell good! I say the clary sage is the stressbuster.

'Just what I need . . . my shoulders get so tight . . . I don't like ylang ylang.'

I joke:

'An aphrodisiac . . . it's not my favourite aroma either.'

She laughs and suggests that would make little difference for her. She has had MS since her early 20s. Her comment makes me wonder about the impact of this degenerative illness on her body image and sexuality. She shuffles from her right side onto her back, wincing with pain. I lower the head of the bed and she finds a comfortable position. She says she is hot and sweaty and needs cooling. A fan lays idle on her bed table.

'Would you like it on?'
'Yes, on low.'

The fan's cool air ripples her nightdress as I give the therapeutic touch. I visualise blue cool waves taking the heat from her. I play Rusty Crutcher's CD *Serpent Mound*. Its haunting drone resonates in perfect pitch with my movements. Afterwards Linda is very still. Slowly she opens her eyes and I see she's on another level of consciousness. She says it was very relaxing . . . her pain remains but it has eased and she feels cooler.

I notice her dry feet.

'Would you like me to moisten them for you?'

She accepts my offer.

'It's been a problem . . . I've had some foot infections. I have some cream in the drawer.'
'You might prefer my reflex cream with patchouli and frankincense added?'

I feel like a tempter knowing her weakness.

'That sounds better . . . umm . . .'

She likes the aroma and appreciates my prolonged foot massage. She has such small delicate feet with long thin toes. Once again, I am the poet in motion shaping therapy with my hands.

Afterwards, I urge her to ensure her aroma-stone does not run dry and that she can choose her own essential oils as she wishes to suit her mood – and that I shall write that in her notes. We make an appointment for reflexology on Friday. She asks if I can leave the curtains round her and would like some more 'relaxation music'. I take her hand as I leave and feel the connection between us. Through our touch we shifted from strangers to a sense of intimacy. I did wonder if I would feel self-conscious treating another therapist but it was wonderful working with her . . . indeed I feel she enhanced her own treatment by being so positive.

I am intrigued why Linda doesn't like ylang ylang. That evening I burn the oil in my aroma-stone at home and appreciate its sweet exotic aroma. Moncrieff (1970 – cited by Lawless 2002:194) comments:

> The writer, working with odorous materials for more than twenty years, long ago noticed that . . . ylang ylang soothes and inhibits anger born of frustration.

That sounds a perfect remedy for someone so young living with multiple sclerosis and its ravaging impact on her life. Creating the essential oil mix can either be a very complex balance of factors or simply an intuitive response that stems from experience.

Reflection

I wonder if my paternal action of inquiring about a single room was justified without first asking Linda if she would like me to act for her. Did I take control away from her? It is all too easy to render disabled people as incompetent and act in their best interests thus further undermining their competence (Charmaz 1983). Yet she didn't want to make a fuss. Perhaps she has learnt that it doesn't pay to make a fuss and risk being labelled as a 'difficult patient' (Kelly & May 1982) and its predictable consequence of being rejected. It is shocking to suggest that staff do label people negatively in a hospice, where expression of anger and despair are encouraged. Perhaps there are less than subtle distinctions and social judgement made between people dying of cancer and those living with a chronic illness such as multiple sclerosis.

Four days later

Linda has been to the general hospital for an intravenous pyelogram (IVP)[8] this morning. She has not moved into a single room. Over lunch I read her notes. Her pain management has been reviewed. She is now on methadone 30 mg, diclofenac 50 mg and mexilitene 150 mg (increased yesterday from 100 mg tds). In the past, she had been prescribed amitriptylline for neuropathic pain. I had felt her pain was neuropathic yet Gladys (staff nurse) thinks Linda's pain is due to her urinary tract infection radiating through her pelvis and down her left leg. She is prescribed trimethoprim for her infection.

Linda's notes inform me that multiple sclerosis was diagnosed 12 years ago and that she has a 17-year-old daughter, Zoë. Yet otherwise, the notes are silent about the impact of her disability on her life except that sexual relations with her husband had ceased some time ago. Such comment disturbs me – it feels remarkably intrusive as if putting her on public display. And yet on another level it acknowledges her as a sexual being, something I rarely see reference to within patient notes. Sexuality is integral to the person's identity and is a major factor in their perceived sense of loss of self (Charmaz 1983). Linda had thrown me the cue when discussing ylang ylang when we had last met. I hadn't pursued the cue, treating it as a throwaway remark and a laugh. I suspect she wouldn't have wanted me to pursue it. Yet maybe I liked to interpret it that way because I am uncomfortable talking with women about their sexuality. Kralik et al. (2001:185) in their study of sexuality for women living with chronic illness, note:

> Women wrote of the discomfort shown by health professionals when talking about sex and sexuality. Such discomfort was not conducive to women disclosing their experiences and in some instances effectively closed off any further communication about sex.

I wonder if other staff explore this with her or whether it is avoided. In a similar vein, Lemieux et al. (2004:634) explored with 10 people receiving palliative care their views on sexuality. They note:

> All but one of the subjects interviewed in this study were unanimous in their views that sexuality and the impact of their illness on their sexuality should be addressed as an integral component of their care. It had been discussed with only one of the participants.

Interestingly, the one participant who did not feel it appropriate to discuss sexuality felt that practitioners should sensitively discover whether patients

---

[8] IVP is an intravenous pyelogram to investigate the kidney and urinary tract.

wanted to discuss it or not. These studies by Kralik and Lemieux et al. note the therapeutic impact of the study on the participants in creating a space whereby the participants could talk about sexuality. Lemieux et al. (2004:634) cite one of their participants:

> At least whatever has been on my mind actually came out – I was able to talk to somebody about it – like you. I think that I have made my point and it makes me feel good that I have offered whatever is on my mind and told somebody. Lighten my load.

Kralik et al. (2001:181) similarly share a respondent's perspective:

> With the telling of my story came a huge release of the flood of emotions and fears that I live with day to day but don't share with anyone else. The research not only gave me permission to share the burden of chronic illness but also to have my story acknowledged and valued.

This quote reflects the general perspective of people that sexuality is integral to their identity as men and women more than the sex act. Lemieux et al. (2004:634) note:

> For patients in this study, sexuality was an important aspect of their lives, even in the last weeks and days of life. Sexuality encompassed many things but was centred on emotional connectedness. Their experience of sexuality changed over time, from expressions that usually included sexual intercourse prior to the disease, to one of intimacy through close body contact, hugging, touching of hands, kissing, 'meaningful' eye contact and other non-physical expressions of closeness and companionship. These expressions were a key component of their quality of life.

Linda lies on her bed with her back to the door. Her eyes are closed as I go to see another patient. As I move, she opens her eyes and catches my own . . . *meaningful eye contact*. Am I responding to her sexuality? She reciprocates my gentle smile and waves. A smile, a wave . . . *non-physical expressions of closeness*? I think so. Reflection brings them into view. Linda is tired and uncomfortable but is looking forward to the reflexology.

The aroma-stone is dry. She didn't ask the staff to replenish it but neither did the staff observe it was dry. My frown is deeply furrowed at such carelessness. Linda's passivity reflects her learnt patient behaviour not to be demanding. As I said before, she doesn't like a fuss and yet I feel her intense frustration. I say:

> 'I have read your notes and plotted the pattern of your pain management.'

She laughs as she tells me her story of getting big boxes of methadone from the chemist. She requires regular breakthrough doses besides her regular medication. I note that she is not on any neuropathic pain analgesia? She says she was on gabapentin but it didn't suit her, but she now feels she may have to go back on it. She identifies her pain as sciatic that overlays her normal pain.

We dwell together like conspirators plotting what oils to add to the reflexology cream. I ask her if she likes 'playing'. She laughs. She enjoys engaging in 'oil talk'. She likes the aroma of neroli. I suggest vetiver? She smells its deep earthy smell and agrees. I say the vetiver is the earth. I use it to ground people; to connect them to the earth. As Davis (1999:308) notes, its Indian name means 'oil of tranquillity'. It is helpful for anyone experiencing anxiety, stress, depression or insomnia. It will also help with her muscular stiffness.

I suggest a 'top note'? Maybe pettigrain. Again she agrees. Worwood's (1999:242) description of the spiritual quality of pettigrain seems particularly suited to Linda:

> The spirit of pettigrain is embodied in gentle strength, encouraging positive resolutions and outcomes at difficult times. It enables us to see ahead and forge a link with our inner truth, understanding that in our personal truth comes strength.

I do not know how Linda feels about her multiple sclerosis. She hides her surface signs even as I intuitively probe her body signs without disturbing her apparent calm surface. I imagine that a disease like multiple sclerosis hangs heavily over an uncertain and disabling future and that such thoughts drain one's positive energy. Pettigrain's message is about finding self within the now and resting with that truth. I also imagine that complementary therapy must be a powerful comforter, especially for someone like Linda who is also a therapist.

I note the strong aroma.

'Is it too heady?'
'No, it's good.'

I ask:

'Do you like the sound of water?'

She does so I play her Rusty Crutcher's CD *Ocean Eclipse* . . . cascades of gentle waves breaking on shores recorded during the longest total eclipse of the sun. Evocative music written with a deep reverence for the spirit.

As I apply the cream onto her feet, I notice the hard skin on her big toes although Linda says she takes good care of her feet. Her toenails are a rich vermilion colour. A red mark rests along the sciatic line. She had picked some hard skin. She closes her eyes and I take her through my relaxation routine mindful of the noise of the busy day that drifts behind the pulled curtains that separates us from the outside world. I listen as two nurses, one an experienced care assistant, the other a student, go to Susan in the next bed to turn her position. First they catch up with their news as they talk over her and then, with uncertainty, consider how best to use the sliding sheets. One nurse calls Susan 'darling' . . . and then 'sweetheart' and then 'darling' again. I feel a frown ripple across my brow. They are kind to Susan but is she simply disembodied? She has lost her name. She has difficulty communicating because of the cancer that has spread to her brain from her primary breast cancer. I sense the way nurses distinguish between patients, because when they move across the four-bedded ward, they call Andrea by her name 'Andrea'. Unlike Susan, she is independent and able to communicate. I wonder if Susan notices the distinctions. I wonder if she minds. A distraction from Linda's feet.

Linda's breathing changes as she sleeps. When I finish, she is very still. It is a few minutes before she opens her eyes and moves back into this reality. I encourage her to drink some water.

As a way of compensation to Susan and working out my residual irritation I find Erica, the nursing student, and suggest she offers Susan a hand massage. She tells me that she is a trained holistic therapist but lacks confidence because she has not practised for the past two years since becoming a student nurse.

We go to Susan (I call her Susan) and ask if she would like a hand massage. Her eyes are alive and she eagerly accepts. I ask if she likes lavender? She does, so we add a drop to 5 ml of sweet almond carrier oil.

Afterwards Erica says how rewarding it was to massage Susan.

'Did Susan enjoy it?'

She did.

'Does she have dry feet?'

Erica exclaims:

'She does . . . I am on tomorrow afternoon, maybe I could do her feet then.'
'I am sure Susan would appreciate that.'

I am pleased because I have opened up possibility for both Erica and for Susan. Yet I ask myself why other staff do not use such simple treatments as hand massage when patients like Susan derive so much benefit. Such an act is such a powerful expression of caring, of paying attention to someone who can only lie in bed. Touch is such a powerful connection to another person, both on the physical level and also on the level of spirit – it helps dispel fear and nurture stillness in the aching spirit.

Perhaps I should have asked the staff to be more mindful of noise when other patients are receiving complementary therapy and to consider whether Susan appreciates being called 'endearing names'. But I don't. I avoid the issue, not wanting to engender conflict – but in doing so I again sense a failure of responsibility only partially relieved by my intervention with Erica. The failure to deal openly with conflict is made more difficult by the culture of niceness that pervades the hospice and blights the therapeutic team. It is intriguing to draw comparison between myself and Linda. We are both unassertive, both contained by the unspoken hospice culture, both anxious of some unpleasant consequence. It feels strange because normally I wouldn't describe myself as unassertive.

Later, at the shift report, I ask the gathered nurses if they explore sexuality with Linda? The general response is that it is not relevant to her care. I am struck dumb. The literature on sexuality rings true. Linda's care is framed by her *presenting* symptoms and that sex is a taboo topic.

Four days later

Linda has moved into a single room. I glance round the door. She's on the phone and does not catch my eye. A few minutes later, I glance again. This time her bed is empty. I suspect she is in the toilet. Did she get there by herself? I am conscious of not knowing about her mobility.

Michael's wife

Waiting for Linda to return I talk to Michael's wife in the room across the corridor. I had met her last week. Michael is not doing so well. She says it will be a sweet release when he 'goes' for both of them. It is hard for her to watch him struggle. Such profound conversations snatched in corridors between moments. Genuinely asking people how they are can unlock a welter of emotion. Perhaps that's why some practitioners do not communicate concern through eye contact, so as to avoid the consequence of the ensuing emotional work. Yet how would Michael's wife have felt if I had not communicated my concern in my eyes and in my words when she was so full of emotion? Perhaps she would have rationalised that I was busy, and thankful for the care given to Michael. To be caring *is* to be mindful of self in relationship with others, even those who we casually pass in the corridor. The smile, the soft eyes, the wave, the touch, the spoken word, all signs of intimacy that soften the dull ache of despair and nurture the spirit of the other.

A few minutes later

Linda walks back to her room. She walks awkwardly as if her pelvis is rotated. I give her a few moments to settle before I glance again into her room. She beckons me in and I sit in the chair beside her bed. She is relaxed and thankful for her time in the hospice.

'It was what I needed.'

Her pain has also settled.

'You have your single room?'

She laughs.

'Yes, the doctor came to see me and said it was noisy in here. I agreed and said I'm not as rested as I hoped. He arranged for the single room and I was moved in half an hour . . . I have brought my essential oils in.'

We dwell in a mutual world of aromatherapy. I ask about her mobility.

'I have a relapse-remitting form of the disease. I have attacks and regain about 80% of the loss, I never get back to what I was before.'

'You seem so accepting of the disease?'

'I get great support from my husband and daughter. I am a passive person and don't really get angry. What's the point? Better to live for each day.'

Indeed.

Two days later

I share my experience of working with Linda with Gladys (staff nurse) in clinical supervision. Gladys had met Linda when she was first admitted to the hospice in 2000 for pain relief when she commenced methadone. Then her mobility had been severely compromised. On this admission, Gladys feels that Linda's behaviour is incongruent, for example asking for breakthrough medication when eating a Danish pastry. She feels Linda is abrupt and unfriendly. Gladys is clearly hostile to Linda's plight. I wonder if Linda reads Gladys's hostility? How can she not? I find myself speculating why Gladys has such difficulty with Linda. Perhaps Linda is addicted to methadone and that we haven't seen this because of our 'palliative care' lens, where such issues are downplayed because of the 'dying' tag. Perhaps Linda exploits our lack of understanding. Perhaps, perhaps . . .

It is intriguing to observe how some patients, like Linda, evoke feelings of anxiety and hostility in carers as if they present an existential threat. It is as if a grey mist descends to obscure the caring sun. Gladys has judged Linda as manipulative and unfriendly. She shares this with other staff and Linda is viewed as a 'bad' patient. Kelly and May (1982) write of good and bad patients, where good is defined as a consequence of interactional pattern rather than anything inherent in the patient's behaviour. Johnson and Webb (1995) term this social judgment, that Linda has transgressed some unspoken rule and poses a threat to normal hospice life. The idea that 'caring' can unwittingly heighten rather than ease suffering is deeply shocking and a stark warning of the need to be constantly vigilant of our practice. I sense *the dark side of nursing* whereby caring is diminished (Corley & Goren 1998). Perhaps Gladys should be labelled as a 'bad nurse' for her failure to care? Once again I sense the tension between being human and being professional and the significance of knowing and managing ourselves so we can be available to the person needing care. As it is, Gladys is locked into her hostility and is not available to Linda. Radiating rejection, she isolates Linda and reinforces her loss of self. Yet her behaviour is also self-alienating. Perhaps putting her into the four-bedded ward was a form of punishment? How is it the doctor could so easily move her into a single room? Gladys simply says he was easily manipulated, reinforcing Gladys's negative view of Linda.

Linda accepted me but then I didn't resist her. Indeed the opposite, I was deeply interested in knowing and responding to her. Perhaps being a man, and a man who is deeply interested in her, I responded to her sexuality. The touch of my massage, the playful choosing of oils, the eye contact, the smiles, the intimacy. Of course it is difficult to know that such an interpretation is true. I know that Linda is likely to have an impaired body image and diminished view of herself as a (sexual) woman. As a therapist, I need to develop a strong sense of my own sexuality in relation to others. I need to be mindful of accepting of such dynamics, indeed of integrating it into my practice.

Trevor

Friday February 28

A stillness pervades the early morning. As I drive I watch the dawn expand, pulling back the night screen. A dark edge of cloud merges with the pale blue on the eastern horizon from whence the sun will emerge. I sense it rising behind the screen, indeed small holes are ripped in the cloud canvas, revealing hot lava. Leafless trees line the road, sentinels to mark the season. And then the sun is up above the cloud, like a Buddha in its golden orange splendour radiating its profound love across the landscape. Such energy ripples through me.

Trevor is 71 years old. He collapsed at home and was admitted to hospital. A brain scan revealed metastatic cancer. No sign of the primary site. He is unable to communicate, his right side is paralysed, and he is doubly incontinent. His face is turned towards the door; facing towards his 'good' left side. I kneel close to his face.

'Hello Trevor, I'm Chris, one of the nurses here.'

His mouth says:

'Hello.'

I take his hand and feel his response. I continue to hold his hand and sense the deep sadness in his eyes. His right eye is sticky (we were informed he has an eye infection). I clean the eye and help him drink some tea. He nods affirmatively in response to my inquiry about sugar.

A television blares loudly. It is the news. I ask him if he is listening. He is. The news is a helpful distraction from his predicament. Another nurse suggests that Trevor turns down the noise as it disturbs other patients. It seems a fine balance to get the noise at the 'right' pitch. Linda found noise intrusive, Trevor finds the noise connects him to his normal world. Perhaps lack of noise confirms his isolation inside a bewildering new world. These are the signs I read. He accepts a spoonful of porridge . . . he chews it for ages, suggesting the texture is not easy for swallowing.

Christine (staff nurse) brings his medication; eight small 2 mg dexamethasone tablets, an attempt to ease the brain swelling to enable some recovery of function. I sense that would be of great benefit, because events have been too quick for him, leaving him bewildered. He also has two capsules – lansoprazole and fucithin. His swallowing is impaired, so we dissolve the dexamethasone and I give it via a syringe.

The lansaprazole can be given as a liquid, although the resultant mix is thick and sugary, reminding me of the smell of candyfloss. I imagine it must leave a sweet sticky taste in the mouth. It is 30 ml, and takes a considerable time to give him.

By the time I finish giving the medications and have helped Trevor to drink some ice cold water to rid the imagined sweet sticky taste, I have been with him for nearly two hours. Time slips by in the drama of the day. Yet it is difficult to leave him. The sadness in his eyes is haunting. I set up an aroma-stone with benzoin, vetiver and frankincense. The resins swirl together in harmony, emanating a strong sense of earthly and spiritual connection. Worwood's (1999:193; 254) descriptions of benzoin and vetiver might have been written for Trevor.

> Benzoin can be a pathway to understanding when all is confusion. It can assist in the choices that must be made with the heart, and be the softness needed when all contact with the self has been lost, helping guide us home to that place within, the inner sanctum of the soul.

> Vetiver stops the swirling of the mind, the turmoil of unanswerable questions. In many ways, vetiver helps us to remain calm when unsettling events affect the spiritual self, and when facing adversity. Gently, and without disturbing the creative forces, vetiver steadies and calms any inner disquiet and in that calmness may come the answers we seek.

I suspect Trevor's mind is crowded with dark thoughts and his despair is a muted cry across a barren landscape. Perhaps benzoin can be a pathway to a place of stillness within the confusion. Does he lie here asking 'Am I dying? Working with Trevor, we need to be inspired, and tune into the mysteries of the soul, and see that our work is soul work; to help him find some inner peace as he approaches his inevitable death. If just for this reason, we must connect to the spiritual dimension of care, then the use of these oils has tremendous value. Frankincense is my spirit protector, both strengthening the spirit in times of adversity and easing the spiritual torment. Perhaps that is why I use frankincense so much in my work.

Agnes (care assistant) helps me wash Trevor's body. Perhaps I should say his body was the focus of our attention. I feel strangely conscious of my hands, and feel the warmth that such self-consciousness brings. Perhaps I am the nurse in the film *The English Patient*, about to caress the burnt and broken body.

I have become more mindful of touching someone; transforming the mundane task of washing into a profound act of caring. That quality of doing something is transformed simply by being mindful.

So as we wash Trevor I am mindful of the way I caress his skin in slow sweeping movements of my hands. His body is in good shape, firm and tanned. He is clearly a man who prided himself in his appearance. He is wrapped in a large incontinence pad – no signs of incontinence. We decide to use a Conveen and a smaller pad held by Netelast pants in case of faecal incontinence. A small pressure graze is evident on his right buttock – the side he leans towards. We use some Tegaderm as a second skin. We dress him in t-shirt and jogging trousers in preference to pyjamas – more dignified even though he will remain in bed. I spend more time with him holding his hand, that I sense comforts him and helping him drink some iced water. He drinks well via the straw and I sense the fighter inside, that despite the overwhelming trauma and despair, he will not sink passively. I imagine I am a refuge for his brokeness. Perhaps it is simply human sympathy in the face of such despair. Perhaps I am a Buddha who holds the hurt child. That feels good if I am mindful enough.

Later, I am surprised Trevor is alone, expecting some family about him. I know his wife has had several strokes. Sharron is his nurse this evening. I tell her about the wound, empty urine bag and his sadness. She knows him. He was a florist. She says he is a lovely man. It is painful for her to see him like this. She senses my concern and reassures me that she will look after him. And she is right, I am concerned for him and project that concern into my talk. Sharing my concern with Sharron is mutually supportive for it allows her to share her concern. A community of caring, where we are available to each other in our common cause. We can carry heavier loads when we share.

In the evening I write a poem for Trevor:

> I gaze your eyes for signs
> To reveal the self trapped inside
> To hear your spirit sing its song
> Of life
> I sense the sadness within your sigh
> I sense the despair in your muted cry
>
> You hold my offered hand
> Our physical connection never imagined
> Just a few days before
> As you went about your daily chore
> Life's turning
> Has no predictability
> Now you are cut down
> Like a broken flower
> That you might have tended.
>
> The oils swirl to open your heart
> Nutrients for the battered spirit
> Torn apart.

Kristin

Friday March 21

Lorraine grabs me as she leaves Kristin's room.

'I have just been telling Kristin about you . . .'

Lorraine pulls me into the room to meet Kristin.

I have read Kristin's notes – she is 51 years old. Her breast cancer has spread to her lungs. Her notes spilled out her distress and panic at what has happened to her.

She pats the bed next to her inviting me to sit with her. She has greying spiky hair and an impish smile.

'What can you do?'

Always the tradesman I lay out my range of therapies. She likes them all. I suggest we decide later this afternoon after she has returned from day care. She may even get a treatment in day care.

She blurts:

'Do you want to see the cancer?'

Before I can respond, she pulls down her grey shirt to reveal her left breast bubbling with recurrent cancer . . . red, lumpy, swollen, angry, fascinating. I have no words.

'Shall I wear my wig or shall I be my real self?'
'Your spiky grey hair is cute. Very impish.'

She laughs.

'I'll be my real self then shall I?'

I nod and smile. Her wig hangs on the back of the door. Long, blonde, highlighted – so different to her short cropped hair.

'Better put some make-up on first.'

She moves to the mirror and adds some bright red lipstick. The red smear seems incongruous but I am touched by her childlike manner. I wheel her to day care.

Around 3pm

I see Kristin through her open door lying in bed. She catches my gaze and beckons me.

'Are you coming to see me?'

I smile.

'Yes.'

She reveals more of the story of her illness and treatment. She finished chemotherapy six weeks ago. By then the cancer had become aggressive and filled her lungs.

'Two years ago I was told I had a few small lumps that they could manage. And now this, nothing seemed to work. I have refused further treatment. The game is up. I just want some quality time now . . . I don't know how best to spend that time . . . doing things, going places or what?'

'I can't give you any advice but saying that I would try and live each day.'

'You know that you are going to die one day but to know it's actually happening is frightening . . . I am frightened.'

Again I sit in the quiet of the afternoon with someone facing the impermanence of life. Kristin tells me she has three children . . . one is married. The other two cohabit with partners. No grandchildren.

'No chance of that now.'

Tinge of regret. I sense the loss. I ask about her work – she worked right through her chemotherapy but feels she must give this up now so as to spend more time with her family.

Kristin shifts the conversation.

'I have this awful sensation in my left ear. If only I could get rid of it.'

'Perhaps reflexology may help your ears. And then perhaps a facial?'

'That sounds wonderful.'

'I'll set you up an aroma-stone first . . .'

We work through my blue aromatherapy box, sniffing the oils and exploring what each oil can offer. She is enthusiastic, feeling positive that she likes this approach.

We chose frankincense to help deepen her breathing and for its spiritual dimension and calming effect on the emotions; benzoin for its warm and smoothing properties, and conscious of its ancient reputation for 'casting out devils' (Davis 1999); and sandalwood because it blends well with the other three oils and for its spiritual dimension. Kristin is enthralled by the descriptions although confessing that she has no religious faith. Yet she does wants to find a spiritual place to rest. I then add rose, grapefruit and a drop of juniper berry to my reflexology base cream. The mixture has a beautiful yet subtle aroma. I inform Kristin that the rose is very feminine sensing that her appearance has always been important to her.

She says:

'You are very perceptive.'

I smile.

'Not really . . . I can tell from the photograph on your locker.'
'That was Eric and me at our daughter's wedding taken five years ago.'

I explain the grapefruit is an immune booster, and works well with rose and juniper berry to help the body get rid of toxins. Grapefruit is also an antidepressant – what Davis (1999:134) describes as:

sunny oil, non-sedative and enlivening.

Kristin likes this description because she doesn't want to be miserable and her normal nature is sunny.

I play Rusty Crutcher's *Chaco Canyon* . . . its haunting tones and echoes vibrate through the stillness of the room.

After the reflexology, Kristin is very still. She continues to remain still after her facial so I continue with therapeutic touch, with the intent of reducing the heat and pressure in her chest. Afterwards I sit on the edge of the bed and hold her hand. Slowly she opens her eyes . . . they are filled with tears.

'I didn't want to come back . . .'

I hold her hand as she cries . . . yet there are laughs as well . . . bittersweet tears.

'I have been to some other place . . . and it's hard to come back to reality.'

Again no words as I sit and hold her in silence. She is so vulnerable at this poignant moment. A tidal wave of compassion crashes through me. Healing is so powerful.

A few minutes later Stella, one of her friends, arrives – she is full of warmth. She says that Kristin, herself and another friend were known as 'the glam gang'. I can see why – they are both very attractive women. Cancer can be so mutilating, tearing through the beautiful body, leaving its passage scars on both body and mind. Stella asks Kristin who did the facial.

'Chris did.'

Stella gazes at me, surprised, and I feel both amused and valued. Such moments of lightness penetrate the mist of despair and sense of awkwardness for her friend when she remains so 'glam'. Doing a facial gives Kristin some 'glam' back . . . to be pampered. To feel the oppressive heaviness lift from the forehead and the ears have lost the ringing ache. Kristin notices and is surprised.

'I didn't cough either!'

The 'girls' chatter and I move away. I say I will see her on Monday.

Three days later

George (the music therapist) is playing music to Kristin and her daughter Vicky. It is very soft yet haunting. Minimalist yet captivating. I move away to visit some other patients. Kristin is struggling. Her pain medication has been remastered over the weekend. She is not comfortable, as if she is toxic . . . her body feels poisoned. She feels it is the drugs and not just the residual impact of the chemotherapy. Her ear is again causing her grief. And within her, the existential angst ripples, that she cannot fathom or resolve. She says she is hot. Lying on the bed in her fluffy pink dressing gown opened at the chest revealing her wounded breast. She senses the cancer in her lungs constricting her. The fear of breathlessness on the edge.

Vicky says George's music was beautiful. An oasis in the desert. Sun emerging from behind a dark cloud. Glimpses of beauty within a desolate landscape. Stillness within the storm.

Kristin would like some therapy, whatever I feel would be appropriate. I have an Enya CD – she likes Enya. Vicky moves to leave but I say it's OK to stay. As before, I give Kristin reflexology and therapeutic touch. Vicky shares her intrigue as she watches me . . . the intricacy of my hand movements as if watching some great skill and visual poetry. The artist at work and that is how it feels. Sculpting the soul.

Next day late in the afternoon I gaze at Kristin as she rests on her bed with her eyes closed. She must sense me because she opens her eyes and waves. I kneel by her bed. She is tired but more relaxed. The heaviness has gone from her chest. She describes the therapeutic touch as like a door opening and shutting on her . . . wafts of cool breeze taking the heat and pressure away. Her daughter, Vicky was amazed by the treatment – both she and Kristin think that the red lumpy area under Kristin's nipple was whiter after my treatment. I am intrigued by this possibility. The healing power of these therapies is a mystery I must simply flow with.

Kristin had again felt the treatment transported her to another place. Although tired she is more still. I ask:

'You are still going home on Thursday?'
'I think so but am unsure how I will manage.'

She feels her breathing is less easy. I tell her that I could feel the cancer in her chest and that it is likely to continue to grow and constrict her. She knows . . . and knows it will finally take her breath away yet she feels less panicky.

Kristin feels more in control since her admission. She is now able to plan her funeral and manage her panic attacks. Whilst acknowledging that being at the hospice has been a sanctuary for her to explore her fears, I sense that she scratches the surface and the depth of her fears have yet to be fathomed. Perhaps the depths are not a place she either wants to or needs to go. One great benefit of body therapies is opening a space whereby Kristin can reveal aspects of herself. So, as I massage her, I ease the surface tension, enabling her to go deeper into her thoughts and feelings. My touch eases the suffering. Listen to the words of Blackwolf and Gina Jones (1996:184–185):

> Give the gift of touch. Touch understands and is understood. Touch is the harmonic healing the grieving spirit craves. A gentle touch on the back, the shoulder, the head, the hand tells the receiver more than what can be expressed. Hands held can quickly heal and bind together more than months of psychotherapy. Touch is the great gift of self that offers immediate renewal and certain connection for both the receiver and giver. Allow yourself to heal, to touch. Simple. Momentary. Revealing. Touch brings a unity of spirit to ease the pain. Give or receive the gift of massage. The painful memories are stored in your muscles. Touch them. Honour them. Release them. Heal them. Honour your body. It is as important a part of who you are as is your spirit. Remember, we live in two worlds. Then experience the peace that follows. It will close the circle.

There are days and there are days . . .

Three days later

I arrive at the hospice around midday. All the beds are full. Kristin's name remains on the whiteboard. She hasn't gone home as I had expected. Two days ago, Dr Brown informed her that her condition had deteriorated considerably and she would most likely die within a few days. She became very distressed with this news, not quite believing that she had come into the hospice to gather her strength and was now going to die here. Events have overtaken and over-whelmed her.

Steph, a care assistant, is running a bath for Kristin but is called elsewhere. She asks me if I can bath Kristin? I gladly accept but would Kristin want me to bath her? I ask if she minds? She's agreeable . . . she's looking forward to a jacuzzi bath, to feel fresh and clean despite her fatigue, and that Vicky will help me. Eric, her husband, is silent. He struggles being with Kristin.

Kristin pulls off the sheets to reveal her naked body except for some small pants. Dignity – what dignity? We enjoy the moment. Her small reconstructed and ulcerated breast against her larger left breast. Such contrast. She stands and pulls on her pink dressing gown for her journey to the bathroom. Her two syringe drivers purr the diamorphine and midazolam into her. In the bathroom, Kristin says:

> 'Eric could not have been in here . . . if he's rude he does not mean to be.'

She refers to his reaction to my bathing her. But I had not picked up any resistance to that idea but I can empathise that it must be hard for him to see her as she is, to see her dying and perhaps to be seen by another man. Yet Kristin is so natural with me. No inhibition even as we laugh at the loss of dignity. Perhaps dignity is not so much the physical exposure but a mental construction. How can she feel dignified when she is reduced to such a state of affairs? Eric encourages her not to bath because she has such fatigue. But she insists – she knows the bath will relax and cleanse her. She stands and moves into the wheelchair, putting on her pink dressing gown.

In the bath, I massage her small scalp with shampoo, teasing her with a variety of different Indian head massage movements She delights in this. She then lays back and enjoys the jacuzzi for a few minutes. Drying herself she laughs at her 'chicken bottom' already red from the bath seat. She has lost two stone in weight.

Back in her room, she settles in bed, Eric and Vicky about her. She is tired now. She accepts my offer of some therapy later this afternoon. Shortly afterwards I meet Eric in the small kitchen and walk back with him. He tells me a bit about his work and his feelings being here. His job is very demanding within an expanding company. Long hours. Being off work now is hard for him because of work pressure. He struggles to reveal his feelings. He really doesn't know how to be, as if it's beyond his grasp. I say that this is probably the most difficult thing he has ever had to face . . . and he says it probably is.

Later, a young woman sits by Kristin's bed. She is visibly upset. In contrast, Kristin seems serene. She is Tania, Kristin's hairdresser. Kristin says that Tania's mother died at the hospice eight years ago.

I break the tension by saying what can we do with Kristin's hair? Tania says how well it has grown since she last saw her despite the fact it's now grey. I suggest some mousse and some different colours? We laugh and play, the gloom lifted for Tania. Tania goes to join the family in the garden. Alone, Kristin tells me Tania's story – she was in Australia when she heard the news her mother was dying. She could not get back in time to see her and still carries that guilt with her. Being here at the hospice is upsetting in that memory besides seeing Kristin.

Kristin has been holding court, saying goodbye to her friends.

'I have so many friends . . . they are all so upset but I'm strangely OK.'

She feels at peace saying goodbye and comforting her friends.

I kneel by her bed. We explore her bad news . . . she says she was devastated on Wednesday. Then the syringe drivers were set up. She seeks reassurance she will not suffer, although she does not feel as if she is dying. She finds it hard to believe that she might die in a couple of days.

I give Kristin reflexology followed by a facial massage and therapeutic touch (TT). As I finish the facial, Eric enters the room. He stands by the door as I work the TT for about 10 minutes. He asks if she is asleep. I say no – but she may be somewhere else. He says he knows what I mean. Kristin told him about the first treatment. She says she can hear us. Eric says he will leave her to rest and protect her from other visitors for an hour.

It is time for me to leave. I am reluctant because I am in a sacred space of stillness where I dwell with this woman. I have found her spirit rhythm and flow with it. I kneel by her bed and hold her hand. She smiles as I stroke her freshly washed cropped hair. She says how close she feels to me. I say there is a huge space in my heart for her. I won't see her this weekend but hope to see her on Monday. She says she will hold on till then.

The family are congregated in the lounge. Eric says to Kristin's mother:

'This is the man . . .'

and to me:

'This is Kristin's mother.'

I respond by saying:

'Your cake in the kitchen is creating sensation amongst the staff!'

Yet I am conscious what she must be feeling, sitting here at the hospice as her daughter slides towards death. Vicky asks what I have done to her mother. I explain the treatments yet mindful of weaving healing illusions or mystifying my work. I sense I give them a sense of peace that I am helping Kristin find a stillness within the unfolding chaos. Vicky says to her grandmother:

'This chap has done wonders.'

I say that Kristin is at peace and it is they that have the hardest work to do. Eric acknowledges this. Now I dwell with the family, conscious of being available to them.

Three days later

A magic Monday morning. A deep orange sun climbs over the horizon. I had watched it disappear last evening. Mesmerising beauty that stirs the soul.

At the hospice two red candles are lit. My first thoughts go to Kristin but no, two other patients . . . one death merges into another on the rollercoaster of death. In Kristin's room Vicky has been sleeping in the chair whilst Paul, Kristin's son has slept on the floor. They greet me. Kristin seems asleep. I just wave.

Later, Eric arrives. He went home last night as Kristin seemed stable. When I ask how he is his face crumples into tears.

He apologises.

'I don't usually cry.'

He reflects how people were attracted to Kristin. I can sense this in my own attraction. There is a small girl quality to Kristin that is attractive, disarming, almost naïve. Some staff felt she must have brain secondaries because of her childlike quality. I wonder at the way people pathologise all aspects of selfhood.

Eric finds the waiting hard after Kristin had been told she would die at the weekend. Now it is Monday. She hasn't died. At the shift report some staff feel she may last for weeks. Now the waiting. Eric feels he can't get on with anything. He can't work or safely drive. Life on hold. Such predictions seem fraught with difficulty when proven wrong. Eric laments:

'Kristin's only awake now for a few hours each day.'

It is as if she is withdrawing from the world. The corridor is a waiting room – a place of transition between the social death and the body death.

We sit around the table in the corridor outside Kristin's room. Eric and Vicky pick out their favourite photographs of Kristin. They are sentimental, remembering past times – a photograph of Kristin in Tenerife.

'She loved the sun.'

Vicky reflects on her decision not to have children and that Kristin wanted grandchildren. Tinges of regret seep into and threaten the sentimentality. Vicky says:

'Mum was only 19 when she had me. I grew up more as friends than mother and daughter.'

Vicky bends on the wind of her grief; a slender reed facing the storm. Walter (1999:62–63) notes:

Photographs are a powerful locus for remembrance . . . people rarely look at family photos together without sharing memories.

And so it is. I am drawn into the family as they laugh and cry their way through the pile of photographs. The photographs are a medium of continuing their relationship with Kristin even before she dies, as if she lives in the photographs.

Kristin is awake. She holds my hand and is pleased to see me. She seems serene, a word used in the shift report, as if she is slightly detached. I ask:

'How do you feel inside?'

She is feeling at peace. No pain. Eric had said that Kristin keeps seeking reassurance that she will have no pain. Her diamorphine has been increased to 40 mg. I informed him that midazolam may take the edge off her memory. The dose has been increased to 10 mg over the weekend. Kristin asks for a treatment later this morning. We agree eleven o'clock after her wash.

Kristin is relaxed after her wash. Her family have moved into the garden to give her some space. She lies in bed. Her breasts are exposed. She does not like to wear a nightdress. Her left breast looks angrier than before erupting with the cancer. Do I imagine it's worsening? I have not so consciously gazed at 'it' before . . . previously averting my gaze as if intrusive on Kristin's sexuality. Her ear has 'popped' again and bothers her. I suggest some peppermint or spearmint on a gauze swab? She likes the spearmint and feels its immediate benefit.

Following reflexology I give therapeutic touch, visualising strands of light sweep Kristin's body, cascading cool rays like a waterfall. It is utterly sacred. I am shaken. As I finish, Kristin's mother enters the room with Kristin's sister, Pauly. She is distressed to see Kristin 'out of it'. I attempt to reassure her that Kristin is simply relaxed, in a place of stillness and love. I feel Kristin's mother's lament; her anguished cry. A mother to lose her beautiful daughter.

I had not met Pauly before. Meeting people in fleeting moments. She moves her mother away – they are going to get some food. Alone with Kristin, I say goodbye, holding her hand as she thanks me. I kiss her forehead and leave.

I am late for a university appointment. Feeling the pressure of time is an unusual experience and deeply frustrating. To dwell with another requires patience where time melts into insignificance. Yet in the real demanding world this can be difficult. Would my 'appointment' appreciate my lateness and my reasons? As it is I apologise, saying I had been held up at the hospice. They are forgiving. Perhaps they sense the sacred furrow that lines my brow.

In the dark evening as I write my journal, I wonder about the wisdom of telling Kristin she would die at a certain time. Was that a good decision? Perhaps with hindsight I might say it was careless because of its consequences even though we think we are doing the best by being realistic. Yet after Kristin had overcome the shock she was able to put herself into order. Her family, however, are left trailing behind her, waiting, waiting . . .

The waiting room

We all wait . . .
Expectant
Waiting for the last breath . . .
Searching for the signs of departure
Of death's train

We all wait . . .
Crowded into the waiting room
Finding some shelter from the gusts
Of death's wind
Waiting marks the social death
A void where we falter
In knowing what to say unable to move on
Or retreat

Waiting . . . I hold your hand
You smile and gaze into my eyes
I feel your soul glow through your gaze
In the stillness of what is . . .
You also wait
And comfort those who tremble.

Waiting is hard
For those who gather about
Whose souls shout
For tender release
Grasping for the sign
Seeking some closure

We all wait
For the train to depart
The track ahead is not yet clear
The red light shines
Yet your death is certain
Only when . . .
Until then we wait . . .

It is not easy to wait and witness a loved one suffer. Yet perhaps it is the family who suffer in the waiting not so much Kristin. Restless they struggle to wait, patience worn thin, anxious to do something. In a world tuned to doing something, waiting might be viewed as a lack of action, simply biding the passing of time. Waiting is in itself action, something positive. For me waiting with the family is action to ease their suffering. Waiting is not a passive thing. Just observing Kristin is an event that changes the situation. Yet carers can struggle with waiting. As Lunghi (2004:374) notes:

> In working with those in long-term care, within a skills-oriented culture, we understandably experience a need to be active in meeting the challenge of another's suffering, loss and decline. Inactively waiting is not considered a viable option.

I draw the family together with Kristin into the present moment rather than waiting for her last breath. I know that Kristin will sense the family are restless and suffer.

Two days later, Wednesday April 2

Eric sits at the table in the corridor. Kristin's room is full of people. Her eyes are closed. I pause from entering the room and dwell with Eric. He updates me with the trajectory of Kristin's condition and treatment. She has deteriorated overnight. Her breathing has become increasingly compromised. In response her medications have been increased. (diamorphine is 60 mg and midazolam 30 mg. She has also commenced Nozinan 12.5 mg.)

Eric feels that people should come out of the room to have a break. I sense it is claustrophobic for him.

After a few minutes, I enter the room and join the family vigil yet I am unable to move to her side even to say hello. I must be still . . . patient for the moment.

The aroma-stone needs replenishing, giving me the opportunity to do something. Moving back into the room I am able to hold Kristin's hand and say hello. She is responsive and smiles through the mist. I speak to her normally, cutting across the lowered tones between the family. I feel the heat of her head.

Outside the room, Kristin's mother is in tears. She wants the family to sit around Kristin and hold hands, to share such a moment. But she feels Eric is resistant. Vicky, the ringmaster elect, tries to mediate, assuring her that Eric won't mind. So many family now gathered, conflict ripples within their collective grief as if the fabric of Kristin's life unwinds and the family are torn apart. I say to Vicky that I would like to give Kristin some therapeutic touch. The family ask to sit in. They gather around the bed and hold hands. Eric holds Kristin's hand and her father holds her other hand. The circle is complete with myself within it. I hold my hands over Kristin's head for seemingly an eternity as I centre myself. I feel the energy pulse through me as I tune into Kristin and then for about 20 minutes I work intensely in the stillness of the room. Kristin stirs and moans as I sweep my hands about her. She tries to say something, her lips slightly parted in a faint smile. I sculpt her body until her etheric field is as smooth as silk. The heat cools and her breathing is easier. To finish I hold her head. Such peace, and without a word I leave the room.

> Then experience the peace that follows. It will close the circle.

> (Blackwolf & Gina Jones 1996:185)

Later, so many of the family thank me and say how much the TT helped them . . . the tension broken, they are relaxed. They can sit and eat lunch. I am astonished the TT had such an impact. Kristin's mother says the memory of that moment will be treasured. We have been touched by some immense presence. But I am breathless. I have opened myself to the cosmic forces yet I feel no need for protection. Indeed I need to suffer and groan in rhythm with Kristin and the family.

Later I return to say goodbye. Eric holds my hand. I say to Kristin that I hope to see her tomorrow morning. I will come in to see her. On my way out I see Pauly in the small kitchen. I pause and hesitate – should I say goodbye? I enter the small kitchen and she moves towards me. Instinctively I move to hold her and she moves to hold me. Her left arm holds my waist as my right arm holds her, gently massaging her lower back. Our faces are so close that I feel as if I might kiss her and feel that she would want me to. It is a raw emotion that sucks us into a whirlpool of love and grief where boundaries have lost their edges.

Next day

I have slept badly, haunted by the idea that Kristin is suffocating under a midazolam blanket when I want her to be free. I sensed yesterday her presence trying to reach through the mist. Yet I also know she feared the suffocation of her breath.

As I arrive at the hospice Kim intercepts me and says Kristin has died. The family have gone. Kristin is laid out in her room. The family have requested she not be moved until midday. She lies so still and pale. The head of the bed is elevated. A daffodil by her right ear. Her teddy bear shares her pillow. Her eyes are slightly open. Her lips slightly parted. The aroma-stone has been turned off so I switch it back on knowing the frankincense will help to release Kristin's spirit.

Sitting by her side, I take her hand and perform the *essential phowa*; visualising a powerful light and presence showering rays of love until Kristin melts into the radiance. Wisps of energy leave her mouth. Her hand is still warm. I gently ruffle her hair and kiss her forehead. Woe is me. I ache so much. Can I simply dwell here? But I move away and wish her a good journey. Outside the room, the whole unit seems deserted. The train has departed, the waiting room is empty. A silence pervades.

Lindsey knows I am suffering and offers comfort.

I ache through the day but I am not sad. I simply ache and cannot put words to the ache. Now, as I write the ache swells. I sense it is love trapped inside me. Its intensity is a new sensation perhaps because I have spent so much time with Kristin and her whole family compressed into these past few days. Just 14 days. I can sense the intensity of this work on a day-to-day basis; how I might be overwhelmed by love and its consequences; how Christine sometimes feels she has no more to give, when she gives so much. I can see how people may need to keep a distance and yet I have no choice. Giving cannot be conditional. Kristin touched something deep in me, some place few patients have touched before. Truly a love story.

On deeper reflection, I see my grief bubble through my container. Once again, I have kidded myself that I do not absorb the suffering of the other as my own. Certainly I teach students of the need to create a space so we do not absorb the other's suffering or we might become overwhelmed. I can visualise the space but such a space also creates a potential distance. Sangharakshita (1999:55) offers a perspective:

> They are keenly conscious of the suffering of others, but they don't suffer them-selves as others do. If one were literally to experience the suffering of others, it would be completely incapacitating: it would be too much. If one gets too personally caught up in someone else's predicament, one can end up simply joining them in their suffering. One needs a basis within one's own experience which is so positive that even though one is fully aware of other people's suffer-ing and one is doing what one can to alleviate it, one is not overwhelmed by that suffering.

Wise and compassionate words to guide me yet, in the moment I swept the space away and embraced Kristin's suffering. I am pleased that I feel as I do. I know the poignancy of grief. It reinforces my sense of caring – to have dwelt so intimately with Kristin and her family. It is as if I have also embraced death and feel more comfortable with my own mortality and impermanence. For grief itself, I do not feel shock, anger, or denial. Perhaps a tinge of sadness but I smile in my thoughts to Kristin, that she has found some peace after her continual suffering for the past two years. Perhaps acceptance, in that death is a normal part of hospice work. But that is more of a rationalisation than true acceptance. I suddenly sense that I do not understand what acceptance means. But perhaps, most significantly, is my understanding that grief has a poignancy and beauty . . . that grief's ache is truly an ache of love.

> Once we experience the pain fully, we are free to open to its meaning. We are ready to catch another rising current. From this opening of our spiritual wings, we are able to move onto the soft breeze of joy.

> (Blackwolf & Gina Jones 1996:186)

I write Kristin a poem:

A love story

Sweet lover with broken wing
where do you dwell
now that the last breath has melted away?
Do you dwell within the sky
Where the deep red sunset fades into the darkening blue?
Have you found a still place
Beyond the suffering . . . ?

Yet the suffering did not dampen your soul
It glowed through to the end
Through the suffering
Through the drugs that took the edge of fear
Through the dark nights with children by your side
Through the sigh of angels wings . . .
A glow that burns bright in me . . .

I close my eyes and see your smile
Such a beautiful smile;
Your eyes so full of warmth and love
That touched my soul;
Your soft hand folded in mine
As we trip across the raw edge of emotion

We danced across the healing space
To ease your suffering
To move you beyond the body decay and lost dreams
Into the still place
That rests deep within each of us

And in this quiet evening I dwell alone
Yet your presence aches deep within
Perhaps you will visit me in my dreams
I will look for you
And when we meet
I will return your smile with love
That is ever yours.

Twelve days later, Tuesday April 15

Today is Kristin's funeral. It feels a long time since her death. She has been constantly in my thoughts. How will the day unfold? The crematorium chapel is packed. People have to stand crowding in from the back stretching down the isle. I am the lone representative from the hospice. Yet I ask myself 'Do I represent the hospice?' I think not. I am here to dwell with Kristin's sprit as it floats between us. The music plays to mark the family entrance. The music is by Enya – *Watermark*. I smile at the recognition of the music I first played her. Some comfort.

I share the pew with four women – they cradle tissues in their hands to mop away their tears. Kristin was much loved. They do not acknowledge me in any way wrapped up as they are in their individual and huddled grief.

First the woman priest. Then the funeral director ringmaster. Kristin carried high in a white coffin borne by four men dressed in formal dress suits. The family trail the coffin and move into their allocated rows. Eric's eyes red from crying. Vicky supports Paul – his lament for his dead mother rings around the chapel. It is a poignant and haunting sound. In contrast, Kristin's parents appear calm on the surface. But I know, as one would know through countless journeys, that contained grief lurks just below the calm surface waiting to burst.

The service is quickly over. Vicky reads a poem she wrote for her mother . . . she makes it to the last verse before dissolving in tears. This time Paul supports her. Then one of Kristin's colleagues recollects Kristin at work and home. The effort to be amusing and lighten the burden of grief . . .

Talk of 'red lipee' reminds me of when I first met Kristin in her room.

The hymns were chosen by Kristin. Her body is given over, the purple curtains are slowly drawn in symbolic gesture. As we file out, *Lady Marmalade* blares out across the emptying space. I know it was her favourite song and an act of defiance yet it feels incongruous and diminishes the spiritual edge. I am the last out. I wonder if this is symbolic of my 'outsider' or professional role – not one of the family or friends . . . still the carer? The funeral director ushers us on. The crematorium man is tidying the prayer books along the pews. The next priest stands at the door waiting to let the next lot in. We file out past the woman priest. I shake hands and compliment her on her fine singing voice. I think how nice it would have been to have a choir.

The family are scattered in the forecourt. Eric is close to the door. He thanks me for coming, evidently pleased I am here. I hold his hand and my other hand moves to the small of his back . . . symbolic support. I am so conscious of touch. Paul likewise is pleased to see me. I hold his hand but I sense he is lost and so hug him. I feel his ache ripple through and touch my own ache. I say:

'You're wearing a hospice badge.'

He laughs. The badge comforts him as if the hospice itself has spread its arms to embrace him.

Vicky, her long hair partially braided, looks beautiful. I hold her and she kisses me. Then Kristin's mother and father and Pauly, Kristin's sister. We greet and she kisses me on the cheek. Like old friends. It is reassuring. I stand and talk with her. Her four children are close by. She says she is not spiritual at all, yet the time in the hospice touched her deeply . . . that it was spiritual. Someone else moves to talk to her and I am alone, slightly lost. People mingling, leaving for the wake being held at the hospice.

I give Vicky my poems but say I won't stay and intrude. Vicky insists, she says Eric wanted me to be there. I must be generous. I meet Stella again and the third member of the 'glam gang'. We chatter, but most of all I dwell with Vicky, reminiscing about Kristin's dying, memories of those past days – the humour, the anxiety, the way the tension burst when people were struggling with the waiting. Vicky shares Paul's struggle how he could not deal with it when Mum was first ill and how only towards the end did he engage . . . hence his grief now . . . his guilt about not being there for his mum . . . the white coffin . . . Kristin's style statement! The Enya music . . . how mum had never heard of Enya before . . . and yet how she loved the music. The family played the *Watermark* track repeatedly the last night until she died . . . Kristin's struggle with her breathing – 'that was awful' – how Kristin waited for the morning to die when the nurse opened the curtains to let in a stream of sunshine that fell on Kristin . . . a beautiful moment. Vicky is sorry she has not contacted me but wants to stay in touch because Kristin asked that she did. I am pleased I touched her soul and eased her journey.

Reflection

I sense my relationship with Kristin took me beyond myself into new landscapes of caring. I challenge myself – could I have been more available to her and her family? How does one judge that? How does one measure the degree compassion is unconditional? There is no measure beyond the experience of it. It is like asking if spirituality can be measured. It is ineffable. Perhaps it can in the degree of lightness and energy I felt. Sometimes I would trip out of the hospice floating on a wave of love. I realise that compassion is both energising and liberating because any trace of self-concern melts into nothingness as it becomes increasingly unconditional.

I ask myself – did I find the perfect pitch between intimacy and distance? At no time did I sense resisting Kristin or containing myself. In that sense I could be intimate with confidence without ever feeling overwhelmed. But I am cautious of being self-congratulatory; of submerging myself in a narcissistic twist. The holistic practitioner acts out of concern for the other rather than their own concerns reflecting a tension between arrogance and humility. Yet, as Blackwolf and Gina Jones urge us – we must wear our regalia with pride, to be proud of who we are and what we stand for. This is imperative for self-esteem and confidence.

> It is time to express yourself. It is time to find, validate, and celebrate your true essence, your truest self.
>
> (Blackwolf & Gina Jones 1996:3)

Anne and Gay

May 23

I arrive at the hospice just after 10.30 am. Gay, one of the secretaries, and another woman pass me by. I say hello and faintly wonder what Gay is doing here. On inquiry I discover that she is Anne's daughter and that Anne is now close to death. I move down the corridor and enter Anne's single room. Gay, her sister Gwynne, and their husbands greet me. Anne's breathing is laboured and noisy despite the glycopyrinate in one of the four syringe drivers. She is conscious and tries to talk from time to time. I say:

'It must be hard for you to sit and listen to Anne's breathing.'

In response, Anne mutters something from the bed. Gwynne says her mother's hearing is keen. I become acutely conscious that I haven't greeted Anne. I take her hand and say:

'I'm Chris, one of the nurses.'

I feel a flush of anxiety to be exposed as so careless.

Gay asks me if I can help ease her mother's distress. I am caught on the spot and feel my panic rise – how best to respond? Perhaps therapeutic touch (TT) or a hand massage? I suddenly feel claustrophobic and say to Gay I will be back in a few minutes.

Gathering my composure I return and suggest TT, mindful of the way TT had helped ease Kristin's family's suffering and connected them together with Kristin. The tension in the room is palpable – a mixture of suffering and expectation. I am struggling to keep this tension at bay so I am not again overwhelmed.

I use my breath as first aid to recover my composure and give Anne TT. As I do, I visualise the movements of my hands as the wings of angels coming to comfort and ease Anne's suffering. After about 15 minutes, Anne tries to say something but I cannot make it out. I sit by her side and gently massage her hands using my stock reflexology cream mixed with the essential oils of patchouli, frankincense and juniper berry added. The family comment on the beautiful aroma. After about 10 minutes, I ask Anne how she feels. She slightly turns her head, a faint smile, and says:

'Lovely'.

The family's tension bursts . . . that Anne could have said that. There is such a stillness and subdued joy in the room as I slip out to set up an aroma-stone with the same oils.

When I return, Gay is alone crying at her mother's side. I move round to comfort her, holding her back as I kneel by the chair. I feel her anguish released. Anne dies about an hour later. The family have gathered in the lounge. They feel my response to Anne transformed the death scene and thank me. Now as we dwell in the aftermath of Anne's death the stillness continues. I feel it deep within me as if it is something quite profound. I must admit I am astonished at what happened in the room with the family – how Anne's breathing and colour changed, how she became calm and the way the tension burst and the anxiety dissipated. Gay's husband felt that as I stroked Anne with the TT he too was also being stroked and felt this calmness. Perhaps an angel did visit. The mystery of TT in working with the whole family, as if the healing had enveloped them as they sat around. The alchemist's art of turning lead into gold.

I am left feeling utterly light as if I am floating. Words seem inadequate. Later, Esme, one of the Macmillan nurses, finds me and says Gay will hold the smell of the oils I had used close to her heart, remembering and cherishing the smell associated with her mother's death. I hadn't thought of using oils to leave a memory but it makes sense; these oils are spiritual and help turn the moment of death scene into a sacred moment. Perhaps I can give Gay some cream to hold the memory into the future.

Two weeks later

I visit Gay at work. She is tearful but reminisces positively about her mother's death, especially the way I had shifted the tension in the room and the smell of the essential oils. I gift her a pot of the cream I had used. She unscrews the lid and exclaims:

'That's it, that's exactly the smell!'

More tears, but tears of gratitude. A memory box of smells to bring comfort and evoke poignant memory of her mother's death in future times. It is as if her mother's spirit and the aroma have fused and thus Gay will always have her mother close by.

Reflection

Sometimes I become anxious if I lose control of the situation. Perhaps this is inevitable considering the unpredictable and emotional situations I find myself in. Perhaps I absorbed the anxiety in the room and the expectation from the family that I could transform the bedside scene from distress into something serene. Anxiety feeds upon itself and yet, astonishingly, the situation was transformed.

Some days later, I reflect on this experience in clinical supervision. It is affirmation that I could transform the swirling anxiety into healing with astonishing results. I needed someone to tell me that because I was haunted by my anxiety. Working with life and death the anxiety of messing up is ever present. It is part of the job and so we need to learn effective ways to manage it, both internal ways through centring ourselves, and external ways through support systems necessary to affirm our worth.

Callum

July 11

Callum sits in the corner of his room. I have been informed that:

'He has been difficult to get on top of . . . restless, agitated.'

I kneel before him and say:

'Hi Callum, I'm Chris.'

He looks blank and then after about 30 seconds speaks.

'I can come in tomorrow with my son and measure up if you let me know what needs to be done.'

At first I can make no sense of his words and then I understand. He was a carpenter. Is this the way his agitation works itself out? Yet the word 'agitation' immediately labels him – I must be sensitive to who *he* is, not simply an 'agitated person' that risks framing my reference for seeing him.

Silence.

Patiently I wait . . . and then he says:

'I can't stop here. I've been here for four days and must get home.'

I ask him who is at home. He stands and shows me the photograph on the window ledge. In it, he stands with his wife Rachel and their five grandchildren. The youngest, held by Rachel is just a few months old. I say the little girl, she looks about four, is cute. He says:

'She's the apple of my eye.'

Such poignancy. Such connection.

Dwelling with him in silence cuts through the 'agitation' to reveal his deep despair that, from time to time, spins into apparent 'confusion' as if he returns to a part of his life when, as a competent carpenter, he was the master of his life – in stark contrast with the helplessness he now feels.

Julie (care assistant) enters and asks Callum about lunch. At first, he says he has no appetite. I imagine his stomach is full of sorrow. But she persists.

'Fish and chips?'

She shows him and he changes his mind.

His talk flips back into him and his son coming to work here. Julie gently reminds him that he is at the hospice. He apologises that he didn't know what he was saying. It seems his despair is on the cusp.

We leave him to eat. Kirsty (staff nurse) fills me in with Callum's history. He recently retired as a carpenter and was hoping to move to Spain. Callum's cancer is very advanced, a mesothelioma diagnosed about three years ago. He knows he is dying. Callum has worked hard and now his dreams are crushed. Kirsty tells me how he followed her about one day and again I could sense his regression, that Kirsty became a safe place to shelter from the storm, a kind of surrogate mother. The question now facing the team is how best to help him? Perhaps being at home surrounded by his familiar life would be best? Kirsty is uncertain because she doubts the ability of Rachel, his wife, to cope. Clearly emigrating to Spain is not an option.

Rachel and her sister arrive. She is just like the photograph. On the surface, she is contained, easy going. As I sit with them, she reveals her distress and exhaustion. She is full of stuff she needs to let out. I can *feel* Kirsty's words.

She says:

'He wants me here 24 hours.'

I can see the way he has attached himself to Kirsty in Rachel's absence. Like a frightened boy drowning in the sea of despair he needs to be comforted. I feel anxious because we talk over him as if he wasn't there. He says nothing.

Wanting to be helpful, I suggest to Callum a foot massage might be relaxing? He accepts.

His feet surprise me. They are soft for a builder. He further surprises me by relaxing quickly. Within a few minutes a muffled snore permeates the room. I gaze at Rachel and feel her smile lift my energy. I too smile.

I move into reflexology, working along the spine and balancing the chakras. I work the head, lungs, and the diaphragm. After 30 minutes he has not stirred. He is asleep. I beckon Rachel and his son Martin, who has arrived. They have been drinking tea. Rachel visibly relaxes seeing Callum so still. She says:

'It's like magic.'

I take her hand and say:

'It must seem like that.'

We pause and still holding her hand, I say:

'Your hands are dry.'

She says:

'They are always like that.'
'Let me massage them for you?'

Her subdued smile radiates through the gloom. Holding her hand is an invitation to intimacy, a gateway to opening a healing space. Like a prop to ease the burden of her suffering. Like an olive branch of peace.

I mix patchouli, frankincense and juniper berry essential oils into the reflexology cream. She likes the smell. She relaxes into the massage and through my hands I feel her anxiety melt and stillness radiate through her body. Afterwards I gift her some massage cream to nourish her dry hands and perhaps more significantly to nourish her spirit. Applying the cream with its aroma will evoke the healing she experienced with the hand massage. I know this through my experience with Gay.

Later, in the sun-drenched courtyard I sit and reflect on Callum and Rachel. Lives torn apart. The soft sound of the water fountain is very calming. I write my notes and read his history. The notes spell out his physical deterioration and worsening mental anguish. He resisted admission because it meant accepting he was poorly and hospice meant death. Murray Cox (1988:11) helps me put things into perspective:

> Sometimes the patient presents with finely chiselled, clearly delineated symptoms. At other times he conveys a baffling sense of the swirling, inchoate, undifferentiated affective surge, he uses many words to try to describe this sense of turbulence, but chaos often seems to get nearest the mark.

Callum's cry across the wasteland 'I am chaos!'
Do I hear him well enough?

> The psychotherapist lives at the point of his patient's disclosure and has a persistent sense of being 'on the brink of something more', as though he is a surf-rider who always wonders if the next wave will carry him further still. He is poised at the unfolding invitational edge of experience that flows out of previous experience. The here-and-now and the there-and-then are inextricably interdependent, and the therapist's task is to facilitate the patient's increasing self-awareness, so that their sense of inner chaos changes and what was originally perceived as inexplicable and capricious, gradually becomes coherent and purposeful.

(Cox 1998:11)

I am a surf-rider who tunes into the rhythm of the wave and rides its length. Callum's chaos is a large wave to surf!

Maya (staff nurse) seeks my advice. She is uncertain about using midazolam with Callum. I give my opinion that midazolam would be a blanket to suffocate him, that his deep despair needed to surface rather than be dampened down. I say:

> 'I don't know what's *best* . . . touch would be *my* way of being with him, holding and comforting him whilst also easing Rachel's anxiety.'

A brief pause and then I say:

> 'Perhaps a small dose of midazolam might take the edge off his fear?'

My words surprise me given my resistance to sedation. Maya remembers an earlier conversation with me when I had challenged her attitude to midazolam. Now she is more mindful of using midazolam too quickly as a way of easing her anxiety to 'fix' Callum's agitation. We acknowledge it is hard to watch someone in emotional turmoil. It is also difficult to resist the family's plea to do something to calm him. At such times, these conversations are vital.

Yet, 30 minutes later Callum remains relaxed after his reflexology. I kneel by his side and call him. He stirs and opens one eye and then closes it. It feels like a miracle to bring him to a place of stillness. Rachel tells me how he was meticulous about his appearance. Designer suits with the tags still on them and now this. It is hard for Rachel to see her proud man reduced to rubble.

Dr Brown has heard how effective my touch was in calming Callum. He asks my advice in managing Callum's agitation. I caution against going over the top with midazolam and suggest we ask the staff to give touch. Dr Brown agrees. He too is doubtful about using neuroleptic drugs.

I am surprised to be consulted simply because he has never asked my views before. I have always felt invisible to him; that the use of complementary therapies is not within his medical gaze. As a consequence, I work in the margins of mainstream hospice care and feel that complementary therapy is viewed with no more than a benign tolerance to help people relax.

My experience with Callum reinforces the significance of appreciating the pattern of his life and strengthening my empathy as to what he is thinking and feeling, rather than seeing him from the perspective of his presenting agitation. Of course, I can't know what he is thinking and feeling. Previous experience gives me a clue yet I must be careful not to think I know and close down possibility. The mindful practitioner is always open to possibility and one's own reactions – it is the essence of wisdom. The key to empathy is compassion. For only with compassion can we truly see the other beyond our ego's grasping. Compassion or love; the healing energy to ease suffering. It is as if Matthew (1995) speaks to me and all healers citing St. John of the Cross:

> Their gaze (the gaze of healers) engages what they see and affects it – 'for God to gaze is to love and to work favours'. These eyes are effective: 'God's gaze works four blessings in the soul: it cleanses the person, makes her beautiful, enriches and enlightens her.'

Three days later

In the quiet afternoon Kirsty sits in Callum's room with a small girl on her lap. Her name is Lisa, the 'apple of his eye'. She gives me such a smile just a few feet from where her granddaddy lies. I wonder – does she know he is dying?

Callum breathes heavily, his skin pale and waxen. I sense his death is imminent. Rachel sits and holds his right hand. Martin holds his left hand. I greet Rachel silently. Her smile is tired. I meet Lisa's mother Vanessa and Nathan, her father, Martin's brother. The room is crowded and heavy with the suffering. I move away for the moment.

Callum has been persistently restless. The night staff had tried a hand massage but he resisted so they resorted to repeated doses of midazolam until he was subdued. Kirsty had given him several foot massages over the weekend when he became agitated that helped him become calmer. However, a syringe driver with midazolam 20 mg/24 hours was commenced. It is now increased to 30 mg. He was also prescribed increasing doses of haloperidol but this was reduced as he started twitching. Now, he has just has been given an injection of midazolam 5 mg for 'breakthrough agitation' that has knocked him out. It seems this progression is inevitable. Have we fallen into the sedation trap?

I wonder why Callum resisted the hand massage from the night staff? Perhaps at night his fear is greater and he felt he was being restrained? Perhaps he did not like his hand being held, it is not to everybody's liking. Knable (1981) says that 70% of patients found handholding a positive experience. Perhaps Callum is one of the 30% who did not? The staff were mindful to pick up the signs and stop but they did not offer the foot massage. Perhaps they were busy or felt inhibited? Perhaps they were irritated with him and he sensed their lack of compassion? Yet Kirsty's foot massages support the therapeutic benefit of this touch. I feel validated yet despondent that he has suffered this onslaught of sedation.

On my return, Rachel is now alone with Callum. I kneel on the floor by her side. She informs me of Callum's deterioration. She is tired but must keep going. She says Callum was angry that his diagnosis took 15 months. She is also angry but has let that go for the moment. Maybe after Callum has died she will make a complaint – not for herself but to stop it happening to someone else. How often have I heard these stories of anger and conflict that cloud the mind and stain the memory?

Callum's head is tilted slightly back. His breathing laboured with his mouth open. Such pale lips. A large ulcer is visible on the side of his mouth. I use the tea tree solution to clean his mouth. I set up an aroma-stone with neroli, lavender and frankincense to help ease the tension and infuse the room with a sense of calm.

Rachel is anxious about Callum's breathing with saliva pooling at the back of his throat making him choke. I raise the bed head and Kirsty commences medication to dry his secretions. The noisy breathing is not easy to bear. Rachel is upset at Callum's mother. She is 91 years old.

Rachel says:

> 'I phoned her and told her Callum was dying – I asked her to ring him and say goodbye . . . but she didn't and now it's too late . . . that would have made such a difference to him.'

I sense the regret and bitterness . . . why is death so often a time for family conflicts to leak out of their containers? For an hour I just kneel there on the floor supporting Rachel as I so often do as death approaches. I deliberate whether therapeutic touch may help Callum's breathing and ease both his and the family's suffering. I remember the benefits of TT on the whole family with Anne's and Kristin's families. However, I decide against *doing* any therapy because he seems settled, his suffering is masked, although I sense his torment bubbles beneath the sedation blanket.

Later, on reflection, I feel I should have given Callum TT. It would not have disturbed him and may have brought him and Rachel comfort. It seems inexplicable that I didn't. A wave of irritation submerges me.

Reflection

On the train to London I read:

> Generally speaking, we regard discomfort in any form as bad news. But for practitioners or spiritual warriors – people who have a certain hunger to know what is true – feelings like disappointment, embarrassment, irritation, resentment, anger, jealousy, and fear, instead of being bad news, are actually very clear moments that teach us where it is that we're holding back. They teach us to perk up and lean in

when we feel we'd rather collapse and back away. They're like messengers that show us, with terrifying clarity, exactly where we're stuck. This very moment is the perfect teacher and, lucky for us, it's with us wherever we are.

(Pema Chödrön 1997:12)

Sometimes I read something that takes my breath away. *This very moment is the perfect teacher and, lucky for us, it's with us wherever we are* – in a breath the perfection of mindful practice. Being mindful creates a space where we can let go these feelings of discomfort and see them for what they are. Yet in order to dwell with these feelings we must also be gentle with ourselves, not to judge ourselves harshly but as Chödrön suggests, to see these feelings as teachers so that the energy of these feelings can be converted into compassion for ourselves and for others. The corollary of Chödrön's words is that comfort is good news and feelings of joy and satisfaction are also messengers yet, how easily we can take such feelings for granted rather than see that they too are opportunities for learning and affirmation.

Two weeks later

The care team gather at the monthly clinical audit meeting[9] to review Callum's care. One significant point to emerge was our struggle to understand and respond to Callum's agitation. I pose the question whether Callum's agitation was a manifestation of what Kearney (1997:63) describes as *soul pain*:

> The experience of an individual who has become disconnected and alienated from the deepest and most fundamental aspects of himself or herself.

Kearney (1997:62) suggests that soul is something distinct as if I have soul rather than I am soul. He describes soul as:

> A dynamic entity, often personified in the feminine form which, while being at home in the deep mind, is constantly moving back and forth between the surface and the deep, weaving a web of images in a restless longing to bring depth to all that is superficial and to bring what is superficial into depth. Soul is the living connection between the surface and the unfathomable and meaning-rich depths of who we are.

It is difficult to accept the idea of soul as some entity. Perhaps the soul is another name for the deeper self in contrast with the surface self – for surely self cannot be split. Perhaps the mind is only ever superficial; where communication is through conscious thought. The deeper self communicates through other forms, for example, glimpses, images, and dreams.

Kearney (1997:65) suggests that soul pain manifests itself in a number of observable ways:

- In the way staff use certain language – for example – 'anguished'
- In the way physical symptoms do not respond to treatment because of the body's connection with deeper consciousness

---

[9] Clinical audit is a multi-professional reflection on clinical practice with the aim of knowing and ensuring best practice as part of formal quality assurance.

- In the way people like Callum experience this sense of flight from the cause of soul pain – reflected in restless and agitated behaviour
- In the way sufferers experience a sense of 'hopelessness' and 'helplessness'

Callum *fits* with each of these manifestations. Kearney further notes that soul pain can also be recognised by the response of carers to the sufferer's soul pain; that they absorb this soul pain and experience an urgency to find a solution for it as if finding a solution for self. Kearney (1997:65) says:

> Soul pain can also be recognised by the feelings and behaviour patterns it awakens or 'constellates' in us as caregivers. In the presence of soul pain, we too are confronted by an insoluble problem. His pain which we cannot control triggers our own ego survival reactions. At a surface level, we too 'fight', that is, we never give up: we continue to try new treatments or administer bigger and bigger does of painkillers and tranquillizers. In other words, we do, we do, and even when we do not succeed, we go on doing.

And it was this sense of 'fight' that was expressed at the clinical audit, together with feelings of helplessness and guilt that somehow we had failed Callum. We had worked through a range of drugs without really touching this pain. It was the defeat of the hero. Kearney describes the Greek myth of Chiron – the myth of the wounded healer. He contrasts between the *heroic struggle* to fight to the death using the modern weapons of medical technology, and *the descent* – the letting go of the struggle by finding meaning in the dying experience. Longaker (1997:11) calls the journey of descent *a fall into grace*. Callum remained trapped in the struggle.

I sense the way the ego wraps itself around the surface mind. Afraid of letting go, it fervently clings to desire and attachments, fearing its own loss. To face death is to face self in utter loneliness. So the ego puts off this task, even in the face of imminent death. Yet the wrapping becomes inadequate and fear bubbles through.

Callum suffered and we might sit about speculating about the cause of his suffering. We might say his ego struggled to control the deep fear that spun him into agitation. As his grip on control slipped, so he slid into the abyss: a dark unknowing and frightening hole of death. Longaker (1997:43–45) informs us:

> When we're faced with the reality of dying we may also be facing, for the first time, the emotional process of letting go our attachment to life. Understanding and working through this emotional pain, like every other task of dying, becomes a huge problem for us if we have never learned how to let go gracefully throughout the many losses in our lives.
>
> When we're dying, there is nothing from our former life we can grasp on to for security. When our mind and body gradually begin to disintegrate in the process of dying, we are faced with the ultimate experience of 'losing control' – with its accompanying uncertainty, disintegration, and fear – revealing our deepest vulnerability. Thus any reaction or emotion a dying person expresses is *perfectly understandable*, given the emotional pain, resistance, fear, and extreme vulnerability which usually accompanies the dying process. *(italics my emphasis)*

Reading the words *perfectly understandable* is a huge challenge because we grope about trying to understand his confusion and agitation. Of course, there is no logic. It is, as Longaker suggests, his existential angst revealing itself, as if leaking out of a tightly closed container. No longer able to be contained it leaks from the edges.

My effort to understand Callum's anguish – that he cannot see the path of the descent because his fear makes him flee into dark corners where he cowers. His only escape is not to flee, but to dwell and work through his fear even at this late hour. To find the gate to the path of the descent he needs a guide to take him gently by the hand and shine a light for him to see. As Kearney (1997) suggests, the guide might use a variety of tools to assist in this work; image-work, meditation, bodywork, art therapy, or other therapies. The guide is someone who shines a light through the dark void to show the way, who holds the hand, and encourages the effort to let go of resistance to find another way than clinging to fear. For sure, no one can know the actual way. Kearney's notion of *soul pain* offers me a powerful image for my practice. It challenges all practitioners to find ways of enabling people with whom we work to find ways of communicating with the deeper self so that people like Callum can be helped to connect and find meaning in their deeper fears. As it was, the drugs subdued him yet what torment rippled within him until he died?

Penny

Friday 25 July

A beautiful woman lies on the bed. She is pale and thin, her long grey hair cascades about her. She greets me with a warm slightly sad smile. I say I'm Chris and she seems perplexed; her son is also Chris. On her locker stands a photograph of a young man with a woman. I ask:

'Is this Chris?'

She says:

'No – it's my daughter and her partner.'

I ask Penny if she is married? Her lip quivers.

'My husband died just over two years ago . . . I nursed him through his cancer. It helped me for what I'm experiencing now. He died peacefully so I'm not afraid of dying or death. Perhaps one thing I hoped for was some time for myself after his death. I'm only 61 but it wasn't to be.'

A poignant smile but I sense her aching heart. Such a gentle woman, like gossamer thread, almost ephemeral in her manner and faded physical presence. She continues:

'My daughter also had cancer but she overcame it . . . she can't have children though as they had to take away her reproductive parts.'

Perhaps a tinge of regret that she has no grandchildren. I ask how she is?

'The cancer in my lungs makes me breathless . . . I feel it creeping up.'

A familiar pattern.

'I am told you are constipated?'

She agrees. She is taking Movicol but it hasn't worked.

She would love her feet massaged. I switch the television off and draw the curtains. The bush outside is almost inside the open window, its red leaves glistening with the rain. The room becomes as dark as the sky. I switch on the bedside lamp and a soft glow permeates the room. It is very still.

Penny likes the aroma of patchouli, frankincense and juniper berry essential oils mixed into my reflexology cream. As I apply the cream I feel slightly uneasy and I don't know why. It is a perfect setting. Perhaps because I had felt such an immediate powerful connection with her I expect too much of myself? Feeling uneasy is a sign of being wrapped up in my own concerns, even if I cannot quite pinpoint the cause. Feeling uneasy suggests resistance. Chödrön (2003:40) reminds me that:

> Resistance is the fundamental operating mechanism of what we call ego, that resisting life causes suffering . . . clinging to our narrow view . . . resisting our unity with all life.

Resistance blocks the energy flow and limits my healing potential. I place my hands along the soles of her feet and centre myself, focusing my love to melt my uneasiness, tuning into her until I become one with her. Slowly I am learning to surrender and flow with the mystery rather than try to control it. As natural as a flower opening to the sun. I guide Penny through my breathing and visualisation ritual, moving the white healing light through her body. I ask Penny to sense how good the white healing light feels, encouraging her inner smile to broaden, releasing the endorphins to ease her physical and psychic pain. And, as I work with her, I too smile through my soft closed eyes and visualise the light radiating through both of us. It is such a pleasurable sensation I want to stay with it.

Bloom (2001:97) notes that:

> The true inner smile is a warm, caring and watchful sensation that is most easily started in the heart and the eyes, and which is felt through the whole body.

As I work her foot reflexes I visualise moving the hard faeces along the colon . . . gently, slowly, moving them on. I visualise her constricted lungs soften under my persistent thumb easing the strangled alveoli, I visualise the cancer cells exploding with the warm healing light. I finish by holding her feet visualising Avalokitsevara, the Bodhisattva of compassion. With each in-breath he fills me with his deep compassion and with each out-breath I transmit this healing energy through my hands to flood Penny's body.

Afterwards she is very still . . . slowly she opens her eyes and softly smiles. The hint of sadness in the corners has melted. I ask her is she would like the music left on.

She points to her heart:

'No – the music is playing in here.'

Such a moment of pure love. I kneel by her bed and hold her hand. I thought carefully before taking it, conscious of intrusion, of overstepping my mark. Permission sought with my eyes – would she like me to hold her hand? She welcomes the intimacy. She says the massage was very different to the massage she received in the day hospice. She didn't feel as if she was fitted into a busy schedule. Here time evaporated into timelessness, where earthly concerns melted into the sacred.

Five days later

Penny's discharge is delayed until Thursday so she can have a blood transfusion. She says:

'The foot massage you gave me last week was so beautiful.'

She laughs:

'I managed to open my bowels . . . I passed a small thing like this . . . *(indicating with her hands)* . . . it was like giving birth and such a relief.'
'Did you name it?'

She laughs again:

'No, but I should have done.'

I ask:

'Would you like another treatment this morning?'

Silly question really as her face breaks into a joyous smile. I offer reflexology between her hourly blood observations. I kneel by her side and we pass the time talking about the meaning she gives to her illness and our lives . . . it is at times, cheerful, poignant and sad. She has a tragic recent life.

'Yet I had many good moments . . . I had such a good marriage.'

She says she had a visitor last evening, a good friend. She was so tired but felt she had to see this person.

'I was thankful when she left.'
'Is talking to me tiring?'
'It is but I love to talk.'

I sense the urgency to talk to fill her life with as much meaning as possible.

The first four quarter-hourly blood observations are completed without incident. I ask Penny whether she would like the curtains pulled to close out the dull grey sky. She says yes but declines the lamp so we are shrouded in a half-light. The soles of her feet are so pale suggesting a deep lack of energy. As I finish she is startled as if waking from a dream . She had heard the sound of water.

I read through Penny's medical notes. They reveal her medical history, the endometrium cancer in 2002, the failed chemotherapy, the lung spread and her refusal for more aggressive chemotherapy preferring some quality of life before she died, a 'palpable liver edge' suggesting liver spread and probable reason for her abdominal pain and nausea.

Kirsty (staff nurse) says that the tightness Penny felt in her chest melted away during the treatment and that she can now breathe more easily. I like the idea of reflexology unwrapping tight knots and releasing energy.

That evening I write a poem:

Sometimes (beyond the everyday)

Sometimes I find myself along the fine
   edge of stillness
Within the passing of a moment
As if my eye was caught by a passing
   glance,
Perhaps a spider moving across the
   floor
That makes me realise there is something
   more
Beyond the grinding motion of
   the everyday.

Sometimes I am distracted within the
fractured day
By the sharpness of this fine edge,
So fine I could cut my soul
Like a diamond polished to reveal
Its beauty that lies just below its surface
   peel
Beyond the staining guilt of the
   everyday.

Sometimes I close my eyes and drift
   along
The fine edge of stillness as if a dream,
As if I were simply strands of gossamer
Caught upon a gentle cosmic wind
   that blows
Upon my ripening harvest, that dances
   and flows
Beyond the confining logic of the
   everyday.

Sometimes I pause amidst the incessant din
And see a gentle light stream somewhere
from a distant place deep within;
I am a moth attracted to this radiant light,
My wings flutter caught in the delight
Beyond the conforming pulse of the
   everyday.

Sometimes I am caught in a karmic wind
That spirals me across desolate horizons
Towards a land of ache and angst
Where the sharp edges of tongues cut deep
Within the mortal coil to disturb my sleep
Beyond the fine edge of stillness I seek.

Sometimes I just gaze at the beauty
of a crescent moon burst forth
and feel my true nature ripple along
   the stillness edge;
Sometimes I gaze upon a sunset of
   brilliant hues
Of reds and oranges against an array of
   darkening blues
Beyond the blistering pressure of the
   everyday.

Sometimes I pause and think of you
The delicacy of a flower opening to the
   morning sun
Its beauty revealed in slow motion
To those who would only see
the fine edge of stillness, a space to fly free
Beyond the stifling cloak of the everyday.

Three days later

Penny attends day care. She looks good, colour in her cheeks, energised and positive about going home. I am mindful of my strong attachment to this woman, perhaps due to feeling poignant because Iris died a year ago yesterday.[10] It is good to remember and honour our practice. I work out my poignancy in a poem:

> Little bird with broken wing
> Your breath expired,
> Your body fell to the earth,
> Your words – am I dying?'
> Linger on the last breath
> And vibrate through time,
> Your smile breaks through the mist
> Like sun shining,
> I bathe in the warmth of your spirit.

Seventeen days later, Thursday August 19

Back to work after two weeks' holiday. The fine weather continues. Penny has been readmitted from home. She has gone 'off her legs'. She tells me she could not get out of bed to go to the toilet. Spinal cord compression has been ruled out. She says that last Tuesday in the day hospice she could not rise from a dining chair. She felt caught in the spotlight when people urged her that she could do it but she couldn't and needed help.

'I felt very undignified.'

These words trigger her tears . . . these losses . . . losing her mobility and her dignity . . . needing help to go to the toilet. This proud lady brought to her knees. She can face death but the dying process eats her away. The pace of her deterioration literally has taken her breath away. But she is determined.

'I am going to eat and build up my arm and leg strength.'

As we speak, in front of her, her meal goes cold but she says it doesn't matter. I sense her courage and yet I also sense she is overwhelmed and she knows it. Penny has a tablet in her hand that Maud (staff nurse) has given her this morning because she was so upset. Maud felt Penny needed something to take the edge off her anxiety. I say I could give her reflexology later. She says:

'That's good but don't wake me if I am asleep . . .'

Later, she is asleep. She looks ragged, exhausted, lying on the bed, very pale and drawn. I would like to treat her but respect her wish and reluctantly leave.

---

[10] My relationship with Iris is described in *Being Mindful, Easing Suffering* (Johns 2004b).

By the nurses' station, a young woman asks for Penny. It is her daughter. I catch her eye and know we will meet soon.

Two days later

I phone the hospice to ask if Penny would like me to visit and give reflexology. Penny is not so well but yes, she would like me to visit. She looks much better sat up in bed. She is pleased because she made her will this afternoon.

> 'The day's been bit of a rollercoaster. I was sick this morning. In the end they gave me an injection . . . just a slight sense of nausea persists.'

She enthuses about the will-making, pleased to put her affairs in order, reflecting on the probate after her husband died without a will.

> 'The "will man" was very empathic.'

I sense the significance of caring at every level, how everyone who touches her can make a difference. Echoes of Frank's (2000) *remoralisation.*

Towards the end of the reflexology, she opens her eyes, looks and smiles at me, seemingly surprised as if she has awoken from a dream. She closes her eyes again and surrenders to my touch, yet the smile lingers on her face. Afterwards I pull back the curtains. The sky is a deep blue. Such beauty outside us and such beauty within us. She says the treatment was wonderful. She is not so spaced out as before but feels transported to another place beyond the immediate suffering.

> 'It complements my other good experience today – making my will.'

I say I will visit her again over the weekend. She is conscious of imposing. I say it is my choice.

> 'My daughters would want me to visit and offer my care.'

In response she says:

> 'I would like to meet your children.'

In dwelling with the other I widen the circle to reveal who I am, my world beyond the therapist's tag, an invitation to deepen intimacy.

She thinks only her daughter will visit. She talks about their closeness and the lack of intimacy with her son.

> 'More a sense of duty visiting.'

She is tearful talking about her daughter who survived her own cancer . . . she grieves the loss of her relationship with her daughter and anticipates her daughter's grief. The maternal instinct – being anxious for her children.

Kneeling by Penny's side, I hold her hand. I say with a depth of eye contact.

'You are a beautiful person.'

She smiles and says that is a beautiful thing to say. I want her to feel cared for, loved . . . that she might surrender into my valley of love. She mentions Ivan, his death and how he is in her heart, with her. I say he is probably in the room with us, watching, waiting, caring. She feels that is a nice idea. It comforts her. And so we dwell in this small room as the shadow of death looms ever larger yet it does not diminish the light. Penny is booked to go home on Tuesday but I can see her slipping away like Kristin.

Incarcerated in this hospice side room is Penny's dark night. The way forward is unknown, and though she faces it with equanimity it is not without a sense of fear. The image of being with Ivan comforts her and gives the uncertain future a focus as if a desert mirage giving her a sense of somewhere to go that is necessary to move forwards positively. Matthew (1995:64) in his commentary of St. John of the Cross, says:

> So, night brings a knowledge of our truth which eases us of our self-importance and releases us for total love. Ultimately, it is bringing another person (quoting St John of the Cross) 'in the midst of darkness and pain where love is present, the soul feels a certain companionship and inner strength' which accompanies her.

I imagine my love is a clearing where Penny can dwell and find a certain companionship and inner strength to prepare for the journey ahead and rest in the *dark night of the soul*.

Next day

Passing the hospice, I drop in to visit Penny. I am intrigued how she feels after yesterday's reflexology. Karen her daughter sits by her left side. Her partner David lies across the bed. I say:

'I'm Chris . . .'

and as a way of justifying my presence I add:

'I've been giving your mum reflexology.'

Karen says:

'Mum's been saying how good that's been.'

And then her tears spill.

'My mum and I have always been so close . . .'

Words drift between us and I struggle to comfort her, acknowledging how hard it is to watch her mother gradually slip away.

She blurts through her tears:

'I have been getting her room ready downstairs at home, it's lovely but now this . . .'

She is bereft as she senses losing her mother.

Penny is groggy after taking diazepam this morning when she had felt anxious. Although Penny had seemingly accepted the inevitability of her death, her deterioration and realisation that death is imminent has sent shock waves through her. Her equanimity has been jolted out of rhythm. Death, the great mystery play.

Yet Penny is not asleep. Her eyes are closed but she grimaces with pain. Tummy ache, her abdomen now swollen into a hard ball. She has eaten some custard this afternoon, her first food today. Karen gently rubs her mother's abdomen to ease the pain but it quickly worsens.

Karen tells her:

'Chris is here.'

I go to arrange analgesia. Karen follows me along the corridor saying her mother is howling. A syringe driver is commenced with diamorphine. Another marker along the dying trajectory. We can relieve Penny's physical suffering with increasing medication, but not her anguish as she hears her daughter's lament. The fabric of illusion torn away to reveal the stark reality of palliative care. Nowhere to hide. The spirit naked. Karen faces a lonely dark journey. I offer her therapy but she declines, she doesn't want attention taken away from Penny. The vivid shapes of palliative care woven in familiar patterns.

Two days later

Blue skies with whispers of cloud. The breeze subdued in the quietness of the afternoon. I drive to the hospice between fields of harvested corn that reflect the coming and going of seasons in the cycle of life. However, such reflection would be of little comfort to Karen.

In Penny's room Karen is being comforted by Sally (care assistant). David sits across the bed impassive. I wait in the background for the scene to play out its tragic drama. Karen cannot be comforted. And over the next two hours I dwell with Penny and Karen. Penny drifts in and out of sleep or perhaps clouded consciousness, it is difficult to distinguish. She has more abdominal pain and Kirsty sets up a second syringe driver with 10 mg diamorphine to supplement the driver with 20 mg diamorphine, 10 mg metaclopramide, and 5 mg midazolam. Penny asks for the toilet, but cannot pass urine on the slipper pan . . . perhaps her swollen abdomen pressing on her bladder. When she wakes, she cries:

'Karen . . .'

and then cries:

'Now.'

Karen thinks she is crying for death to release her but I cannot tell. Penny's eyes are wide open and strange. Karen says Penny sees goblins.

Perhaps if I close my eyes I will see them too . . . but they are elusive.

When Karen takes a break, I give Penny some therapeutic touch. As I move my hands down across Penny's body I murmur *Om mane padme hum* – Avalokitishvara's mantra. Does it help? Karen feels it does, she feels the healing energy infuse the room. I sit and hold Penny's hand, gently massaging her hands and communicating healing touch. When Karen takes another break, I sit alone with Penny and say my goodbyes wishing her a safe journey.

I find Karen and David sitting in the courtyard bathed in the late afternoon sun. It is very peaceful. I feel the warmth of the sun touch the surface of Karen's deep gloom. She says it is beautiful here, she feels cared for here but she also knows that when Penny dies she will feel utterly alone. I hear her cry across the wasteland:

> Little bird
> Your mother must soon die
> your anguished cry caught on the breeze
> your gently flowing tears spill into the dark void
> Where you feel love is ripped from you
> Yet it lies deep within your heart
> I cannot ease your pain
> But hold you close all the same.
> The sun goes down on your love
> You face an artic winter of despair
> your heart cleaved in two
> you will search for the lost part
> where your mother's love lies;
> Can you see she flies with angels
> in chariots of golden dust?
> Close your eyes and feel her softest touch
> So her love may melt the grief that consumes like fire
> And bring light to let the future grow.

Driving home, I feel alone. Perhaps I could have stayed but where does one draw the line? Penny died peacefully in the early hours of Sunday morning.

Reflection

Penny's *fall into grace* was disturbed by Karen's cry who could not be consoled. Perhaps it was Karen who needed midazolam? The good death script torn yet revealing its fallacy. Could we have helped Karen more? I doubt it – she needed to lament yet be held without constraint. Penny felt cheated to die so young at 61, but she could accommodate her loss of earthly life in the knowing that she could be reunited with Ivan, her husband. Penny had nursed her husband through a long illness and eventual death. She described his death as peaceful, which gave her strength to face her own death. My intimacy with Penny reflected in the number of times I 'popped' in to see her. I accepted an unspoken responsibility to be available to Penny even though she did not ask for it. As with Kristin, the continuity of relationship and therapy feels vital. Putting myself in Penny's shoes I would want continuity of therapy as a sacred space where I could dwell in peace and love and ease my suffering. Yet I am not Penny. Intimacy can be demanding. My compassion leaves me vulnerable and yet my vulnerability is protected by compassion. Compassion knows no boundaries although I sense a 'professional' line that should not be transgressed.

> I drew a line to separate you from me
> but I kept tripping over the line
> and hurting myself . . .

Perhaps it's not so much a question of drawing a line but erasing the line altogether?

Luke

Friday September 5

Luke greets me by informing me he isn't comfortable and needs to pass urine. He wants to use the urinal bottle sitting on the edge of his bed. He doesn't have the energy to stand. With my help he slowly moves his six feet plus frame so he can pee. Unsteady, he leans his heavy yet withered body against me. I take the strain. Back resting on the bed, relieved, he relates his illness story – the way the cancer spread from his bowels to his lungs and, in his words:

'It's not long once it reaches your lungs.'

He reads his death sentence. Silence. I wonder whether he seeks reassurance that this is not true or confirmation that it is. Not knowing him it is difficult to say. I affirm. He does not pursue the thought.

He is 57 years old and diagnosed with liver and lung metastases from his primary bowel cancer. He was admitted yesterday to the hospice with uncontrolled vomiting. Quickly his vomiting and pain has been contained with 60 mg metoclopramide and 30 mg diamorphine via a syringe driver. No longer distracted by these physical symptoms he faces the reality of mortality. In the poignancy of the moment, I twist Bob Dylan's lyrics in my head:

'It's all right ma, I'm only dying.'

I ask him whether he wants to wash this morning?

'I had a bath yesterday that exhausted me . . . I didn't enjoy it . . . I'll wash at the bedside later.'

He is keen to have a foot massage, anything that might relax him. But first he will have some breakfast.

'Poached egg on toast please.'

I give him the nebulisers that lay on his bedside locker and go to fetch his breakfast.

He has some chest pain that I diagnose as indigestion. He has had a triple heart bypass operation for angina in the past. The small neat scar down his sternum a constant reminder of past wars. A call to Dr Brown who visits and prescribes an antacid. The pain quickly evaporates. Drama over, we return to the mundane issue of his dying.

Audrey, Luke's sister, arrives. Her husband died of cancer earlier this year. I wonder how she feels seeing her brother like this. No giveaway signs – she is composed but concerned as elder sisters probably are to their younger brothers.

I ask:

'How are you?'

She smiles and says she's fine; the ubiquitous greeting. Her eye contact averted from my soft inquiring eyes as if she might lose her composure under their gaze. But, for the moment, I do not pursue my inquiry. There will come a moment.

Luke's breakfast is cold and only partially eaten. I clear away the tray and ask if he's ready for the foot massage? He is and settles his long body into a comfortable position. The massage is a revelation for him. It deeply relaxes him. Shortly afterwards, Lorraine, his wife arrives. She is elegant and sun-tanned. She says the tan is just from the back garden.

Later Luke is asleep. Lorraine comments:

'It's the first time I've seen him sleeping without twitching.'

I say:

'I do relatives as well . . .'

but she rejects my offer, not wanting to detract from Luke's care. Later she changes her mind and sends me a message via one of the other nurses.

'Yes please, if you have time.'

Perhaps putting her 'on the spot' with my offer when we had just met had invaded her space? Adjusting her space, she can now accept.

After lunch Luke again sleeps. I suggest he has some peace. Lorraine muses that he now sleeps so much of the time. I feel the sadness in her voice as if, in sleeping, he is slipping away from her. She says:

'It's been so hard caring for Luke as his condition deteriorated . . . it's such a relief he's here in the hospice.'

His stay is planned for one week although I sense he will die before then. She is exhausted but will persevere as spouses must.

She surrenders to my touch as I work her feet with slow firm movements. I imagine I am sculpting a fine bowl where she can put her sorrow and rest a while. I smile as her face relaxes. As I finish Luke begins to twitch and groan. Lorraine is distracted, upset to see him suffer even as I encourage her to close her eyes and let go of the tension she holds within herself.

Luke is tense, and his tenseness ripples within him, bubbling to the surface from hidden depths even as he sleeps. Gazing at him, I realise how little I know him even though I have dwelt with him for most of the day. He knows he is dying. He told me that death is a mystery that is hard to contemplate. I really identify with that idea especially when the person, like Luke, professes no faith to hold on to. I sense his existential or spiritual loneliness as he struggles to find meaning and acceptance. Meaning in life or meaning of death? Acceptance of what? Obliteration? When people have no faith I endeavour to create a sense of reverence to touch and nurture his spirit so it can emerge and bloom even in the shadows. So, in the quiet sunny afternoon with the patio doors opening onto the small garden where the ornamental heron watches over us in the shade of the small tree, we dwell together and feel the mystery.

Reflection

The experience is elegiac, a song of mourning with Luke and Lorraine in creating sacred space where we can dwell in the suffering and sorrow. It is not trying to quell the sorrow but live through it, learn from it, and emerge through it more enlightened. The profound nature of palliative care emerges like the early morning sun radiating through the gloom. It has a strange paradoxical dark beauty. I must learn not to jump in too quick to offer a relative therapy before I have read the signs and tuned in appropriately. In my haste to be helpful and available I stumbled.

Paula

Across the corridor
I wonder if Paula would like a foot massage.
She seems so lost sitting in her chair
Her body tilted
One side stricken
Her mind searching for words
Her mouth seeking expression
Exasperation!
I kneel before her
And touch her despair and sadness.
Her daughter sits on the bed
Just 19.
What does she think and feel?
No give away signs.
Like a rag doll Paula is helpless.
As the brain tumour bites ever deeper
Paula waits.

Sitting on the floor at Paula's feet, my hands gently massage her feet as I try to comfort her. I sense only despair that won't lighten. In truth I feel uncertain whether I help ease her suffering but I must believe that somewhere in the dark gloom I have touched and nurtured her spirit. To find the sun. Is there more I could do? I know that the massage will have comforted her enough. I must rest in that knowing.

Further reflection on 'the good death'

Monday September 22

The sky is pale blue with scattered clouds tinted peach by the sun that has yet to emerge. As I drive, I glimpse the sun through holes punched into the bank of cloud low on the horizon. I am also reminded of Buddhist practice; moments where enlightenment might be glimpsed through the dense cloud of the ego's chatter. Such moments are beacons for I sense deep within my Buddha nature. Healing practice is like punching a hole into the dense cloud that suffocates Paula's spirit. If I were her, what would I want? A perilous question because I could never fathom what she is suffering. Limits to my empathy. However, I think most of all I would want to be loved, in all my human frailty, so I was not alone on this journey.

At the hospice I listen to the conversation between Kirsty and Christine after the morning shift report. Kirsty says:

> 'Tony died yesterday . . . it was really beautiful . . . he got twitchy which put me in a dilemma. Beryl (his wife) wanted him to be conscious. I gave him some midazolam 10 mg about one hour before he died . . . he was having periods of apnoea and then he would open his eyes . . . he had his arms outstretched . . . Beryl was holding one hand and Terry (his daughter) holding the other . . .'

Such conversations reveal the caring team's quest to ensure the 'good' death and the potential conflicts both within self and with the dying person's family. Tony got twitchy and immediately Kirsty reached for the medical solution despite Tony's wife protestation. Kirsty has some image of a good death she strove to realise – *he got twitchy which put me in a dilemma*. Perhaps Kirsty knows the family will be distressed if Tony is not 'peaceful' despite their protestations for him to be conscious. It raises the question – do staff sedate for their benefit rather than for the patient? Lawton's (2000:120) words are confrontational:

> As Fagerhaugh and Strauss have pointed out, sedation 'puts the patient into a living sleep with drugs and thus constitutes an imposed social death (1977:162). In removing a patient's sentience through sedation the last vestiges of their personhood are also erased; aspect of person and self which involve patient's ability to 'act', choose and make decisions for themselves. It seems important, therefore, to explore the extent to which such a practice is actually done for the benefit of the dying patient him or herself.'

And in the unspoken background – what does Tony feel? I wonder what Tony would have wanted. Without doubt, an institutionalised image of the good death where the person drifts off peacefully in a climate of family together-ness, is a powerful background for hospice practice. McNamara, Waddell, and Colvin (1994) comment from their study on the threat to the good death within hospices:

> Nurses speak of the need for excellent standards of care and adequate symptom control. They aim to provide holistic care and comfort to both patients and families and work towards providing an environment where the patient may die peacefully and with dignity. (p1504)

> Nurses validate the good death experience by recounting stories where 'the family were all involved', where 'the patient fell peacefully asleep forever', and where 'the patient made a tape of farewells to her family'. Some dramatise the event. One nurse added a setting of the sunset and a wilted flower. These events become ritualised: rhetoric and powerful imagery work to reinforce shared meaning. One nurse did, however, relate how, in many ways, there has been a backlash against 'all the warm fuzzies' as she called it. This is, in part, due to the stories that do not fit the patterns of the good death. (p1506)

Words like 'beautiful' both embellish and reinforce the idea of the good death as a practitioner ideal. Where the stories do not fit the pattern of the good death, practitioners seem to take it personally, expressed as failure, guilt, and distress. It is futile to imagine that practitioners can always create the good death. Of course, the idea of a 'good death' also suggests a 'bad death'. But I sense it is not helpful to think in these terms.

Perhaps it would be better to think in terms of knowing and easing the other's suffering. The more the other's suffering is eased the better the death is likely to be for that person. As a practitioner, I tune into and flow with the other's wavelength. Their suffering is not my suffering and I must accept that sometimes their suffering cannot be easily eased as with Paula. Consider Elizabeth's plight.

Elizabeth

Elizabeth is 46 and has breast cancer with liver and bone metastases. She was transferred from the general hospital where she was admitted unconscious probably due to sudden steroid withdrawal. She has been ill since her last chemotherapy treatment. Talk that she has been 'rude' to staff and is irritated by the slightest noise. A night staff nurse had actually written:

> 'I have been unable to explain such a sudden change in her personality.'

I want to shout:

> *'Perhaps she is simply fearful and projects that fear – why do we take it personally and let it offend us? Why should we expect patients to be **nice**?'*

I am indignant at the hospice culture of niceness. Are people blind to themselves? I don't shout, yet I feel my frustration leak out along the edge of its container. It has a bitter taste.

Elizabeth's head is tilted to the right side on her pillow. A barely-eaten bowl of cereal in front of her. Her hair is sparse, indicative of recent chemotherapy. Her face thin and jaundiced. She washed her hair three times yesterday trying to wash out the hair loss. Her wig on the locker reminds me of Kristin and stirs up quietened emotions. I am also reminded of a recent conversation with a cancer ward sister about a woman wanting her hair to fall out quickly because she couldn't stand the threads of hair everywhere . . . in her mouth, on the pillow. The sister felt that it is not the hair loss that is so distressing as much as its falling out. And so it seems for Elizabeth.

After gazing at her for a few moments, I knock gently on the door. No response. Moving closer, I say:

'Hello Elizabeth.'

She opens her eyes and smiles.

'I'm Chris the complementary therapist.'

She says she attends day care and appreciates the hand and face massages that Sam (therapist) gives her. Elizabeth's talk is fixated on her swollen legs and reduced mobility.

'I've got to get walking and need this lymphoedema sorted out . . . my partner is returning from Bristol and could take me to the hospital to see the therapist. I've mentioned this to Kirsty who's left a message on the therapist's answer phone . . . I'm anxious to get fit for my next chemotherapy.'

Elizabeth is quite determined and I see that I must help her achieve in this endeavour. Distracting her, I suggest perhaps a gentle foot and lower leg massage may help using some essential oils known to benefit fluid retention and toxic build-up and to help her relax. Perhaps therapeutic touch might ease her persistent kidney pain that she scores 3 to 4 on her pain chart? She accepts the 'bait'. I lift the quilted bedcover. She says:

'It's very pretty – like the hospice itself.'

Mindful of the shift report talk I say:

'We weave an illusion of prettiness perhaps to mask the real nature of the place.'

Elizabeth tunes into my comment. She is under no illusion and is interested that I had picked up on the hidden meaning in her quilted bedcover comment. I wonder if I should have played up the illusion rather than pull the mask away. Perhaps because I had tuned into her I could say that. I am certain she appreciates my authenticity rather than pretence, beguiled by the illusion of 'pretty'. Perhaps that's why she's rude because she suffocates under a 'duvet' of 'pretty' illusions? Interesting thought.

After the massage and therapeutic touch, Elizabeth is relaxed although the kidney pain has not eased. She resists my offer of analgesia.

> 'I don't want to take analgesia in case it clogs up the liver. I've taken a quarter tablet of DF118 on five occasions in the past three days.'

Words that reflect her need to be in control. She wants to talk about her son, who is 19, studying at Bristol University. His pictures through different ages stand along the window ledge. She laughs.

> 'He won't like seeing that . . . it's hard for him . . . he won't talk about his feelings . . . his stepmother's also got bone cancer.'

Although I do not surface the thought, I sense she asks me to speak with him, to help him release his feelings.

Elizabeth had a mastectomy in 2000. In June this year she had oesophageal bleeding and bandaging. Her notes reveal:

> 'Elizabeth has looked on the Internet and is aware that oesophageal varices may be a result of portal vein occluding.'

The liver cancer at work obstructing her venous and lymphatic flow from her lower legs and making her jaundiced.

After lunch I go to say goodbye. Her pain has gone. She feels relaxed and felt the therapeutic touch helped considerably. Could she have some more treatment on Wednesday when I next visit? No news about the lymphoedema therapist . . . a look of resignation. I sense her frustration being unable to make these things happen yet we can work with her. Staff need to understand her frustration and need for control and not absorb her frustration when it breaks out as apparent rudeness and react like critical parents. In not understanding her, staff risk increasing rather than easing her suffering. In doing so, we fail her and ourselves. OK – it may not be easy to journey with some patients like Elizabeth but who said palliative care was easy?

Trapped in an ethos of niceness staff are at risk of not being authentic, of weaving illusions, of creating environments dedicated to masking the horror of death and dying. Conforming to a perverse norm is a repetitive pattern that stifles the spirit of both patients and staff.

Two days later

The jaundice in Elizabeth's eyes has deepened – a deep yellow that gives her a feline appearance. Her first words are that she doesn't want therapy. I can see that she is tired. I know the lymphoedema therapist rejected seeing Elizabeth because treatment was pointless and outside her work area. I understand the therapist's need to draw boundaries about using available resources in the best way but a palliative attitude would see the treatment as justified from a psychological perspective rather than just from a narrow physical perspective. Irrespective, Elizabeth feels her legs are more comfortable. I say that with the therapeutic touch she can just close her eyes, that it requires no effort on her behalf. She says:

> 'I'll leave it up to you.'

I am in a quandary, not wishing to impose my therapy but neither do I want to push her to make a more decisive decision. Uncertain I change track and say how pretty her sky blue nightdress is. Teasingly I say:

> 'Does it match your eyes?'

She smiles and opens her eyes wide. They are deep brown against the jaundiced white. More forthcoming she says that her 'kidney' pain only slightly aches (2 on the pain scale). She also has some pain in her bottom because she is unable to move in bed. I sense her sadness and apathy, that she has no energy and like many other patients, the thought of therapy is exhausting even though it requires no effort and would be deeply relaxing. I suspect she knows she is dying, that things have turned against her and perhaps feels therapy is futile despite its positive impact on Monday.

Reading her pattern I decide to leave her to rest for the moment and explore the situation with Kirsty, who feels Elizabeth has let herself go – normally she is very particular about herself but she hasn't washed for two days and she resisted Kirsty's effort to change her nightdress this morning.

Later, in the afternoon, Elizabeth asks me if I gave her a treatment this morning when she slept. I smile and say I didn't want to impose. Her comment intrigues me, because her question suggests she would have liked the therapeutic touch. Did I read her wrongly? She says Peter, her partner, is coming in soon and will help her get out of bed and walk. Beneath the fragile mask she must keep trying.

I say I will see her tomorrow and offer her another treatment. She thanks me for popping in to see her.

Next day

I hesitate by Elizabeth's door – should I impose myself for I sense that my presence does impose something on her when she prefers to be left alone or that she feels the burden of resisting me even as I emphasise 'no pressure'. I decide to pop in. She is awake and looks very comfortable turned on one side. She smiles and says hello. I say:

> 'You look very tired.'

She says she is. I ask if she walked yesterday. Peter had got her out of bed and walked her with her zimmer along the corridor last night. She closes her eyes to dismiss me. I wish her well for her discharge tomorrow and leave.

However, outside the door I am bothered. I share my thoughts with Kirsty who also feels we struggle to get alongside Elizabeth. Elizabeth intends to attend her chemotherapy appointment tomorrow and get her Hickman line flushed. She insists she's going for the appointment. The decision to give further chemotherapy was made last Friday but she has deteriorated. Is it appropriate? Would it not be futile?[11] Maybe, but if she insists then perhaps the doctors need to give her every chance. I know Elizabeth's partner Peter struggles to accept that Elizabeth is dying and will clutch at every straw. I would be honest and say it's futile but still offer the opportunity. She will suffer more not taking the opportunity than if she did. Hope outweighs the discomfort of the chemotherapy in her precarious state. But all of this is speculation. Tomorrow is another day. As Kirsty suggests, we need to get alongside Elizabeth and support her in her decisions even if we struggle to accept them. Having Kirsty available to talk things through is vital to chew over the doubt that taunts the mind and twists reason.

Louise

September 23

Louise is a 58-year-old Caribbean woman who lives with her sister. She has a sub-acute bowel obstruction as a complication of her carcinoid liver that has metastasised to her liver. She has a bad taste in her mouth. She holds a vomit bowl in which she spits out the toothpaste together with a stream of green vomit. I suggest an aroma-stone with black pepper and camomile essential oils might help settle her digestive system?

'If you think it might help dear then anything's OK by me.'

She smiles and takes my hand.

'Thank you.'

I remove the cardboard vomit bowl and fetch another, some warm water to wash her hands, and a mouthwash to rinse her mouth.

The next morning Louise is feeling much better. Her pain and nausea better controlled. She regulates her eating to manage the symptoms.

'This morning I had a boiled egg . . . I really fancied that.'

---

[11] Futility is a technical term to refer to treatment whereby it is ethically justified to withhold medical treatment if it would not improve the quality of life of the patient.

The aroma-stone is missing. She says they took it away. She feels upset because she had really benefited from the aroma.

> 'It was very refreshing . . . I could inhale it and feel it soothe me . . . it took away the pain and nausea.'

Of course, whether the oils really took away the pain and nausea is unknown. However, the fact she felt it did is important.

> 'Could you have asked to keep the stone?'
> 'I don't like to make a fuss . . . they're busy and other patients need them.'

Louise's voice is apologetic and subdued like a child afraid of censure. Do you hear these voices in your practice?

Cindy (staff nurse) doesn't know why the aroma-stone was stopped. She isn't even aware that Louise had one. I feedback Louise's words to Cindy and say I will replenish the aroma-stone. As Cindy is Louise's nurse, I am slightly astonished that she didn't know about the aroma-stone. Does she not read the patient's notes? My comment 'it was written in the notes' received no acknowledgement. Further evidence of the peripheral role complementary therapies have in everyday practice despite their therapeutic acknowledgement. Perhaps I should expect this rather than be astonished. Perhaps if a therapist worked every day then nurses would be more mindful of complementary therapy treatments. As it is, Louise gets the message that staff are careless. Perhaps it would be better to offer no service than a partial one? I am pleased I confronted the situation without projecting my frustration.

After lunch Louise again comments on the aroma's benefit but suggests it is less potent than Monday. I had added one drop less of camomile, which subsequently adds to the mixture. She is grateful. You may ask what difference one drop of camomile makes – but evidently it made a difference to Louise.

Next day

Louise's aroma-stone is switched on but has become dry and caked. I replenish the stone as before. She has no pain or nausea and again comments that inhaling the aroma soothes her. This time I ask Frances (staff nurse) to remind staff to *think aroma-stone*. Frances is very apologetic – she has a very positive attitude to aromatherapy but admits it had simply been overlooked. Again I am mindful of my frustration. I am more assertive in challenging the issue – the assertive mantra *tough on the issue, soft on the person*. It's an effective mantra because it teaches me that giving feedback is focused on the patient's care, not a personal issue.

Louise, like so many other patients, is passive and felt unable to challenge the nursing staff on why the aroma-stone was removed. A holistic philosophy to healthcare is centred on a collaborative approach of working with people to appreciate and meet their health needs. As such, holistic practitioners need to actively facilitate patient empowerment, planning with each patient the care they need. Yet the reality despite the rhetoric of empowerment is passivity. Do patients learn to be passive along their illness journeys? Are healthcare practitioners socialised to be authoritative? Undoubtedly the symbolism of becoming a patient seems to strip people of their autonomy and mute their voice. Does Louise fear sanction if she complains? It is a recurring theme through my narrative and presents as a significant contradiction within the hospice culture.

Saturday October 4

From my study window the sky is so immensely blue. Nature has such pure colours to stir the spirit.

Last Thursday Gavin, a student on the first day of the *Becoming a Reflective Practitioner* course I teach at the University of Luton,[12] challenged me about the value of reflective writing. In particular, he was sardonic of its *flowery nature*, especially my allusions to nature. Was it embellishment or meaningful? In response, I drew a parallel between appreciating nature and being caring; that appreciating the beauty of nature is beyond reason as if it vibrates within me, nurturing my caring spirit. I spun it round, suggesting that nursing had hard images of science that needed softening. Gavin sensed what I meant. Marcia, another student, also felt this connection to nature. She had this image of washing up whilst looking out of the window at a rose, and being infused by its beauty; that is was essentially a spiritual connection that transforms something mundane (either washing up or caring) into something sacred. Appreciating beauty in nature is a reflection of holism, that the wholeness of holism is nature itself, that we are nature itself and appreciating a blue sky or a rose is in essence appreciating ourselves. We *simply* have to pay attention and listen with our senses. Yet science is the mind-God and demands allegiance, even ridiculing the soft edges of caring as something girly. The masculine shadow of science darkens the blue sky and obscures the caring view.

Listening tunes me into caring and nature tunes the listening. In his book *Being and Vibration*, Joseph Rael (1993:34) relates the story of his grandmother telling the children that people are made of sound:

> Since people are made of sound, listening is important. It is through listening that you become a true human, and a true human is a listener who is constantly attuned by working with everything that is happening. To become a true human you must become conscious of listening and hearing the voice of the great mystery speaking through everything, through the sound of a tree, or the bird flying overhead, or the wind in the room, or someone breathing, or someone talking, or a moment of silence. The activity of sound is what made the people. It is, therefore, simply through listening, and using that listening and paying attention, that one finds the guidance of the great mystery along the path of life.

---

[12] See University of Luton website for course details at www.luton.ac.uk

Listening is not merely listening to words; it is listening to the sacred vibration or great mystery that exists within everything. When I commented to Elizabeth on her cornflower blue dress and the colour of the eyes she looked at me and smiled as if I had listened beyond the surface of things to touch this sacred vibration. Listening, paying attention – these are the qualities of being mindful, listening with intent to touch the spiritual both within self and other, listening with intent to heal both within self and other. It is beyond any rational idea. According to Rael, vibration evolves in a natural order and is continually moving from East (emotional) to South (mental) to West (physical) to North (spiritual) and to the Centre (the heart). Each direction represents an element of consciousness as represented by different sounds.

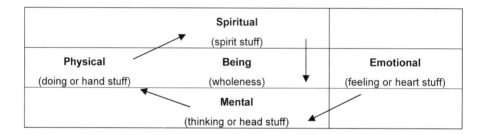

- Being mindful I tune into my feelings and the feelings of the other
- Being mindful I tune into my thoughts and the thoughts of the other
- Being mindful I tune into my actions and the actions of the other
- Being mindful I tune into my consciousness or spirit and the consciousness or spirit of the other
- Being mindful I touch my whole being and the whole being of the other and the oneness of all things

Each level unfolds into the other. The spiritual takes relationship into a transcendental level characterised by wholeness where there is no separate thinking, feeling and doing – there is only being in its wholeness. I have noted that many patients touch this space during therapy. Through vibration, the body transforms itself moving to higher levels of consciousness and in doing so will lift others. Rael (1993:88) notes:

> What is interesting about this lifting energy is that when it happens to us, it also happens to other people who are also being lifted to the next level. If we are being lifted others are lifted as well without necessarily being conscious of the process.

Rael's words are a revelation. I realise that the centring rituals in commencing and completing a therapy are most significant and that healing is a transmission of energy through me. Healing as vibration inspires me to reach deeper inside to feel this connection and use it more consciously within my practice; to *really* feel healing.

This insight is reinforced through reading *The Reconnection* by Eric Pearl (2001). Pearl describes his use of healing touch as vibration and his mission to help people reconnect strands of DNA as a force for human realisation. Pearl challenges me to listen to the person receiving therapy and give less emphasis to technique. This is a tough message because my complementary therapy training was dominated by technique. Pearl's message is clear – focus less on technique and more on intuition. I have come to appreciate that a focus on technique limits the benefit of any therapy. To learn to swim I must first let go of the sides, move out of the shallow end and shed the fear that I might drown.

Ruby

Early morning indigo sky. Such stillness. Ruby arrives at the hospice. She is full of cold, congested, has a headache and feels miserable. I set up an aroma-stone with eucalyptus and lavender essential oils. She loves the aroma and immediately feels its benefit as she inhales it. An hour later, her headache has gone and she breathes more easily. By lunchtime she feels much better. So simple, so transformative. If only I could always be so available and effective.

A playful line:

> Ruby Ruby your name so red
> Misery and cold has gone to your head
> Inhale the sweet release
> Feel your cold and misery cease
> Take my hand and feel at peace.

Joyce

Across the four-bedded ward Joyce packs her bags waiting for her transport home. The effort has tired her and she moves back onto her bed to rest. I suggest she might like a therapy as a goodbye gift? She is very receptive. I give her therapeutic touch for 15 minutes. Afterwards she is very relaxed. She says:

'I had the sensation of coldness running through my body but it was pleasant.'

During the treatment, I listen more mindfully to the rhythm of Joyce's body and break up my learned pattern of giving therapeutic touch. Without doubt, the therapy is different. I am more focused, more intent. I have a stronger sensation in my left hand. I experiment with the distance of my hands from her body until I find the healing distance. I am freer using my hands intuitively although still working from head to feet. No shaking of hands to rid 'negative energy', what Pearl (2001:133) describes as a 'fear-based ritual'. Being mindful opens up possibility and loosens attachment to learnt ways of doing things. I sense the way I have got locked into normative patterns of seeing and responding to practice.

Schön (1983) offers words of wisdom that ring true for my practice:

As a practice becomes more repetitive and routine, and as knowing-in-practice becomes increasingly tacit and spontaneous, the practitioner may miss important opportunities to think about what he is doing. He may find that he is drawn into patterns of error which he cannot correct. And if he learns, as often happens, to be selectively inattentive to phenomena that do not fit the categories of his knowing-in-action, then he may suffer from boredom or 'burn-out' and afflict his clients with the consequences of his narrowness and rigidity. When this happens, the practitioner has 'over-learned' what he knows.

Reflection creates the opportunity to challenge normative ways of being, cure blindness, foster mindfulness and open up the possibilities.

Cindy

Wednesday October 22

Cindy has arrived from the general hospital after spending 12 weeks there. She has refused further chemotherapy for her lymphoma. She describes the chemotherapy as:

'An awful experience . . . now I want my body to recover before any more, if at all.'

As she speaks, her lips tremble as the shadow of death moves across her. She knows that is most likely she will die soon but still has hope. Her abdomen and legs are grossly swollen. She feels the tightness in her abdomen – it is uncomfortable. She is 61 years old. Cindy is receptive to any therapy that I think might help her. I sense her exhaustion and give her therapeutic touch for about 20 minutes. Afterwards, she is more relaxed and feels she can now sleep to recover some energy.

Three days later

Cindy sits in a chair with her legs raised on a stool wrapped in a leopard-patterned blanket. She welcomes me but is cautious about accepting my offer of therapy as her husband and son are visiting. I say we can spend a few minutes? She agrees but will she need to move on to the bed? Again I reassure her she can stay just where she is. All she need do is close her eyes and relax into the therapy. She smiles, closes her eyes and surrenders.

During the therapeutic touch Cindy goes through a range of facial gestures that astonish me; her eyes are half opened and rolled back as if she has died; she grimaces and bares her teeth; her mouth is half open letting out a fine mist.

Afterwards I ask what the therapy was like. She says:

'I was just very relaxed.'

I ask if she had any thoughts. She had but they left her during the treatment. She had no body sensations. She smiles and thanks me. I am puzzled by her bizarre facial expressions. In description, they compare to the extraterrestrial manifestations that Pearl described, as if some other force was at work. I draw no conclusions but leave myself open to possibility. I also wonder about Pearl's claim that just reading and absorbing the messages in his book will raise my own vibrations. Umm.

Three days later

I drop in at the hospice on my way home from teaching at the University. The early shift are preparing to go home. Stella (staff nurse) asks if I am going to see Cindy. She says how much Cindy appreciated my treatments. Cindy doesn't like being touched so the therapeutic touch was ideal. I hadn't known that. I appreciate that Cindy tells the staff how beneficial the treatments are because it reinforces their value. Maybe it will eventually result in fewer dry aroma-stones and more paid therapists!

Cindy has deteriorated although she looks very comfortable in bed turned on her left side taking pressure of her sacral sore. She feigns a weak smile. I can sense she is unhappy.

'How are you?'

She cannot pretend. 'Not so good.'

'I can tell. Are you turning things over in your thoughts?'
'Yes.'
'Do you sense this thing creeping up behind you?'
'Yes.'

I am surprised at my euphemistic turn of phrase but it makes sense to both of us. Cindy is hopeful of recovering her strength but she knows within herself that she is dying.

'Would you like a treatment?'
'Yes please.'

For 30 minutes, I give Cindy therapeutic touch. Slowly, rhythmically, I move my hands across her wasted and swollen body. No facial gestures this time. Her mouth is closed and serene. She seems at such peace. Afterwards she shares how she felt the energy move within her especially down her legs which had been cold but are now quite warm. As before she had moved in a space beyond thought, a place of refuge from the storm that batters her.

Three days later, Halloween

The morning sky is a uniform grey colour wash. Such a contrast from yester-day's clear blue sky with bird feather clouds. Cindy went home as planned yesterday to her rearranged bungalow. She didn't really want to go but did it for David. On the whiteboard the bed-space notes 'Reserved for Cindy' just in case.

November 5, Guy Fawkes' Night

Cindy was re-admitted to the hospice on Sunday and died on Monday. I am tempted to ask about her death, in particular if she was at peace. But I refrain. Sometimes I prefer to dwell in the mystery. I sit by the fountain for a few minutes and say a prayer for her spirit. I never got to know if Cindy had any faith. It never emerged from our conversations. Maybe I should have known that.

Martin

Wednesday October 22

Martin has been admitted to the unit for 'symptom management'. I had met him briefly on Monday, no more than a hello. He is 55, the same age as me. Dressed in black like me. I had sensed his anxiety but did not pierce it – my impression of an emotional cauldron bursting under a constrained surface. Today, I am asked to care for Martin because he is embarrassed to bath with the female nurses. As I enter his room, he acknowledges me but I sense a distance. We sort breakfast out, his medication and plan the morning. Lying in bed he has no pain although his abdominal pain has not been well controlled. He is in transition from fentanyl patches to methadone 10 mg three-hourly on request. He is conscious that he has neglected himself and feels yucky! He would like to trim his beard, bath and wash his hair.

Some time after breakfast he moves into the bathroom. He looks at himself in the mirror with disgust that his beard has got so long and his body is wasted. He has lost around 10 kg. He uses professional barbers' trimmers which effortlessly transforms his beard's appearance. However, the effort draws out his abdominal pain – he describes it as a deep stabbing pain. I give him his methadone.

I have booked the jacuzzi bathroom which Martin anticipates with some pleasure. He walks there pausing to say good morning to the staff congregated for morning coffee. After soaking in the bath for 20 minutes, he is ready for a hair wash. He enjoyed the soak.

> 'Layers of skin have flaked off . . .'

and he feels the warmth of the bath has eased his abdominal pain. Getting out the bath and standing to dry himself again brings on the pain. I give him methadone in accordance with his fentanyl conversion programme and suggest using a heat pack, which he appreciates. He would like some therapy later this morning if I have time.

Adrian, Martin's brother-in-law phones to ask how he is? I find myself caught in a dilemma about what to reveal – the tension between easing the relative's anxiety and respecting Martin's autonomy and rights of confidentiality.

I inform him that Martin has been up, bathed and trimmed his beard, and that we are working to manage his pain adequately. Adrian seems satisfied with this, pleased that Martin is engaging with the world, and thanks me for informing him. I tell Martin that Adrian phoned and what I had said – not a blink of concern. I am satisfied I had not been overly indiscreet. Randall and Downie (1999:69) note that:

> Whilst the obligation to keep information confidential is generally known and acknowledged, and it is clearly described in professional codes of conduct, it is surprising how often information is given to relatives without the patient's consent.

In response I wrote (Johns 2004b:146):

> It is true. I have often witnessed nurses attempting to relieve the relative's distress or anxiety with explanations about the patient's behaviour, as if they are seeking to relieve their own anxiety. Our own anxiety is no rationale for action. As Randall and Downie (1999:71) state – it is easy but not justifiable, when talking to relatives and answering their queries to give them more information about the illness and its likely progress than the patient possesses. Health care professionals have a natural desire to assist the relatives by answering their questions, and it can be difficult to remember that the patient is the person primarily entitled to information about the illness, and that this information should be passed on only with the competent patient's consent.

Perhaps a more appropriate response would be to ask Martin what he would like me to say to any inquiring relatives. This experience makes me more mindful of this eventuality.

As I return to give Martin his therapy, his sister arrives. He enthuses to her about his day; reflecting the importance of physical care and paying attention to small things that make him feel cared for. As a consequence he moves closer to us, less lonely, more animated. Now he is keen for his therapy. As a therapist I have moved away from hands-on nursing care, yet I see that integrating therapy with nursing care makes sense. It honours the wholeness. I am less someone coming in to do something. I cannot think of anything more intimate than helping someone bath – this realisation became so poignant when working with Kristin. I have commented before on the significance and intimacy of bathing another to create therapeutic space (Johns 2004a). In the modern world, staff nurses bathing patients becomes increasingly remote and undervalued. Nurses everywhere may give rhetoric to holistic practice yet in practice nursing becomes increasingly technical and fragmented. Nurses become technicians strutting in the bright light whereas in the shadows, the hidden work of caring takes place usually by nursing assistants. Lawler (1991) coined the term 'behind the screens' hidden from view, and James (1989) reveals the emotional work that is generally viewed as little more than a natural extension of women's roles in society and *ipso facto* unskilled. Yet, as my stories have revealed, emotional work is the essence of care, focused as it is with the meanings people give to their illness experience. As James (1989:19) notes:

Emotional labour is hard work and can be sorrowful and difficult. It demands that the labourer gives personal attention which means they must give something of themselves, not just a formulaic response.

Must give something of themselves. In other words emotional work is intimate and spiritual.

However, in my experience emotional work is not sorrowful. Indeed, I find it uplifting. It is an intriguing question to ask what makes emotional work either sorrowful or uplifting. Is it a reflection of the carer's perspective? As I look back and reflect on my morning's work with Martin, we have dwelt together and emerged through the gloom into a clearing of renewed possibility. It is vital work. I find no sorrow in it or in my other stories. Am I better prepared than other nurses? My intuition tells me that it is related to the spiritual development of the practitioner. Clearly emotional *care* (rather than *labour*) must be valued by the individual. It must also be valued and supported by the team of carers, not merely as a 'nicety' but at the core of the caring endeavour.

I suggest to Martin that therapeutic touch may be most beneficial at this time. Holding my hands over his crown chakra I tune into Martin's vibration until I become one with him. A sense of stillness about us as if we are in a bubble. When I say:

'I've finished, Martin . . .'

he opens his eyes as if startled. I ask him if he had felt anything. He says:

'I was floating . . . I sometimes have dreams where I am floating.'

I ask:

'Was it a good sensation?'
'It was . . . I would have liked to have been there longer.'
'I can come on Saturday afternoon and give you another treatment?'
'Yes . . . I would like that . . . perhaps my feet then?'

I am deeply moved by this healing experience. I am learning to *really* listen to the other's vibrations and become more in tune. I sense that often I merely scratch the surface of the other's being, perhaps because I have been overly concerned with technique. Letting go of technique is liberating.

Three days later

Dressed only in his boxer shorts, Martin lays on top of his bed despite the cold in the room due to the failed heating. Yet he is not cold. He seems 'spaced out'. Two syringe drivers pulse a new concoction of analgesia as we try to get on top of his pain. He says he has been talking to Princess Diana. Is this a delusional state? Is he toxic from the cocktail of medication we heap in our efforts to bring his pain to heel? Is it a reflection of his deeper existential crisis playing out on the surface? Perhaps it is simply true. I certainly don't doubt him. He is perfectly aware of who I am. He asks if I am going to do his feet, remembering our conversation on Wednesday.

I concentrate on tuning into Martin's body, feeling my way across the feet, more conscious of my touch against his feet, more visual, imaging light being channelled through his body. Once during the treatment he jumps up.

'I thought a dog was lying on the bed.'

On the surface, he seems deeply relaxed but something deeper bubbles up. After the reflexology I continue with therapeutic touch. As my hands move about him, so his hands move slowly in patterns over his abdomen as if he is stroking something. It is as if our hands dance together. Afterwards he says:

'That was amazing . . .'

but he says it in such a detached way as if he is somewhere else. Such mystery.

Three days later

Martin's pain is proving difficult to tame. He became increasingly toxic on Sunday. Ketamine and haloperidol were discontinued. He has recovered to some extent from the toxicity although his pain control remains elusive. The room is dark. His eyes are closed. I sit and watch him move his hands in space . . . eventually I touch his arm and say:

'Hello Martin.'

He blinks and opens his eyes.

'It's Chris.'

Suddenly Sharron (staff nurse) enters the room with Martin's mother, his ex-wife and one of his four sons who has just have arrived from Germany. I discreetly exit. Outside the room, Sharron is in tears. She says:

'Did you see that . . . Martin's smile and the way he opened his arms to her?'

I had missed it but I am touched by Sharron's compassion. She really feels for and suffers with her patients. The spark of love is a furnace within her. As Sangharakshita (1990:47) teaches:

love changes into compassion when confronted by the suffering of a loved person.

Love needs to be expressed – perhaps that is the reason I give it so much attention in my words.

Three days later, October 31

Martin is restless, apparently confused. The staff are undecided whether his condition is due to disease progression or drug toxicity. He has had two faecal vomits suggesting a bowel obstruction. Octreotide is given via a syringe driver to help this symptom. Yet he is also severely constipated. Ten days ago he passed a constipated stool but nothing since. Four days ago he was given a per rectum examination – his rectum was empty but the constipation may be higher in his colon and may be contributing to the bowel obstruction? Other syringe drivers pump Nozinan 25 mg and midazolam 10 mg in the effort to quell his restlessness. As always I question this approach to managing anxiety – does it merely dampen his anxiety like a suffocating blanket? Martin is drowsy slipping in and out of a restless sleep, twitching and pulling at things in the air.

On the bed table are two photographs of his four sons. I try to engage him in conversation. He is rational but the effort to focus conversation tires him. He asks to be left in peace.

Gloria, his sister, and Bridget, his ex-wife are with him. Gloria is very distressed at Martin's deteriorating condition. When the women take time out, I give Martin therapeutic touch. During the therapy his legs twitch violently. Bridget comes back into the room and Martin wakes, startled, as if pulled back into this reality. I leave them together but later Bridget seeks me out and asks if I can help Martin be more awake as two other sons are coming over from Germany later this morning. I seek counsel with my colleagues about the current medication regimen. I argue the midazolam could be stopped and the Nozinan reduced by half if only to see its impact on Martin and respond to the family's need for him to be more awake and that being with his family may be the best therapy for his angst right now, especially as we are far from clear about his disease progression. A sympathetic response – but will they act?

The TT has little effect on Martin's restlessness. About two hours later I give him more TT that helps him relax into a proper sleep. Gloria and Bridget are relieved. Later the three sons are around Martin's bed. Martin is awake but drowsy.

I say to the sons:

'It's good to see you here.'

The sons respond positively and Martin raises his arm in a clenched fist salute. The boys acknowledge this with a cheer. It feels like a triumph. The boys talk of their journey . . . the congestion on the M25. They lapse into German as I stand on the edge of this reunion, and it reminds me of the many times I stand on the periphery of families, hovering, being available but knowing my place. After a minute or two, I excuse myself.

In the end room, a goodbye party is in progress for Helen, one of the doctors. I come out and see Gloria and Bridget still sitting in the corridor. I explain the noise is a party to say goodbye. They understand. As Gloria says:

'Life does not stop . . . it goes on . . .'

Her tears flow as I hold her.

Later at home reading *You are the Light* by Sahajananda (2003:83), I am captured by these words:

> The way is not a road but truth itself. Truth is not a definition but life itself, and life is not static, but always moving. Truth cannot be defined because every definition of the truth is like a tomb and only the dead are put in tombs. Life is the way, a journey, a dynamic process, a movement towards the destiny of every person, a destiny in which our temporal state finds its final consummation with God.

These words resonate with the truth of holistic practice flowing with Martin's experience rather than fragment him as symptoms. I sense we have lost him as if he has been put in his tomb. Holistic practice *is a movement towards the destiny of every person* yet, in our anxiety, we clutch at our technical knowing to solve his predicament and take responsibility for his body. Entangled in our own confusion we do not see him. Being attached to knowledge is an ego thing. Again Sahajananda (2003:124):

> The ego is the creation of the human mind through ignorance, and it is bondage from which the human mind has to liberate itself so that it can discover the truth and grace of God.

The grace of God is a metaphor for the sacred mystery within us. To help our patients' movement to embrace the sacred mystery we must embrace the mystery for ourselves and let go of our attachment to knowing, for such attachment is ignorance. Only then can we dwell with the ebb and flow of Martin's suffering as a mystery unfolding. Yet I fear we are out of step.

Five days later, November 5

Martin is alert and conscious although, in his words, 'lethargic'. He has not eaten for days and his bowels remain unopened. His medication is unchanged. He asks if I can give him another one of those wavy treatments and to remind him afterwards to tell me about the after-effects of his previous treatments. During the therapeutic touch he mumbles and moves his hands – I wonder where he is. Afterwards I remind him 'after-effects' but he only mumbles. I say I will see him next week? He murmurs:

'I may not be here . . .'

I wonder in the silence between us if he knows he is dying. But as we dwell in the silence he continues:

'I may be in a nursing home.'

I can only smile at my more sinister interpretation.

Six days later, November 11

I have not seen Martin for six days. He looks pale and gaunt, his beard unkempt, returning to its wild state before he first shaved 20 days ago. He greets me with a firm handshake and asks me to sit with him. His clouded consciousness seems to have passed although he is tired. He is having bouts of faecal vomiting due to his bowel obstruction. In his words:

> 'My mouth is like the bottom of a parrot's cage . . . I'm not eating so the digestive juices in the stomach regurgitate and leave this bitter taste in my mouth.'

I ask if I can do anything to take this taste away? He shrugs his arm past an array of juices but nothing seems to help. His aroma-stone is missing. He says he liked the smell so I will inquire what happened to it and re-establish it. Taste is related to smell . . . so a pleasant smell may well improve the taste in his mouth. Simple logic.

I ask:

'Are there things you still need to do in life?'

He exclaims:

'Yes, so much . . . I want to go fishing, see my sons, go shopping. . . .'

The list continues and then he says:

'. . . but I can't do any of them now.'

I remark:

'I used to love fishing when I was a boy.'

He says how much he loves fishing . . . he throws his arm as if casting his line and hooks a carp, taking the barbed hook from its protruding lip.

'Maybe some videos on fishing?'
'No . . . it wouldn't be the real thing.'

Silence . . . as we ponder the loss of a future.

'As you lay here do you think or feel about the future?'

Martin blurts out:

'Christ, I'm only 55.'

More than a hint of his anger that he is dying.

'I have no means of expressing what that means.'

I say:

'I can't imagine it either, what it must be like waiting for that mystery to unfold.'

I feel sad when he asks if we could sedate him if necessary to cloud his perception. I say we can. It is a poignant moment not least because the staff have found it difficult to move close to Martin to explore such thoughts and feelings. He is cut from his moorings and drifts on strange seas.

I offer therapeutic touch. Martin says he calls this the floaty treatment because that's how he feels . . . as if he floats above himself. But first I re-establish the aroma-stone. Estelle (care assistant) sees me with Martin's notes and anticipates my criticism – she admits to taking the aroma-stone away because she read in the notes that its use was to help ease Martin's anguish and she felt he wasn't anguished.

I am astonished. How blind can we be? Even though he does not express it verbally, his anguish ripples across his being like waves that crash against frail defences. Estelle listens as I tell her about my conversation with him and his anguish that fills the crevices of his being. She thinks that a man to talk with helps him express himself . . . the talk of the fishing . . . and it's true, the connection on this level leads to other levels . . . it relaxes him and opens up spaces where it becomes more possible to talk of deeper darker things. But I am left wondering – is caring such a lottery? It is ominous that Estelle could make clinical decisions about whether to renew an aroma-stone. Her gaze did not see him.

Martin surrenders to the moment and floats away to the strains of Enya that accompany my hand symphony. He is relaxed if slightly spaced out . . . a pool of stillness in the raging current that sweeps him inexorably to the big ocean. Afterwards I sit alone in the courtyard gazing at the water fountain and listening as it splashes across the stones. I close my eyes and practise the metta bhavana meditation, sending Martin love and easing the ache that has swollen deep within me.

Three days later, November 14

A still clear morning. The colours of the autumn leaves are stunning. The shift of colours through green to reds, yellows and brown falling to colour the ground. As I drive I follow my breath, breathing the stillness into my heart chakra, nurturing my compassion for the day ahead. I am a still clear morning.

Arriving at the hospice two candles burn. One is for Martin who died at 1 am. He deteriorated suddenly during the afternoon. He lies in the closed room. I touch the cold skin of his forehead and take his hand. Gathering my energy I practice the *essential phowa*, my closing gesture, guiding his troubled spirit to merge with the light. Martin struggled with death as he struggled with life. It has been a tough yet compelling journey alongside him.

The call home
Not earthbound any more
You can wing your way through the myriad of stars
Casting a line for the gleaming carp
shining in your dark skied eyes
That calls you home;
No one knows what happens at the end of the journey
No one knows where the dead go.[13]

Reflection

Reading through my reflection of being with Martin I sense the way my frustration ripples through the text. Perhaps, because his life was so tragic, I was drawn into his suffering. But that's simply the way it was . . . the way we were. My frustration is my spirit becoming snared in the rubric of symptom management that obscured seeing Martin as a suffering man as doctors and nurses shuffled cocktails of analgesia and sedation, striving to find the right formula to quell Martin's symptoms.

Given the situation again would I respond differently? Naturally I would respond differently simply because I have learnt through reflection yet I can't pinpoint exactly what I would do differently. But then I say to myself as I have said before 'it's good to grieve', for grief reveals both the aching and joyful heart. My grief honours Martin as if a way of touching myself with my own presence, or put another way, that grief is healing. That tears wash away the stains and cleanse the spirit.

I know that embracing the other's suffering may cause me to suffer, to grieve. Being human I am not immune to absorbing the suffering of the other. Kate White and her colleagues (2004:440) recognised the impact of the patient's unrelieved suffering on nurses:

> All the nurses reported that they tried very hard to relieve a patient's suffering and when they were not able to do this there was a feeling of helplessness, distress, vulnerability, frustration, sadness, of being overwhelmed or a sense of failure.

Many patients die in distress, yet this is not 'failure'. Is it simply that the culture of the 'good death' creates this individual and community expectation that suffering can be fixed, hence creating the idea of failure when suffering leaks out? White's work reflects the tension between being human and being professional that Hem and Heggen (2003:4) have highlighted, a tension that suggests intimacy within relationships is problematic. My interpretation of

---

[13] Inspired by Jeanette Winterson from her book *Lighthousekeeping* (2005).

this problematic links with interpreting another clause within the NMC *Code of Professional Conduct* (2002:4):

> You must, at all times, maintain appropriate professional boundaries in the relation-ships you have with patients and clients. You must ensure that all aspects of the relationship focus exclusively upon the needs of the patient and client.

Yet what is an appropriate professional boundary in relationship with a patient? The idea of boundary is problematic, suggesting a separation of self from other.

For practitioners who work in palliative care, whether in hospices or intensive care such experiences are commonplace. Death can become a normal occurrence. How easy to get hardened or complacent. The candle burning reminds me that it was Martin who died and helps me into a place of stillness beyond the chaos of his death.

Through reflection, I confess my suffering. The idea of 'confession' is appealing, not as a stick to beat myself with, but as a soft breeze to stir my spirit in my quest to realise desirable practice. So my suffering is not something to defend against but to open up to. As Thich Nhat Hanh says on his 2005 calendar for October:

> The Buddha called suffering a holy truth
> Because suffering has the capacity
> Of showing us the path to liberation
>   Embrace your suffering, and let it
>   Reveal to you the way of peace.

Maureen

October 31

Maureen is close to death. The lottery is out on her time of death – will she make it through the night? Her brother and sister stand vigil waiting, waiting. The brother says:

> 'She is a fighter.'

Maureen seems peaceful but even so I decide to give her therapeutic touch and set up an aroma-stone. I am filled with such peace doing the treatment that my legs feel very light afterwards. Her children too, seem more relaxed. I explain to them that I have balanced Maureen's energy field and that she is peaceful and in no distress. She has no religious faith, indeed the opposite – she had no time for religion. I would have thought otherwise. I ask if Maureen had any favourite smells. Linda, her daughter says:

> 'Definitely not lavender . . .'

almost anticipating that I would suggest burning lavender in the aroma-stone.

'What smells did she like?'
'None really.'

I add one drop of frankincense and one drop of patchouli to the aroma-stone – no more than a hint of odour. Later they say the aroma is just right, that it adds a sense of reverence. A positive aroma seems significant in creating a reverent and serene environment as death approaches that benefits the whole family. Of course, I choose the oils for these qualities. On a deeper level, the aroma releases the spirit within the onlookers and leaves a positive memory trace of witnessing the dying and death experience.

Such simple acts of creating sacred space with this family. As a therapist it is what I do, but I do wonder if nurses could just as easily learn these skills as part of their nursing role, given their significant therapeutic impact. I wonder if nurses draw boundaries on the scope of their practice that sets limits on their possibilities. One of the care assistants is an aromatherapist, yet she is discouraged from acting as an aromatherapist when 'nursing'. As a nurse might hold someone's hand, I might gently massage it. All practitioners need to expand their repertoire of therapeutic responses to be more available to help patients and families meet their needs. When nurses congregate around the nurses' station and banter I must question their morality, especially when they might be sitting with and holding someone's hand. When nurses say 'there is nothing to do', they mean there are no tasks to do. Perhaps they do not see the spiritual because they do not see it in themselves. Perhaps I might be accused of being *precious* in my own emerging spirituality, yet I do not think so. I hear the 'old school' hospice nurses lament:

'Nurses do not spend so much time sitting with patients. The old matron would never had tolerated it.'

The erosion of values bites deep and wounds the spirit.

Rachel

October 31

Rachel is 43 years old. She has lung cancer with local mediastinal spread. The cancer wrapped around her superior vena cava. Her pain control is elusive. Indeed, she greets me with a complaint of neck pain due to the fact she had fallen asleep with her TV headphones on. Knowing I massage, she requests:

'Can you massage my neck and shoulders?'

Seated in her chair with her feet up, her legs covered by a blanket, she gazes curiously at me. I kneel by her side.

'I could massage your neck but first let's try therapeutic touch?'
'OK, but first I need a fag and some coffee.'

She reminds me of a porcelain doll, very petite with dyed blond hair meticulously groomed, wearing a satin pink nightie. And yet she is already a grandmother. The therapeutic touch takes away her neck pain and wrist pain that she hadn't mentioned. She is now pain free; even the hip and back pain that had persecuted her through the night has gone. She is well pleased and so am I. Sometimes TT is like a miracle. I set up an aroma-stone using marjoram and bergamot essential oils to help ease her stress and infuse the room with a beautiful aroma that she appreciates.

Five days later

Rachel is dressed in black. Again she sits with her feet up. Left hip pain radiates to her back. She says the bed is the cause of that.
    I say:

'You seem down?'

She candidly agrees.

'I'm feeling stressed and anxious.'

The aroma-stone on her locker is unplugged and caked with dried oils. She enjoyed the aroma and would like it replenished. More neglected aroma-stones.

'Would you like some more touch therapy?'

She agrees but would first like a fag. I smile.

'Of course.'

I sort of expected her response.
    She lies on the bed as I play music by Enya. She likes the music and easily relaxes as I work with her using TT for about 30 minutes. Afterwards she says the hip and back pain have eased. She felt heat coming out of her head, which I attribute to releasing her anxiety. She feels very relaxed. A pain emerged from another back area during the treatment.

'I almost had to ask you to stop it was so painful but it then went away . . . it was as if you had drawn the pain out of me.'

Indeed, that is what happens.

I write Rachel a poem:

> The early dawn tinged with pink
> Like flamingos in flight
> Rachel dressed in black greets me
> Her eyes like slits pierce
> Her thin smile softens the edge
> Yes, she would like another treatment
> 'Can I have a fag first?'
> All things in perspective;
> She lay on the bed
> And gives herself to my tender touch
> My hands tingle above her
> Soft strains of Enya;
> Afterwards she felt the heat leave her head
> Anxiety dissipating
> She says 'I almost stopped you . . .
> The pain came from inside
> It was as if you drew it out of me
> And it had gone'
> I smile
> And say that 'touch is a mystery'
> Rachel folds back into the day
> As I move away
> Lighter
> Dwelling in the mystery.

Billie

Friday November 14

Billie is 65 with breast cancer that has spread to her lungs, bones and liver. Her jaundiced appearance reflects her advanced liver disease. She is conscious yet precariously hanging onto life. She asks me for a drink. I raise the back of the bed to help her drink. Just a few sips. The smell of liver disease is about her yet the smell hints of fear. I am told she is peaceful but I suspect beneath the surface she is tormented.

I ask:

'Billie, are you afraid of what's happening to you?'

She looks at me, and her eyes tell me she is.

'Yes.'

I ask if she has any faith. Again her eyes search me out.

'No.'
'What do you think will happen to you?'

She doesn't know what to expect. The great mystery of death stares her in the face. I have pricked a bubble and sense the fear seep out along the seams of the container she has held it fast. Again the question haunts me 'What must it be like to face death?' So often I have asked this question. It seems vital to grasp, and yet there are no answers.

Andrea (staff nurse) asks me how well Billie had taken her drink. I say just a few sips.

'Can she manage oral medication?'
'I doubt it.'

But when Andrea asks Billie if she will have a syringe driver she declines. When challenged with her difficulty taking her oral medication she reluctantly accepts the syringe driver. It is imperative to be proactive with Billie's comfort and anticipate her pain. Andrea asks me what I think about midazolam? I agree a small dose (5 mg) in the driver over 24 hours might help take the edge off the fear. George, the music therapist, has come to play for Billie. I say I was going to do TT and he invites me to work with him. His haunting music creates a sacred space. Billie is asleep when we finish. For the moment she is at peace. Harmonising my practice with George is profound. The energy felt electric. George is able to tune into the person's vibration and find the notes that resonate with that person. It is what I try and do yet the music seems to open pathways for the sprit to fly.

Avril

Across the four-bedded ward, Avril lays on her bed with her back to the ward. She is depressed and struggles to face the world. The management of her nausea has been a huge problem for a long time. Now it is easier but a dark mood has enveloped her. She is 59 with cancer of the pancreas. She doesn't think I can help her. Indeed she doesn't think anyone can help her; that she is beyond help deep within her despair. However, she likes the idea of burning some essential oil. She likes lavender. I mix lavender, bergamot and pettigrain, all chosen for their known mood-lifting qualities. It is a beautiful aroma. Worwood's (1999:242) description of the spiritual dimension of pettigrain creates a sense of reverence and purpose:

> The spirit of pettigrain is embodied in gentle strength, encouraging positive resolutions and outcomes in difficult times. It enables us to see ahead and forge a link with our inner truth, understanding that in our personal truth comes strength.

The idea of reconnecting with our inner truth, that depression is the ego's final defence against threat. Worwood (1999:194) says of bergamot:

> It lightens the shadows of the mind, bringing an awareness that the light will rescue us and take us ever forward to the realms of peace and joy.

And lavender (1999:225):

> When deep sadness covers the spirit like a suffocating blanket, lavender gently lifts the weight. When inner tears fall, lavender gently wipes them away. When depression clouds the psyche, lavender blows it asunder. And with those with worries that trouble the spirit, lavender lifts the veil of despair.

Later, Avril sits on the edge of the bed eating some breakfast. Perhaps she does have some energy or that the oils stirred her spirit. Dr Brown has prescribed an antidepressant yet when Andrea is offered the tablet she denies knowing about it and refuses. Accepting she is depressed is difficult for her. She seems lost, beyond us. I feel drawn into her despair even as I wonder if my response will help to lift the dark cloud that envelops her. Perhaps death will be merciful and release her from her torment. I sit with her for a while in silence. I sense her ambivalence at my presence; one voice screaming 'leave me alone', that she might prefer to dwell alone in her suffering, and the other voice screaming 'help me'. Perhaps the sense of impotence she engenders alienates her even in this healing place. I imagine Avril's silent scream and write a poem inspired by Kate Rusby's song *Falling*.

Silent scream

No one's about to hear my silent scream
You look for me where I can't be seen
Life breath's still strong within me
So tell me why I can no longer breathe?

Here I am falling, but falling to where?
Hold me and take me to where I belong
For I am too weak to make it alone
Let me fly on your angel's wings.

Time moves on and I know it won't be long
And in time I won't fear the day
Yet I sense as you sit there
You do not know what to say.

My body is tired, my body aches
I have tried to grow my own wings
They broke and I drift alone on the tide
Waiting for the ride home.

Reflection

I know people will question the claims Worwood (1999) makes for the spiritual qualities of essential oils. As an aromatherapist I too question these claims. It goes back to that searching question 'How can we recognise the spiritual?' What would be valid rules of injunction (Wilber 1998)? Avril's spirit is blunted through depression and I rather pessimistically sense the oils will have little benefit. Yet experience suggests the therapeutic value of these oils value in creating sacred space and lifting the spirit. I rest in my faith and experience. Sharron Salzberg in her book *Faith* (2002:67) writes:

> (faith) doesn't decide how we are going to perceive something but rather is the ability to move forward even without knowing. Faith, in contrast with belief, is not a definition of reality, not a received answer, but an active, open state that makes us willing to explore. While beliefs come to us from the outside – from another person or a tradition or heritage – faith comes from within, from our alive participation in the process of discovery.

Faith is not faith in something outside of me although it might be triggered by something outside such as Worwood's words – what Salzberg (2002) describes as 'bright faith'. It is only when something is experienced and verified does faith deepen and becomes known. Salzberg (2002:56) writes:

> In order to deepen our faith, we have to be able to try things out, to wonder, to doubt. In fact, faith is strengthened by doubt when doubt is a sincere, critical questioning combined with deep trust in our own right and ability to discern the truth.

Perhaps Salzberg talks of reflection – the sincere, critical questioning in action. Through reflection, we reveal and explore the creative tension where learning can take place – the tension between our vision for practice and an understanding of our current reality. Through understanding and commitment to our values we take action toward resolving the tension until we can realise our visions as a lived reality. In so doing, we sweep away illusion. We verify and deepen our faith in the mystery of caring; and in so doing cultivate our intuition, become more skilful in our actions, nurture our compassion and cultivate our wisdom – so at the end of the day we fulfil our caring destiny and responsibility.

Hebs

Across the four-bedded ward Hebs gazes at me intently, as if saying 'Why haven't you been to see me?' She is a magnet pulling me towards her. She is 71 years old. She was admitted from home 13 days ago very weak. But since then, to people's surprise, she has picked up. She shows me how she can now move her hands and feet. She tells me that she wants to stay at the hospice. I know from the shift report of her domestic strife and the lack of support she would get from her husband.

After her wash, she sits and looks out of the window across the gardens. She would love a foot and leg massage. Her legs are solid due to abdominal pressure. Her skin is very dry. She relishes the light massage using frankincense and grapefruit essential oils. Periodically she opens her eyes and says:

'Lovely.'

My touch and attention fills her with pleasure and takes the edge of death's journey. I imagine such therapy being an oasis in the desert, a place of nourishment and rest for the journey ahead.

I finish as lunch is being served. A different kind of nourishment. Friday means fish and chips. The greasy smell drifts along the corridors. I wonder if people prefer that smell to the aromas I have set up in the ward. Perhaps fish and chips is a real smell associated with living, whereas my aromas are symbolic of the dying journey. The words of Jean-Dominique Bauby (1997:96) come to mind in his story of the *Outing*. Bauby has locked-in syndrome following a stroke and is incarcerated in a hospital. Claude is his scribe – Bauby writes by flickering his eyelids. Brice is his daughter. They have taken him out for a ride in his wheelchair to the beach:

Claude and Brice bring me to a halt downwind. My nostrils quiver with pleasure as they inhale a robust odour – intoxicating to me, but one most mortals cannot abide. 'Ooh!' says a disgusted voice behind me. 'What a stench of grease!' But I never tire of the smell of frying potatoes.

As carers we cannot take anything for granted as to what smells or pleasures people prefer. And when the person is unable to say, then it challenges us to be more sensitive and tune into the other person. Avril could say she liked lavender yet others find it repellent. I do not carry the essence of baking bread, or fish and chips, or diesel oil with me but perhaps I should?

Henry

Monday November 17

A beautiful early morning sky with a vivid red streak stretched along the horizon. Red sky in the morning shepherd's warning. An omen for the day? Billie died at 6 am. Avril insists on going home today. Hebs greets me with enthusiasm anticipating another leg and feet massage. Her oedema is much reduced – perhaps the massage helped? She thinks so.

In a single room I meet Henry. He will be 73 tomorrow. He is also going to a nursing home, as his wife feels unable to care for him at home. He was unhappy with this idea but today he is more philosophical and accepting of his loss; losing his independence, his home and being separated from his wife. His voice is flat reflecting his despair. Yet on a brighter note he accepts my offer of a foot massage. As I massage his feet, he unfolds his life story.

He has lived in the town all his life. He left school at 14 and worked as a nurseryman until the council compulsorily purchased the land to extend the nearby school. He then worked for a local truck company for 30 years in the stores department, a time span broken only by serving in the army during the Korean War.

> 'You left school in 1945?'
> 'Yes, that's right.'
> 'You just missed the war?'
> 'I did that one but I served in the Korean War.'
> 'You must have many memories of that?'
> 'I do . . . of so many friends that got killed.'

After all these years, Henry still feels the horror of war and the sadness of friends dying. It is as if war scarred him for all time.

> 'Were you married then?'
> 'No.'

A smile creases Henry's face.

> 'That came later.'
> 'How many years have you been married?'

'49 years.'
'Tell me how you met your wife?'
'It's funny, really . . . we met by chance. A friend of mine was going to the pictures with his girlfriend and asked me if I wanted to come along as his girlfriend was bringing a friend.'
'A blind date?'
'Yes.'
'And love at first sight?'
'No . . . I didn't take an immediate fancy to her . . . that happened later.'
'49 years – your Golden anniversary next year. What date?'

Henry stumbles to remember the date.

'August . . . August 10.'

I want to say . . .

'Something to live for . . .'

but I do not want to remind him of his cancer and threat of death.
On the window ledge are picture of two girls. I guess correctly.

'Your grandchildren?'
'Yes . . . Corrine is 14 and Laura is 16.'
'Your son's or daughter's?'
'Daughter . . . we only had one child. We don't see too much of them these days.'

I sense a touch of regret in Henry's voice but again he is philosophical know-ing that young people lead busy lives and have no real time for old people. He hopes they will visit him in his nursing home.

Henry is bored at the hospice being unable to move about. His great love has always been gardening. His son-in-law will keep an eye on the garden now, will grass over much of the garden to make it easier to maintain. I optimistically say that perhaps he can potter about the garden at the nursing home. He muses:

'They have a nice large garden . . .'

as if the idea is both appealing and hopeful. I sense the importance of people having something to look forward to as they are devastated by loss. How easy to write Henry off as some sad terminal old man. Yet he is only 73 tomorrow.

We spend nearly an hour reviewing his life. Most often I ask people to close their eyes and relax and listen to music, but for Henry I sensed this need to find meaning in his experience and make connections with his past so he can look forward to his uncertain future positively (Marris 1986). It was not idle chat but significant for me to appreciate his life and the meanings he gives to his current predicament. For him it was time to honour his life and feel acknow-ledged as a person. There is some evidence to support the value of review work with palliative care patients (Pickrel 1989, Wholihan 1992). From a psychosocial perspective the work of Erikson (1982) would see my task as helping Henry resolve the potential crisis of ego-integrity versus despair, the last of eight stages of man.[14] A Buddhist interpretation of ego-integrity versus despair might be yielding versus failure. Yielding is surrendering to what is to come with a positive attitude whereas failure is resistance, a fear of surrender in the ego's desperate attempt to hold onto control and cling onto a separate reality.

Our talk was easing Henry's suffering by helping him find his feet on the path he must travel with greater understanding and resolve. My hand merely holds him whilst he finds his footing.

Later he informs me:

'My legs feel wonderful from the massage this morning.'

Small gifts bring such pleasure for both of us.

Reflection

Once again the first two Burford cues: *'Who is this person?'* and *'What meanings does this person give to their health–illness event'?* structure the healing space. Not knowing Henry does not constrain me giving him therapy. Indeed, it creates a space for the person to share their story. Responding to the cues is not simply collecting information, it is caring, as suggested by the idea of life review. As his story unfolds so are the meanings he gives to life revealed. It is profound work, reflecting the natural intimacy of holistic practice, a world apart from 'assessment'.

Len

Monday November 17

Across the corridor, I greet Len. We have met before on previous admissions. Yet his memory of me is as a staff nurse.

'I didn't know you were a therapist. You had a staff nurse manner about you.'
'Now that's an interesting comment. In what way?'

Len struggles to put this into words.

'Perhaps a manner, even an air of authority?'

He laughs. He makes me wonder how I essentially view myself – as a therapist or a nurse? Clearly he perceives a difference in authority between them. Does my 'authority' shift between roles? Do I present myself in different

---

[14] A recent paper that addresses this issue is Trueman & Parker (2004).

ways? Does more authority enhance or diminish the therapeutic potential? Reading back through my journal I do sense a subtle distinction – that I do tend to be more authoritative as a nurse. I also sense I am more therapeutic as a therapist which leads me to speculate an intriguing equation – the degree of perceived authority is inversely proportional to therapeutic potential. Perhaps it is also partly Len's own perception – that he has learnt nurses are more authoritative than therapists and responds accordingly. Either way, it is clear that health care workers need to mindful of the way they present themselves and in creating therapeutic space. Such moments of insight are vital.

Len is a non-cancer patient who has chronic heart and lung condition that makes him breathless. Usually a cheerful man, he says he has been moody these past few days because he has struggled to breathe at night. Last night he used the oxygen concentrator via nasal cannulae and slept much better. Problem solved and he has recovered his cheerful self. He has complementary therapies in day care on Wednesdays and describes the different approaches of the therapists in giving him back massages, some are gentle and others more vigorous. He prefers the more vigorous approach although grateful for whatever is given. If I have time, he would like a back massage.

I add one drop each of lavender, cypress, benzoin and frankincense to the carrier oil mix of 20% wheatgerm with 80% grapeseed. At first, the lavender dominates the aroma and then it fades into a delightful aroma that Len appreciates. I have chosen these oils for their ability to help Len's breathing, to improve his circulation and ease his stress. As I have noted previously, benzoin has an ancient reputation for casting out devils (Davis 1999, Lawless 2002). And it seems to me that living with debilitating chronic illness is a devil that weakens the spirit. Lawless notes that benzoin warms and tones the heart and circulation, both physically and metaphorically. She cites Maury (1989:57):

> this essence creates a kind of euphoria; it interposes a padded zone between us and events.

A padded zone might refer to mindfulness – the ability to create space between an event and our response. As such, perhaps benzoin heightens the ability to become mindful. An intriguing thought. Len leans across a table supported by pillows as I vigorously yet cautiously massage his back. Afterwards he is tired and sleeps.

Later, I return to ask if the treatment was beneficial. Connie, his wife, says how pleasant the room smells. She says Len's breathing is easier and thanks me. Len just smiles. He is used to Connie speaking for him. Perhaps she compensates for his compromised breathing. He says:

> 'The massage was good, just the right amount of pressure. I felt that as you opened up my muscles so you opened up my breathing space. I feel so much more relaxed.'

For someone with chronic obstructive pulmonary disease aromatherapy massage would seem a vital part of everyday therapy. Perhaps it should be prescribed, shifting thinking beyond pharmacological approaches to embrace a more holistic approach. Certainly Len finds it very beneficial.

Give yourself the gift of a massage.

Russell

Esme (Macmillan nurse) has asked me to visit Russell and his wife Agnes at home. Russell is 79 years old and suffers with lung cancer and liver metastases. Agnes answers the door.

'Don't worry about that . . .'

she says, as I wipe my shoes.

'Russell's upstairs . . . Russell, Chris is here.'

Russell comes downstairs easily. He apologises for not shaving.

'Eight years in the army, we scraped every day.'

Clearly he is uncomfortable being seen as unshaven.

'My little great-granddaughter, she rubs my face when I haven't shaven and says "that's rough Grandad".'

I ask him how he is. He points to just below his Adam's apple.

'It's here, makes breathing difficult.'
'And swallowing?'
'Yes . . . I can't eat hot meat . . . take plenty of this stuff . . .'

he says, pointing to some Ensure.[15] Russell and Agnes unfold their story of failed treatment and his current predicament. He has been suffering from headaches and dizziness, and is sick after taking his 'sicky tablets'. Agnes chips in:

'He hasn't left the house since March.'

Russell continues:

'Just a few minutes in a car and I'm sick.'

I wonder about a syringe driver for his sickness but that would mean a district nurse visiting every day and she only visits weekly at the present time. He has also stopped taking dexamethasone because he feels they also make him

---

[15] Ensure is a high calorie liquid food supplement.

sick. He has lost a lot of weight. He stands and shows me his baggy trousers. He knows he won't get better but his mood does not seem unduly low.

'It's these headaches that really get me.'
'What do you take?'
'I have the morphine twice a day. I take co-proxamol tables for the headaches. They seem to do the job quite well.'

I think to myself:

'. . . *but not well enough because he has constant headaches.*'

Agnes says:

'He has about six each day.'
'What about your bowels?'

Russell grimly laughs.

'Bunged up all the time.'

We enter into an inconclusive conversation about bowel management. He cannot tolerate Movicol and periodically has to resort to suppositories or even an enema.

I wonder what therapy would be most beneficial. I suggest either therapeutic touch or reflexology. Agnes knows about reflexology and shares a story of her daughter's friend who had it with good benefit. However, I feel the therapeutic touch may best help his headache just now.

Russell agrees and relaxes easily in the chair. Afterwards his headache has gone but he still feels a pressure in his forehead . . . as if it is still lurking there.

'I have this feeling all the time.'

He is drowsy after the treatment but feels very relaxed. His wife notices and is pleased. As I go to leave, I ask her how she is. She is stoic and says OK but I sense her tiredness and say I can offer her a treatment?

'Can you?'

I give her my phone number to contact me if they need me and suggest I visit again to give Russell reflexology.
Agnes says:

'Pop in any time'.

She pauses and says how unfair it is, that the good people get taken. She and Russell have no great faith but if there was a God he wouldn't allow it.

'The man next door he's got cancer but is getting over it. Another man in this road lost his wife – she was only 37.'

I have heard this so often before, this muted anger at an erstwhile God that reflects the depth of their suffering, a suffering that feeds upon itself as Russell slowly deteriorates each day, a suffering that is not easily eased. Perhaps knowing others also suffer from cancer helps ameliorate the unfairness. Perhaps that is how Agnes rationalises her anger and despair.

Outside it's threatening rain. The tragedy of peoples' lives strikes me. If only Esme or district nurses could give Russell and Agnes therapeutic touch or massage as part of their role. Yet the Macmillan nurses don't do 'hands-on' care and the district nurses are run ragged. Where is the space for holistic practice?

Monday December 1

Rain pours down outside, yet its rhythm is pure music. Over the weekend, I attended a retreat with Paramananda at Friends of the Western Buddhist Order. Paramananda is the author of *A Deeper Beauty* – a book that inspires my practice. He writes (2001:111):

> To walk in beauty means to walk with an awareness that is open and appreciative of the world around us. When our lives are dominated by an inner poverty we are not able to experience beauty . . . We need to find beauty in the very act of walking.

I might change the words and say 'We need to find beauty in the very act of caring'. Indeed, as I reflect on my practice, I become more aware, more in awe of the mystery and beauty of life, that even in deep suffering, beauty is found in the poignancy and tenderness of the moment, in the deep compassion that suffering evokes and in the responses of patients and their families to caring. It is a transcendence of poverty. Reflection creates this space to pause and appreciate such beauty.

During the retreat, Paramananda read a Mary Oliver poem called *The Deer*.[16] Listening, I was transported beyond the body into a timeless moment of realisation. Mary Oliver's words resonate with reverence about the meaning of being in the world. Can I sit idly by when my love can make a difference to the world? The retreat raises my awareness of *being earnest* and the paradox that to be earnest requires a deep stillness where the vibration of love can bloom and resonate.

My journal plots my *journey* of easing suffering and spiritual growth. I often play *The Journey* by Bliss[17] as an accompaniment to therapy. As a reflection on

---

[16]   *The Deer* is in a collection of poems by Mary Oliver (1990).
[17]   *The Journey* CD by Bliss, see Discography at end of References.

Mary Oliver's poem and more deeply as a reflection of my own spiritual journey I compose the poem *The journey* through the music's six parts.

Inspired by the meditation practice of *Mindfulness of breathing* I write a second poem *The breath* as a reflection on the significance of breath as *spiritus*, in realising my own deeper beauty. Writing poems releases my imagination and nurtures my spirit, for poems and paintings capture something of the ineffable nature of spirit beyond the limitation of words. I am always surprised how art is self-revealing.

The journey

Orange world
Mary Oliver's words ring –
'This is earnest work.
Each of us is given only so many
    mornings to do it
– to look around and love';
In earnest I push through the mundane
To reveal the soft orange glow of
    expanded consciousness
To feel the soft edge of love vibrate
In waves that ripple into the dark void;
So few mornings left.

New dawn
And if I wake into the new dawn
Beyond the dreams that haunt,
I can touch your face
And feel the love burst
Like a torrent set free
From that which contains.

Hymn
Moving away from the tipi flap
Where I sit
The music rises deep from within;
A hymn of love
That vibrates about me;
My hands tingle with awe.

Spring
It seems that I have sat for a long time
In a long winter
Waiting sometimes patiently
And sometimes restlessly
for the new shoots
Of life to spring within.

The journey
Am I ready to move beyond
The known
Into the dark void
Where suffering cries its name
Where blame rules
And love is a mask to hide the pain?

Reflection
I retreat into the soft music of Bliss
And pause between the breaths
To sit on the edge of a deep crater,
To feel the music's pulse vibrate
Stirring the dormant spirit
To that place deep within where love
    blooms
With reverence
        and the soft glow of faith.

The Breath
With eyes closed
I sit and focus the breath;
The first deep breath is a torrent of
    bliss
As if washing away
The debris that fills the abyss;
Such a deep first breath
that is never ending;
a smile across my face
I burst with love
yet pause
And slowly release the breath
Into a still place
Beyond the mind's aching grasp;
The body demands another
    breath
This time softer
Less full
But more sublime
As if inhaling a soft penetrating
    light
That reaches deep into the dark
    body voids;
And again
The slow release into the light
    spaces
Letting go the ego strain
Emptying self
But I know the ego
As the distractions creep in
I can smile at them.

Jane

Wednesday December 3

Two days ago Jane was told that 'there was nothing more that could be done' in treating her cancer that had spread from her breast to colonise her lung, liver and bones. Her right breast was removed in 1992 and her left breast in 1999. She is 61 years old although looks older with her toothless grin. She is deeply distressed by the news.

She sits in a chair by her bed. Her lower legs are bandaged wounds from when she fell on stone steps. I ask if she would like to put her legs up?

'No thank you . . . I like to feel the ground beneath my feet.'

I suspect those words hold a deeper symbolic meaning.

'I am the complementary therapist – can I offer you a therapy whilst I'm here today?'

Silence. Gently, I ask:

'You had some bad news two days ago?'

She gazes into my eyes as I kneel by her side and sighs.

'Yes.'
'How are you now?'
'Better today . . . it's hard to know what to think.'

I sense her tears are close to the surface. What is she feeling, thinking right now? Empathy is so hard. Again I ask myself 'What if it was me sitting there – what would I be thinking and feeling knowing I am going to die?' I like to think I could surrender into the Buddha's light but would I? Would some deep and as yet unfathomed fear of death surface to rip away my Buddha's mask of delusion? Is my faith deep enough?

I respond:

'I know . . . it's something that I too must face one day. Do you have a strong faith?'
'Yes.'

Jane looks at me and smiles.

'Does that bring you comfort?'
'No . . . I have lost faith.'
'Because of what has happened to you?'
'Yes . . .'
'That surely God would not have let this happen to you?'
'Yes . . .'

Reminiscent of a confession, Jane reveals her loss of faith. Such a burden to carry. Such torment to unravel as death approaches. All these years she has had a strong faith and now, at the very end of her life it shatters. Like a crystal glass crashing against a hard place. She is left groping about searching for meaning at a time when she would seek comfort in her God.

I thank Jane for sharing her thoughts with me. Perhaps talking helps her to touch her God again.

Jane is uncomfortable, so Stella (staff nurse) and I help her back into bed. Perhaps there is a paradoxical comfort in physical pain to distract from the deeper spiritual pain.

In the afternoon, I return to massage Jane's feet. Barry, her husband and her GP are at the bedside. They create space for me to give Jane the foot massage. I take her wound bandages down. Her legs are so bruised.

I feel her feet and heels. No pain. She says:

'The vicar has been to see me.'
'Did you talk about these things?'
'No, because of everybody else about.'
'Did it help to talk with me this morning?'
'It did, thank you.'

I gently massage Jane's feet. Afterwards she says it was lovely, very relaxing. Out of the blue, she blurts:

'Am I about to pop off?'

Her question surprises me.

'Why do you ask that?'
'Because of your concentration with my right foot . . . as if you could tell something.'

I reassure her that no such signs were present. She reads me, interpreting any sign as an ill omen. Her fear ripples from her enveloping me. Barry is distant, remote in an armchair a few feet away. What does he feel and think as he gazes upon his wife's spiritual chaos? No signs evident behind the bland smile.

This evening as I write my reflection I am bothered by my conversation with Jane. I really want to help her reconnect with her God, partly I suspect, because I have found my own faith and partly because it's hard to witness her suffering. Yet I wonder if I trample along the edge of a vast crater when I should tiptoe with caution. I do not know Jane and yet we have already plumbed the depths of her despair. Do I really think I can help her reconnect with her God in the face of her fear as she gazes at death's grim mask? The spiritual has a raw edge. Jane is like many people who take their faith for granted as something normal and social without thinking about what it really means to live and die.

Perhaps people like Jane see faith as protection from dying, as an immortality quest? Whilst I am intrigued why Jane would blame God, I know that it is not an uncommon phenomenon. Young and Cullen (1996:134) reflect on one couple in their study:

> They had both belonged to a church but the experience of those final weeks robbed Harold of his faith and nearly did the same for Lillian.

Just as Jane does, I struggle to find meaning in her predicament. Suffering is a mystery, deep, very deep within her, beyond explanation. I must simply flow with her.

Two days later

As I enter the unit Barry is sitting waiting whilst the nurses do Jane's dressing. He smiles knowingly.

> 'She's waiting for her foot massage.'

It is good that the massage had a positive effect. Jane greets me with a wide smile. She seems happier. She says our chat has helped her deal with her crisis. She's also spoken with the curate and let go of some of her angst towards God.

I commence with a relaxation ritual. First, I ask her to concentrate on her breathing – following her breath in and following her breath out. I then ask her to imagine she is surrounded by a warm soft healing light and to breathe in this light. I suggest that this light is God bathing her in his divine love. I do this to help her visualise and sense union with her God, to feel his presence bathe her with love.

After the massage, Jane feels calm and comfortable. She says that half-way though the therapy she experienced a slight feeling of nausea that passed off. I am always intrigued how reflexology pulls out distress from the body. Could the nausea be a metaphor for her resistance to God?

However, my doubt persists to press my brow – do I meddle in things beyond me? To reflect I review myself within the *spiritual traps* (figure 6.2).

I have used these traps before (Johns 2000b:164–166) but using them again feels very confrontational. Do I lay a 'spiritual trip'? Perhaps not obviously but maybe subconsciously my own faith imposes? Does that matter or is that simply my 'spirituality' expressing itself? Being a natural part of me it is not something that can be turned on or off as a technique. The hospice's roots were strongly Christian but this influence has diminished, reflecting society's secular turn. The hospice's 'expectation of a good death' is always an imposition as normal caring behaviour. There is an element of 'idiot compassion' to such behaviour, in particular the avoidance of spiritual talk itself. I feel the opposite of 'idiot compassion' but am I intoxicated with intimacy with death? Do I wallow in voyeurism or sentimentality? Do I fear Jane will pull me into the dark abyss of my own mortality crisis to drown me in its dark waters? Do I have unresolved grief? I grope my way along the edge of the crater gaining

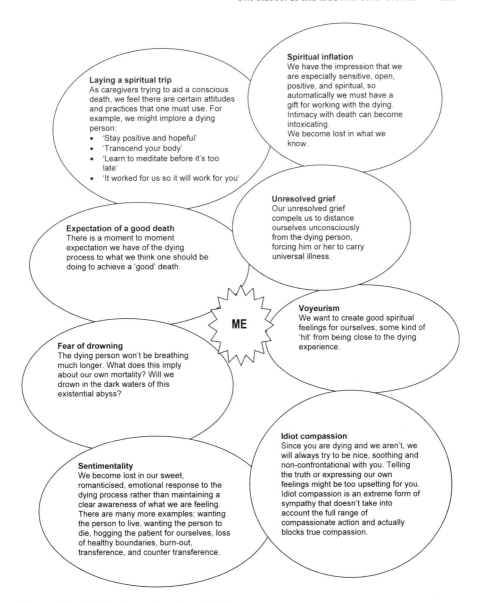

Laying a spiritual trip
As caregivers trying to aid a conscious death, we feel there are certain attitudes and practices that one must use. For example, we might implore a dying person:
- 'Stay positive and hopeful'
- 'Transcend your body'
- 'Learn to meditate before it's too late'
- 'It worked for us so it will work for you'

Spiritual inflation
We have the impression that we are especially sensitive, open, positive, and spiritual, so automatically we must have a gift for working with the dying. Intimacy with death can become intoxicating.
We become lost in what we know.

Unresolved grief
Our unresolved grief compels us to distance ourselves unconsciously from the dying person, forcing him or her to carry universal illness.

Expectation of a good death
There is a moment to moment expectation we have of the dying process to what we think one should be doing to achieve a 'good' death.

ME

Voyeurism
We want to create good spiritual feelings for ourselves, some kind of 'hit' from being close to the dying experience.

Fear of drowning
The dying person won't be breathing much longer. What does this imply about our own mortality? Will we drown in the dark waters of this existential abyss?

Idiot compassion
Since you are dying and we aren't, we will always try to be nice, soothing and non-confrontational with you. Telling the truth or expressing our own feelings might be too upsetting for you. Idiot compassion is an extreme form of sympathy that doesn't take into account the full range of compassionate action and actually blocks true compassion.

Sentimentality
We become lost in our sweet, romanticised, emotional response to the dying process rather than maintaining a clear awareness of what we are feeling. There are many more examples; wanting the person to live, wanting the person to die, hogging the patient for ourselves, loss of healthy boundaries, burn-out, transference, and counter transference.

Figure 6.2   Spiritual traps (Borglum 1997).

insight, learning the lessons. I learn that I cannot be spiritual if I'm wrapped up in my self-concern or accept responsibility for Jane's spiritual needs. Self-concern is a dam that stifles the flow. Jane's spirituality is essentially her business and perhaps I do interfere, however well-intentioned. I sense Borglum's (1997:66) 'long shadow of good intention'. Yet I am essentially responding to her suffering not her spirituality, and her suffering is spiritual crisis.

I need to explore these ideas and doubts with a spiritually-tuned person. We need a multidisciplinary clinical supervision group where such issues can be 'confessed' and explored in safety, facilitated by a 'spiritually aware' outsider.

The value of reflective practice as confessional, for surely holding such doubts that I cannot resolve risks eroding my spirit, just as it does Jane. If we truly value holistic practice, we must ensure we have the resources to ensure staff are able and sustained to practice accordingly.

Four days later

Jane is no longer calm, but angry and tormented, struggling to make her peace with God. Her smile is forced when Barry says:

'Here he is.'

I sense she has deteriorated. Her face is glazed. She resists my offer of a massage. Perhaps her anger won't let me in. She is waiting for her leg dressings. I read the signs and don't pursue my offer. I feel clumsy, feeling the need to help Jane, but mindful that anything I say will seem glib and merely irritate her. Silence for a moment and then I retreat, wishing her well.

Three days later

Jane remains angry. Barry is his normal 'jokey' self, perhaps his way of coping. I mention Jane seemed distressed when she rejected my offer of a foot massage last Tuesday. He says she was having a difficult day. I sense how Jane's mood fluctuates from day to day as she wrestles with herself. I know her oppression lies deep within her as her mind tries to reconcile her dying with a vengeful or loving God. Her ego, deeply threatened, resists reconciliation. I am mindful part of me is steering clear of the stormy water because I do not know how to be with her, I feel uncomfortable yet I also feel uncomfortable avoiding her. Caught in the compassion trap (Dickson 1982). How have I managed to get wrapped up in her suffering?

Three days later

Jane has deteriorated further. Her abdomen is swollen and tight. She remains fearful. She resists syringe drivers because two people in the bed that faces her across the four-bedded room have died. Each had syringe drivers commenced before dying. She would rather suffer the pain than submit to death's inevitability.

I decide to confront my avoidance. I kneel by her side and take her hand . . . she moves her hand away. I both feel and accept her resistance. I know it's not personal. Her fear is like a tidal wave engulfing me. The staff are anxious for Jane to accept sedation. The old nutshell – for whose benefit is sedation?

Her family are gathered. They struggle to witness her suffering. Barry's mask of humour is slipping as if he doesn't know how to be. Her daughter is frustrated at trying to get her mum to accept syringe drivers or at least periodic injections. The tension is palpable.

Later Jane accepts an injection of diamorphine to ease the pain but resists sedation. Does she resist sedation because she fears losing control and the descent into something unknown and frightening? Better the devil you know? We absorb her suffering even as we try to rationalise it. We absorb it because we resist it rather than flow with it. Young and Cullen (1996:132) offer a thought for reflection:

> One particular condition of a good death – not that it should be without pain but that, as far as possible, the pain should be under the control of the patient and that the patient should be to some degree in control at the moment of death.

Perhaps, therein lies the essential nature of palliative care. It is not easy to witness another's suffering especially when the person resists you. Without doubt, appreciating and responding appropriately to *soul pain*, to use Kearney's term for such fear and agitation is the most challenging and controversial practice.

Veronica

Early December

Fallen leaves damp from the rain littered along the verges. Veronica is tucked away in the corner of the four-bedded ward. So quite and curled up it is easy to pass her by. No visitors again this afternoon. She has been blind since September as a result of a brain tumour. She is resting with her eyes closed. I sit and gently hold her hand. Her own hand closes around mine and she opens her eyes . . . she stares at me the way blind people do. She is pleased I give her this time and would like me to massage her hands and play some music but only if I'm not too busy. So typical of her, thinking of others and making no demand for herself. She likes music and in her sensory deprived world I can appreciate that. For about 20 minutes I sit with her and massage her dry hands and stick-like arms. She then closes her hands over mine and thanks me. She whispers:

> 'I mustn't take any more of your time.'

I thank Veronica for letting me massage her arms. I sense the other women in the ward watching me, perhaps waiting for their turn. That's always a problem of entering the ward . . . not that I had deliberately gone in there to see Veronica, just that she caught my attention being alone. The other women both have relatives visiting. One woman says to her relatives:

> 'He's a complementary therapist . . .'

As I leave, I smile at the gathered families . . . they return my smile with curiosity.

I rework my reflection as a prose-type poem, revealing my sadness at her predicament:

Veronica tucked away in the corner,
alone . . .
No visitors again this afternoon;
blind, yet what does she sense
as she approaches death?
What does she see in the darkness?
Perhaps childhood memories?
Or bright lights of spent romance?
Or perhaps regret?
Perhaps I should ask or would I intrude?
I sit with her.
A touch of sadness stirs within
Yet smiled away in the moment.
'Shall I massage your hands,
Play you some music?'
She turns her head towards me
A faint smile
As she folds her hand over mine
'Only if you aren't too busy'.
Her spirit glows
And lifts me beyond the throws of sadness
As my hands respond to ease her.
Even as she dies
she turns her thoughts to others
makes no demand for herself,
So easy to pass by.
She takes me to my still point.

I am touched by my encounter with Veronica. I know virtually nothing about her yet she wore her spirit on her sleeve. Her spirit was an open invitation for anyone to touch although not something that could be touched with the mind. It could only be touched by my own spirit. 'Spirituality' can never be a technique to solve the other's 'spiritual' problem. I pick up the challenge I posted in working with Edward (see page 65). Spirituality is primarily *being* not *doing*. This realisation challenges a scientific approach that spirituality can be known as an abstract entity and responded to with technique, in the demand that spirituality must be accommodated within the 'system'. As Walter (2002) suggests – perhaps the word 'spirituality' is no more than an expression coined for a secular religion as it seems to lack meaning for many of the people I met who had no or little religious affiliation. Indeed, few patients in my narrative had a strong faith. This small part of the world has turned secular. Although Veronica did not profess a strong faith, some patients do yet it often seems to bring them little comfort. Indeed it can torment, as with Jane. I sense that 'existential crisis' may be a more appropriate expression for people who fear death rather than 'spiritual crisis'. I am mindful of my own spirituality, and yet this self-knowing emerges as vital in responding to the other on a spiritual plane. I say it is vital, yet the spiritual realm of care is obscured, as if uncomfortable to know in the secular and scientific culture of everyday practice. That strikes me as a fundamental paradox within a hospice setting. I wonder that if the patient has faith (either spiritual or religious) then that is that person's concern. Maybe my role is to simply inquire if the person needs my help to meet his or her spiritual or religious demand. Essentially, the patient's spirituality is not my responsibility unless it is pathologised within the 'medical model/symptom management' gaze as might be interpreted within the National Institute for Clinical Excellence (NICE) guidelines.

As I see it, the practitioner must be spiritual to see and respond to the spirit in others. It isn't about God. It isn't about meaning. It is simply *Being* beyond the ego's insistent demand for attention. Our minds are full of chatter that obscures the spiritual view. The silence between thoughts gives a glimpse of a deeper spiritual being if the practitioner is mindful enough. Being mindful of our thoughts and bringing our thoughts to rein. Being mindful is akin to appreciating beauty. Like appreciating Veronica as simply beauty rather than an old, blind woman dying of cancer. Appreciating beauty transcends thought and takes me to a dimension of *Being* where I am spiritually aware.

Tolle (2001:10) describes *Being* as:

> The eternal, ever present One life beyond the myriad forms of life that are subject to birth and death. However, Being is not only beyond but also deep within every form as its innermost invisible and indestructible essence. This means that it is accessible to you now as your own deepest self, your true nature. But don't seek to grasp it with your mind. Don't try to understand it. You can only know it when the mind is still. *When you are present,* when your attention is fully and intensely in the Now, being can be felt, but it can never be understood mentally.

When you are present is to be spiritually attuned to the other. *Being* is beyond mind and cannot be envisaged within a conceptual framework. Of course this is the reason why so many people struggle to *know spirituality* approaching it from a scientific perspective. Tolle (1999:16) suggests that when a person is fully present:

> it raises the vibrational frequency of the energy field that gives life to the physical body.

Of course, I know this well through my use of therapeutic touch where I centre myself and massage the etheric body, the energy field closest to the body that is the life force. Yet, as Tolle suggests, bringing myself present within any caring encounter will have a similar effect. If our spiritual presence can enhance patient well-being, is it then incumbent on all carers to develop this aspect of Being?

The idea of Veronica being alone plays on my mind. Alone seems such an evocative word, an iconic word that reminds me of words by Jeannette Winterson's I had used to capture the reflective moment (see page 43) and which I break into poetic form:

There are so many lives packed into one.
The one life we think we know is only the window that is open on the screen.
The big window full of detail,
where the meaning is often lost among the facts.
If we can close that window,
on purpose or by chance,
what we find is another view.
This window is emptier.
The cross-references are cryptic.
As we scroll down it, looking for something familiar,
we seem to be scrolling into another self –
one we recognise but cannot place.
The co-ordinates are missing,
or the co-ordinates pinpoint us outside the limits of our existence.
If we move further back,
through a smaller window that is really a gateway,
there is less and less to measure ourselves by.
We are coming into a dark region.
A single word might appear.
An icon.
Alone

Who is alone –
Is it she or I?
Why might I think she is alone?
True, no one sits by her side
Yet . . . perhaps inside
She brims with memories of relationships
Perhaps she dwells in rich company
Perhaps that is why
She can smile and gently fold her hand
Over mine;
A hand gnarled with age
caresses mine like silk
to ease my suffering
and lift me out of sadness
So I am no longer alone
In the quiet afternoon where we dwell.

I respond to the word *alone*. I wonder – it is I, rather than she who is alone? suggesting my sadness might be more complex than simply a response to seeing Veronica physically alone. I sense an intriguing mystery deep within me but avoid the exploration, at least for the moment.

Being with Veronica – care without words in the quiet of the afternoon. Such experiences remind me not to pass people by; that the most profound work is revealed in such moments I learn that spirituality is seeing beauty in self and others. I learn not to assume that people are lonely simply because they are physically alone. Being with Veronica was both deeply humbling and fulfilling, as if my own spirituality has been fed, so I am less alone. She taught me well.

Two days later Veronica has died. I am told she slipped quietly away. No fuss. Barely a flicker of emotion amongst the staff. Death is routine except perhaps for the more heroic death.

Reflection on grief

This evening, Aimée, my elder daughter, finds Smudge, her hamster, dead. She was curled in a ball as if she died in her sleep. For the past two weeks, we have been expecting her death. Aimée is beside herself with grief. She blames herself for not playing with Smudge, not realising she may have been dead since last night. She knew that Smudge might die at any moment but that has not prepared her for the actuality. We talk about the 'old times' with Smudge and Nibbles, her previous hamster, the way Smudge always used to bite my finger. Tears mix with laughter. Reminiscing about the dead is a positive way to restore the spirit.

That night Aimée had a dream. She had looked in Smudge's cage. Smudge was still there dead but two fluffy balls of baby hamster were running about. The dream was so real for her and reassuring in some way. We bury Smudge next to Nibbles. Charlotte, my younger daughter, writes Aimée a short poem to bury with Smudge:

> Smudge rides in a golden cart
> Away to heaven
> But still in your heart

Aimée takes comfort in the idea of Smudge running around with God even though she denies the presence of God within her own life. Perhaps this enables her to imagine a future with Smudge that could not exist if dying was total extermination. Smudge was never simply a replacement for Nibbles. Indeed for some time Aimée resisted intimacy with Smudge because of Nibble's memory. Yet in time her intimacy grew until her attachment to Smudge became unconditional. Now they lie side by side in the 'hamster cemetery'. I sense Stroebe's dual process or oscillation theory at work as Aimée already moves between contact with Smudge and moving on without her (Stroebe & Schut 1999). She continued her relationship with Nibbles even as she developed a new relationship with Smudge. Her grief for Nibbles never diminished; it was as if her heart expanded to accommodate it, factors congruent with the 'continuing bonds' understanding of the grief process (Klass et al. 1996). Through her suffering Aimée grows with support and understanding from others. Through this reflection I can better understand loss and grief.

Hugh

January 2004

There are some people who simply make me feel humble. Hugh is so open and receptive despite his suffering. I am told he is very anxious. He knows he is terminally ill with his lung metastases. He immediately apologises for his low mood and I can sense his tormented mind. His syringe driver pulses with midazolam 5 mg, haloperidol 5 mg and diamorphine 75 mg. Donna, his wife, fusses about him, his anxiety is infectious.

He laughs when I offer a foot massage, saying he can't bear his feet being touched. I say he will be surprised.

'OK then, give it a go then. I'll try anything once.'

I subdue the lighting and play an Enya CD. Periodically during the treatment he murmurs:

'That's wonderful.'

He eulogises to Donna, his wife, about how wonderful the treatment felt and how relaxed he now feels. They have two children each from their first marriages and a 12-year-old daughter Jackie who is not present.

I ask Donna if she is OK. She parries the question, saying she is fine. I offer her a foot massage. She politely declines.

Hugh chips in.

'You should have one, it will really help you to relax.'

I don't push it as I am mindful that Donna doesn't want to deflect care away from Hugh.

She smiles.

'Perhaps next time?'

Later, as I leave the unit, I see Jackie. She is very pretty and glances me a smile and, just in that moment, I sense the utter poignancy of her predicament being so young as she witnesses her father's death journey.

Later, thinking about Donna I appreciate how much she suffers because of the struggle to manage Hugh's pain. Although he is now pain free, she is unable to relax because it remains a threat. I suspect she also absorbs his fear of losing control, that she herself fears losing control. Meta and Ezer (2003:88) comment from their study of the meaning spouses attribute to their loved ones' pain during palliative care, that spouses:

> Often find themselves experiencing the pain and suffering when their loved ones are in pain.

Meta and Ezer (2003) note that in the face of their partner's pain, spouses feel helpless, a sense of injustice, and fear. This helps me understand Donna's reluctance to let go of her attention to Hugh enough to accept a massage for herself; as if accepting treatment for herself is turning attention away from Hugh and will make her feel guilty. Another recurring pattern through the narrative.

Six days later

Hugh sits with Lea, the complementary therapist in the day hospice, selecting Bach Flower Remedies. He is not sleeping well at night and wondered if Lea can help. Lea suggests white chestnut. Hugh says he doesn't have persistent thoughts. I chip in and suggest he may have thoughts on a deeper subconscious level that he doesn't perceive? Hugh is open to this possibility.

I suggest:

'Perhaps you fear losing control and cannot let yourself go to sleep?'

I pause . . . I needn't finish the sentence, for Hugh knows exactly what I am suggesting. He completes the sentence:

'. . . and never wake up again . . . that's it . . . the fear of losing control . . . as if I am right on the edge.'

I suggest *cherry plum* may be the Bach Flower Remedy of choice (Howard 1995:21):

Cherry plum is for people who fear losing control of their behaviour. They may be on the verge of breakdown.

Hugh realises he can no longer defy death. No more substitutes or bargains. He is stripped bare to face his ultimate future. He stands on the edge precariously looking into the crater. He holds on desperately to prevent himself from falling. Yet he knows that the ground below his feet must inevitably crumble and he will fall into the oblivion of death.

Eight days later, Friday

Hugh informs me he is going home next Monday but is anxious that he won't manage well. I ask:

'Do you want to stay here?'
'No, I want to go home but Donna works part time and being on my own I don't know if I can manage.'

I ask if the Bach Flower Remedies have helped. He thinks so.

'I've been swigging the bottle . . . it must be the brandy! I'm calmer, less fearful of losing control so it's been really beneficial. Thank you. Is it possible to have another foot and leg massage?'

We arrange a time after lunch.

After lunch, I find Hugh in day care sitting in his wheelchair. We find a therapy room and transfer him with difficulty into a reclining chair. He struggles to get comfortable because his bottom is sore. After the massage he is relaxed and finds it easier to transfer back into the wheelchair. He exclaims he has more energy, that the massage swept away his fatigue. He is more cheerful and positive. Therapy is very beneficial!

Edith

Late January

Mary (Macmillan nurse) has asked if I would visit Edith, a 55-year-old woman with breast cancer that has spread to her lung, who is feeling depressed. Today, in the late afternoon, she sits at her kitchen table painting. She says she was going to ring me and cancel the treatment because she felt uncomfortable accepting help, her vulnerability, her 'weakness' on display. Perhaps Mary contacting me had put Edith on the spot, and that, despite our 'good intent', it stripped her autonomy at a time when she is most vulnerable? Maybe I should have contacted her directly.

Paint everywhere, like a child she plays, seeking distraction. Yet the painting is full of colour, wistful, a blue sea. She says she doesn't feel anything . . . just empty inside. She needs to get away from the pressures, maybe go to the sea. Edith, who gives all of herself to everybody has run out of energy. Pressures at home. Life has squeezed her dry.

We sit at the table, her painting between us and gently turn her life over; the way her cancer has eaten into her life and eroded the things in life she most valued. In particular, she talks of the way it has torn her apart from her husband. Her daughter is angry at her so now she feels alone, desolate. Together, we choose her aromatherapy oils. She mentions grapefruit – 'a sunny oil' excellent for depression. A drop of patchouli to help her feel more positive. A drop of rose, to nourish her femininity, 'to touch and stir her spirit' (Worwood 1999:245). The blend is unbalanced so I add a drop of lavender 'to gently lift the veil of despair' (Worwood 1999:225).

She looks up and wistfully smiles at me, her greying hair loosened, droops over her brow.

'What do you recommend . . . am I worth it?'

I return her smile and discounting the negative vibe, I suggest an Indian head massage. I explain what it entails. She says it sounds good.

I gather and clip back her loosened hair. I hold her with my left hand on her brow chakra and my right hand over the alta mater chakra at the base of her skull and centre myself. I feel as if I hold the universe. I hold and contain her vulnerability and imagine that to be held when the spirit is low must be the most comforting experience.

I massage her upper back, neck, arms, her scalp and finally her face. Moving slowly along the pattern of pressure points on her forehead is a moment of stillness and intensity. We finish. She says it was wonderful and is deeply thankful. I have given her something back, some love, some energy to replenish her spirit. I am deeply moved by giving Edith this treatment as if we had fused our sprits. Indian head massage is a most sacred massage in the way it confronts suffering with its intimacy and lifts the stress and sadness from deep within the aching body. 'Touch is the harmonic healing the grieving spirit craves . . .' Blackwolf and Gina's words are a mantra, and as I touch Edith I sense the truth in these words.

I whisper to Edith words that Blackwolf and Gina (1996:100) have given me:

> What sadness grips your heart? What anger must you release? What trauma do you have to dance? Honour the trauma of your Self. If you have been a victim, please find someone qualified to hear you, to help you heal and understand your pain. Look at your experience with the soft focus of ain-dah-ing. See the world, honor the questions, and enter into the dark places. Allow the pain of your trauma to help lead you back into the light of peace and balance. Dance the warrior dance of Self. Heal with your family and community. Wear the blanket of the warrior.

I sense Edith's despair is the loss of love, self-hatred, an alienation from one's soul or what Blackwolf and Gina Jones describe as ain-dah-ing – your home within your heart, Ain-dah-ing is the place of peace and freedom from fear of dying. Without fear love can flourish. Touch given with deep compassion helps the receiver find a way back into their heart and touch ain-dah-ing where fear melts in the face of love. My hands across the body are a warrior's dance to stir the spirit. My message to Edith – remember you are a warrior!

Nine days later

As I drive to the University, I am mesmerised by the dance of the bare trees as they swirl in the wind against the rolling grey sky. A dervish dance, apparently chaotic rhythm yet perfect harmony, bending and flowing to the wind music. The tree naturally gives way to the forces and yet, so often, people like Edith, resist life's forces and snap. The practitioner needs to appreciate the rhythm of the dance so as to synchronise rather than resist the dervish dance, what Newman (1999:227) describes as the rhythm of relating, by compassionately listening to the words and especially the silences between the words where empathy and connection become possible. Newman describes this as synchronised talk dance. She says:

> Such synchronisation has an effect of making the interactants feel good about what they are doing and about each other.

And when the gusts and storms that blow are the patient's mood and talk, the practitioner, like the trees, must bend in the wind in graceful dance without resistance or else she too will surely snap. Then the connection is lost and caring perishes on the wind.

Richard

February 5

Richard was admitted yesterday. His notes reveal he has suffered from emphysema for eight years. Now he has lung cancer. As I put my head around his door, I find him standing using the urinal bottle. My apologies. A few minutes later, he is sitting in a chair connected to an oxygen concentrator via nasal cannula. He is breathless yet talks continuously. He is dubious about complementary therapy. He doesn't see how it might help him. He feels able to cope with the cancer unlike his wife who is really struggling and would *really* benefit from some therapy.

Linda, one of the care assistants, joins us. Richard has clearly connected with her. She says the therapies might be beneficial. I explain I simply massage his feet. He responds:

'Now that sounds good.'

He likes the smell of the patchouli and frankincense mixed in my reflexology base cream. I explain the patchouli is to help nurture positive thoughts.

'I could do with some of that then . . .'

and the frankincense will help his breathing and ease his anxiety. He approves. After his reflexology he feels so relaxed, that his mind was taken off his breathing and he could breathe normally. The chest pain has also gone. He is amazed.

He didn't much like my music (Rusty Crutcher's *Chaco Canyon*). He tried to visualise a beach but could only think of Great Yarmouth on a stormy day! Some time ago, he had been taught to breathe using visualisation. Already he is talking and joking again. Perhaps this is his way of coping but he has seen another way with the massage.

Five days later

I share my experience with Richard with the palliative care students I teach[18] as an example of reflective writing (from my journal notes rather than the polished narrative presented in this text). They pull out four significant issues:

The first issue is 'knowing him'. In the few minutes between meeting him and giving him the therapy had I got to know him well enough to respond appropriately? The art of connection and empathy – Who *is* this man? What meaning does he give to his experience of being here at the hospice and dying? How is he feeling? What things are important to help ease his suffering and the suffering of his family? Cues that guide me to appreciate his life pattern.[19]

Part of his pattern is his incessant talking and laughing. What does it reveal about him? Perhaps it is too easy to assume he is anxious about suffocation and death. Although it is a pattern well known to me I must keep my mind open and resist making assumptions. I can work with him without applying a label. It is enough to flow with what's unfolding.

---

[18] BSc Palliative Care programme at the University of Luton, www.luton.ac.uk
[19] Burford reflective cues – see page 14.

Another aspect to his pattern is his resistance to complementary therapy. His past hospital experience has been in a technological environment. Perhaps he simply resisted the unknown. Perhaps I simply hadn't explained to him well enough what I could offer. Perhaps he felt put on the spot and needed time to consider. A stranger walks into your life and says:

'I am a complementary therapist – would you like a therapy?'

Barely time to take breath.

The last issue was his need to be 'comforted'. Most striking was his attachment to Linda, the care assistant, because she saw and responded to him as a vulnerable and frightened person. He regressed because he did not have the resources to cope. Linda's response was maternal, a therapeutic parental response to the hurt child, someone he could 'hold on to' and feel safe as the gathering dark clouds threaten doom. She is good at doing that.

On my way home from the University, I drop into the hospice. Richard's stay has been extended – he was due to go home tomorrow but his condition has *deteriorated*. Deteriorated – a euphemism for imminent death. Syringe drivers have been set up and pulse diamorphine 35 mg and midazolam 5 mg into his suffering body. Through the open door to his single room, I see his bed surrounded by people. As I enter into their domain, they pause to look at me. Richard greets me and informs his family that 'I am the foot man', words that I immediately associate with a Beatles song . . .

'Here comes the foot man goo goo gee choo.'

Richard guesses that I have come to offer a therapy and declines as his family are here. These people are his wife, daughter, son-in-law, grand-daughter and another woman I don't place. However, his daughter says it's time for them to go, recognising that dad would benefit from more therapy. They leave and Hettie, his wife, and Richard breathe a sigh of relief. It's tiring for them to entertain. Hettie is very tired.

'I haven't slept for five days since Richard has been in here.'

I ask her:

'Did you have some therapy today as arranged in day care?'

She replies:

'No, I didn't . . . it didn't happen.'

She rationalises this failure as staff being busy but I note an edge of frustration in her voice and body gesture to be let down. In the moment it is easy to offer and in the busyness of the next moment it is easy to be careless. Trust is so vital if we are to journey with the person under such traumatic circumstances.

When trust fails, despair exacerbates. I don't pursue the issue but offer her a foot massage after Richard. Perhaps I compensate for the broken trust, a healer of trust but I know I can help her and must do so. She accepts my offer. As I prepare for Richard she wraps herself up in a duvet in the recliner to rest. She removes her shoes and socks as if in anticipation.

I play Richard *The Journey* by Bliss. He says:

'Ah yes, this is more my type of music, more melodic.'

He quickly relaxes, knowing the routine. As before, he holds the tension in his feet. Slowly each foot relaxes until he is totally relaxed. His feet are warmer than previously, especially his right foot. His legs are emaciated as if the muscles have caved in on themselves. As before, his breathing settles into an easy natural rhythm in tune with my movements. I finish the reflexology with healing touch, simply holding his feet for two minutes as I channel healing energy through my hands into his body.

He says:

'Wonderful, Chris . . . this time, the music took me into outer space. I could see patterns and shapes.'

He talks and laughs. Hettie looks at him incredulously and gives me a 'knowing' look. I recognise a pattern whereby onlookers struggle to accept notions of the mystical. I want to know more about his space trip but resist my curiosity because of Hettie's reaction.

I mention the warm feet and ask if he has a chest infection? He says he has. I ask:

'Are you taking antibiotics?'

He is. He is amazed that I could tell that from his feet. He looks at me inquisitively. I simply say:

'Your feet were warm.'

He cracks his side with laughter at so obvious an answer when he had expected me to reveal a hidden sign. His laughter makes him breathless! The moral being – that *too* much humour is not good for you.

Hettie has such small feet. I apply the cream to her lower legs as they are very dry. She too likes the smell of patchouli and frankincense. I commence with relaxation when, after a couple of minutes, Richard says he must call the nurse.

'I'm meant to inform her when I have the nebuliser.'

Despite the noise of the nebuliser, Hettie is very relaxed. She doesn't stir amidst this noise and interruption. Her eyes are closed. My compassion for this exhausted and suffering woman smiles across the distance between us. My gentle and rhythmic hands tune into and dance with her, easing her suffering and energising the spirit. Eventually the nebuliser is finished and a deep stillness falls across the room.

Afterwards there is a different mood in the room. The tension has eased. Hettie is sleepy but the strain has evaporated from her. Her headache has eased but not completely. In knowing Hettie and the way she responds to him, I now know him better. On the surface is the mystery of the unknown unfolding in unique yet recognisable patterns that, like deep ocean currents, ripple through the experience.

Gill

Two days later

I have been seeing Gill at her home for the past 15 months following her mastectomy and removal of 15 axillary lymph nodes, seven of which were cancerous. We have journeyed together through chemotherapy and radiotherapy. Now, we journey with persistent chest pain where the saline pouch valve seems to be snagged, severe hot flushes attributed to her hormone therapy and our constant traveller depression. Yet always, in defiance she shows me her brave smiling face.

As I give her reflexology, I play some music I like very much from the film *Angels of the Universe* by Sigur Ros and Hilmar Örn Hilmarsson. She felt the shifts in the music's rhythm fragmented her experience and that the violins, soulful as they were, made her feel sad. Gill affirms Richard's experience that tuning into vibrations that resonate with healing is vital so the body can become whole and heal.

Richard and Hettie

The next day, Friday February 13

Hettie is cutting Richard's hair. As usual, he is laughing and talking. He declines therapy because the family are visiting at 5.30 pm. Hettie challenges him.

'You have plenty of time!'

But he resists her pressure. He needs to finish his haircut. Hettie retorts:

'That's only two minutes.'

He continues:

'I need my nebulisers, then the commode and wash below, and tea . . .'

In response to the rising pressure, I say:

'No pressure.'

I sense the irony that my role is to relieve pressure yet create it as if the offer becomes an expectation. Yet Hettie knows how tense Richard is and how the massage eases it. She gladly accepts my offer of a foot massage. She says how much she benefited from the last therapy.

Richard's chest is no better despite the antibiotics for his chest infection. Perhaps their prescription helps the family feel something positive is being done to ease the breathlessness. Perhaps they do help yet Hettie's shake of the head and downward gaze reveal her resignation.

Hettie relaxes in 'her' corner, her feet already bare and raised on the recliner. I mix frankincense and pettigrain into the massage cream. It is a gorgeous aroma, more feminine than the previous patchouli/frankincense mix.

She laughs.

'I need that.'

Hettie purrs her approval. I say the pettigrain is a good stressbuster, implanting the suggestion so she will think that, and heighten the placebo effect. Davis (1999) says it is useful for insomnia linked to loneliness or unhappiness rather than anxiety. It is an essential oil I hold great faith by. As I apply the cream I ask:

'Have you managed to sleep?'
'Not really.'

She tells me about her son Ed. He is 35 and also has cancer. He is in London today to see if any further treatment can be offered after two re-occurrences. Hettie is not hopeful. I ask if he has a family. He has a two-year-old son. Hettie cries and I feel her intense suffering through my hands. I can only mumble about how cruel life can be. No music as background just the murmur of conversation between Richard and Sophie, his daughter, and the background hum of the oxygen concentrator. At one point, a volunteer noisily serves his supper. Yet Hettie is relaxed and sleeps. I am mindful of my reaction to the noise. Part of me feels irritation, that more respect is needed, but another part of me recognises that I now dwell within this family; that the therapy is part of the unfolding, evolving whole, that whilst sacred it must never become precious. Such realisation softens my irritation. A smile replaces the frown.

Afterwards, Sophie says:

'We can accept what's happening to Dad because the emphysema started eight years ago so we've lived with his steady deterioration, but with Ed, it's much more painful . . . but we stick together as a family and as a family we'll get through this.'

The family inhabit the hospice. Their nomadic camp. I debrief with Doreen (staff nurse) and discover that Ed is booked to have a blood transfusion at the hospice on Monday. She, rather euphemistically, describes him as 'not well' and says he may be admitted.

Later, as I am leaving the hospice, Hettie smiles and says she feels good. Richard is happy about this and says he will be waiting for his therapy when I next visit on Monday!

Hettie and Richard travel along a roller coaster of emotion. I begin to tune into the way each thinks and feels, appreciating the family pattern of managing the unfolding drama of Richard's death and the darkening shadow of Ed's illness. I press buttons to reveal and release the feelings locked within the brave masks. I offer myself as a container to hold the despair. I must understand their beliefs; reinforcing positive beliefs and challenging negative beliefs yet all the time being mindful that in dwelling with the family my role is to support their family's caring not substitute it.

Hettie is exhausted but she cannot let go no matter what it costs her. It is both her burden and her joy to ensure Richard's comfort. Without doubt, Richard's positive comments about the massage help to ease Hettie's suffering. The more he suffers the more she does as she absorbs it as her own. So the more his suffering is eased so it is for her. It is a basic equation.

Later at home I write Hettie a poem.

Hettie

She curls in the corner
as if a refuge from the unfolding and unyielding crisis
her feet naked stretched along the recliner
await my touch
she gives herself to this moment
a cool breeze fans the room
from the open window
cool yet refreshing for the gasping breath
that relentlessly pulls away his energy
each breath an effort.

Outside the window is another world
obscured from thought
where trees dance in rhythm to the breeze
where bare branches pirouette
where blackbirds chirp their song;
inside we care caught on the tide of each breath
a drama unfolding towards death.

Breath
I say to her
concentrate on *your* breath
follow each breath in
follow each breath out
let go of your fear and relax into this moment
easier said when husband and son are dying
yet for this moment she does let go
her tormented body drifts into a moment's sleep
and when she wakes she sighs and smiles
and maybe she hears again the blackbird's song.

Edith

Monday February 16

It is a mild day. The sky a grey wash as if a heavy blanket to subdue the spirit. I imagine depression is like that. It has been three weeks since I visited Edith. She greets me warmly at the door. More colour. She wears a long blue dress. She shows me the painting she had started when we last met. She had painted a desert and the sky with the stars twinkling but with nothing else and then she painted the oasis, her refuge . . . symbolising that she had found a place to recover. The desert, a place of solitude but also beauty, a place where she needed to go despite the pain to find herself. Now she is coming out of the desert but has she learnt the lessons? She reads me a poem finding expression for her despair. She says she meditated looking out of the window listening to the birds. It reminds me of Hettie's poem being able to hear the birds amidst the shriek going on around. A connection between experiences.

> It may be that some little root of the sacred tree still lives.
> Nourish it then, that it may leaf and bloom and fill with singing birds.
>
> (Black Elk – as told through John G. Neihardt 1988:274)

She asks for a reflexology treatment and afterwards I sense her depression lift like grey clouds parting to reveal the blue.

Richard and Hettie

At the hospice, I meet Hettie leaving Richard's room en route for the kitchen. She is tense. It has not been a good day. Ed has been admitted but he is poorly, in pain and very tired. Richard is wound up. Hettie pleads:

'Go and see him, he is expecting you.'

Richard says:

'I need you.'

He tells me he is so taut with seeing his son so poorly

'I could smash the wall . . .'

The sheer intensity of pain is hard to bear . . . to observe such suffering. I move through it and give reflexology as we listen to Rusty Crutcher's *Ocean Eclipse*. I have chosen this music because it has the sound of the ocean lapping the shore. I thought it might take Richard to the beach again. His feet are swollen with oedema. His right foot is tense as I massage it and then it gives way as he relaxes.

Forty minutes later

He says he is relaxed . . . that he couldn't believe that possible after the way he had felt. He thinks it is a miracle and perhaps it is. He says he was on the beach at midnight, a place where he used to take Hettie and the children when they were small to see the moon and walk along the beach during the night. It is a place of great nostalgia that comforts him. He also experiences many shifting colours.

Later I give Hettie reflexology and play the same music. She wakes from the therapy with tears streaming down her face. At first I thought it was because of Ed and Richard but it isn't. She dreamt she was on the beach at Deal where they used to go when the children were small. The whole family together. It is 2 am. Richard has got them up to see the moon and walk the beach. . . .

Hettie is tearful yet the dream comforts her. I sense a deep symbolism in the dream but I resist interpretation . . . just let it be. Yet I am intrigued by Hettie dreaming what Richard had visualised. She still has not slept except for short snatches. She is deeply distressed with Ed's condition, helpless that he is in such pain, fearful that he is going to die.

Reflection on suffering

In my search of the 'suffering' literature I discovered Elizabeth Harrison's paper *Intolerable human suffering: the role of the ancestor*. Harrison (2000) considers the nature of intolerable human suffering in her literary criticism of *The Salt Eaters* by Toni Cade Bambara, guided by Toni Morrison's characteristics of 'black art', in particular the role of the ancestors – who are benevolent, instructive and protective, provide wisdom and timeless. In the book, suffering for Velma became intolerable because she had lost touch with the ancestors.

I interpret the ancestor as the connection with our roots. For Hettie and Richard this is rooted in their extended family. Sophie suggests the family will hold together. For Edith I am uncertain of the roots of her depression. Edith's suffering was intolerable and she retreated into depression as if she has become alienated from herself and from her community. As Younger (1995:53) notes:

> In suffering the realisation of one's aloneness becomes most acute. First suffering alienates the sufferer from himself or herself, then it alienates the sufferer from others.

Harrison (2000:8/9) emphasises the importance for carers to acknowledge the ancestor:

> Skill and compassion are of little value if we fail to respect the relationship between the client and his or her ancestral system and develop the care plan based on their direction. We should assess suffering with care, and take extraordinary efforts to understand the patient's story from within the limitless boundaries of his or her own culture. In the process, we should seek information about the client's ancestral system, a way of being in the world that determines the ability to survive unbearable suffering. If the ancestral system is weak or absent, the trajectory of human suffering may not be favourable. We will not, however, be able to affect that path, nor

re-build a weak or absent ancestral system, until we are able to answer the question: what does the sufferer have to hold on to?

I am drawn to the metaphor of *the mooring*. The person is battered by the storm yet her ancestor system moors her to the pier. For Edith, her mooring has snapped. She is tossed on a raging ocean out of control. As a carer I become her mooring, her surrogate ancestor, until we can regain the pier and reconnect once again.

Harrison's and Younger's work helps me to position myself in the other's suffering, in contrast with much of the nursing literature on suffering in its 'scientific' quest to know suffering as something universal and abstract that obscures rather than reveals its nature. Suffering is ineffable; deeply subjective and unfolding. I can map it along a continuum from surface suffering to deep suffering marked by increasing alienation from self and others, a shift from love to hate where, at some point it becomes intolerable:

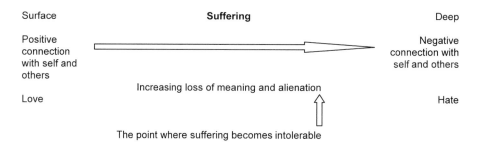

Surface suffering is a ripple of existential restlessness typified by a range of feelings such as craving, jealousy, lust, boredom, anger, dislike, frustration, emptiness, etc. Such feelings are viewed as normal for most people. To some extent, such feelings are all markers of alienation or a non-acceptance of self although contained by positive connections. However, at some point along the continuum, the alienation becomes self-conscious and the suffering breaks free from its container, its moorings, and spirals into a void where such words as worthlessness, hopelessness and despair capture the feelings being experienced. It is a loss of control and hatred.

For Edith, shifting the metaphor from storm to desert was helpful, for a desert is a place of solitude, stillness and beauty where perhaps one can dwell guided by the carer-ancestor and reconnect positively to self as the first step to connecting positively with others. I take Edith's hand so she can connect positively with me. It is the healing relationship whereby she can grow through her suffering to find new meaning amongst the debris of her life, to find new ways of being.

Halldórsdóttir (1999) identifies three challenges that face the sufferer:

- To find a way to express the suffering
- To find meaning in suffering
- To open up to the healing light of love

These challenges are my challenge as a therapist and healer. As a therapist, I am a clearing where the sufferer can dwell and find a voice to express her suffering. In dwelling with the sufferer I became conscious of myself as ancestor. But who are my ancestors? I sense the presence of Buddhas and Bodhisattvas. Ancestors are faith, and through faith I can let go of the hope that is a craving for attachment, an escape from anticipated despair. Faith is the route to the spiral path of liberation from the endless turmoil of suffering. My stories have seen so many people cling to hope. People fear that if they let go then the void of despair will swallow them. Yet with faith, there is another way. Sophie had faith the family will sustain them. Edith, seeks faith, reaching for something meaningful, purposeful, rather than clinging to what has already been lost. Her art was her reflection, her dwelling amidst her suffering and through it emerged possibilities for new ways of being. It is a similar thing for my writing.

I write Edith a poem:

The breath of love

The desert stretched before her
until it touched the edge of each horizon;
she asked herself 'is life so barren,
suffering so endless?'
She had an urge to go away
yet she was stuck in this place;
without boundaries to contain her.
She felt she would fall
into the yawning void
that opened before each tentative step.

Suffering renders the soul bare
when it becomes intolerable;
Hear her cry for lost ancestors to hold her
and cleanse the stain,
to ease the sigh that weeps
from her torn and blistered mouth;
Love heals the soul to bear
the strain of life's load,
yet love is so easily swept away on a
careless tide
to reveal the hurt inside.

She felt his love radiate across the
    dark chasm
yet she was uncertain
what this love might be,
she who felt so dark where
even a faint glow might blind her;
wrapped in this love she felt the
    healing power
so she could smile again
the weight lift from her tormented spirit
that had lain, torn.
amongst the debris of her life.

She reached out to touch his face,
to feel the space between them,
to traverse the dark void
where her life had enfolded into
    a nameless oblivion;
Could she unwrap herself
into the warm light of love?
She wriggled to loosen herself
from the hook that bound her to
    misery;
Her lip bleeding,
she swam again in life's rich
    current.

She closed her eyes and dreamt;
She was on a deserted beach
walking the shoreline
where the deep blue sea met the
    shimmering sand;
gentle waves lapped her naked feet
sun's rays caught her brow
as she paused to gaze at the sparkled
    water.

She bent to gather driftwood
in shapes that mirrored her tortured
    soul;
looking up . . .
she brushed away the loose strand
    of hair
and felt again the breath of love move
    within her,
she gasped to feel alive again
for love to her *is* life.

Richard and Hettie

Monday February 23

Richard is tense. He resists my invitation for therapy because he does not want to compromise his comfortable position in bed. However, as an ancestor, I confront his resistance. I know he needs my help so I insist. Caught by my insistent smile he capitulates. Afterwards he is very relaxed and deeply appreciative. The Native American flute music makes him think of Peru, remembering a television programme. No beaches.

Four days later

Hettie watches helplessly as Richard panics to catch his breath. A sputum plugs his airway. Eventually, with the help of nebulisers, he manages to shift it. Her tears reveal her suffering. She suffers to watch her loved one slowly disintegrate toward death. Richard is exhausted. No effort to resist. Again, the reflexology takes him into a deep relaxation.

Afterwards, he feels that layers of pain have been peeled away as he was transported to a place where he could dwell without fear. As the light of the day fades, he talks about what is happening to him and Ed, his son, that they will both die. Talk between men who are connected. As he says:

'I would love to spend time in the pub with you.'

Affirmation that I dwell within this suffering family. *Dwelling with* is the ancestral connection as gradually I merge and become one with them with intimacy and without resistance. Perhaps it is the quintessential holistic relationship.

Three days later

Richard and Hettie are behind closed doors with Daphne, the social worker. Time hangs in the air.

Later I discover Hettie making tea in the small kitchen. Her eyes are strained from crying but she also laughs.

'That was good to get all that into the open.'

I feel her relief as walls of silence have been broken down. Why is it so difficult for people who have spent a lifetime together to talk about dying, death and loss?

Duhamel and Dupuis (2003:116) offer questions the practitioner might use to strengthen the family's ancestral roots:

• What has been the hardest thing for your family since you were told about the transfer to palliative care?

- What is helping you most in coming to terms with this situation?
- Which one of you is having the hardest time coming to terms with this stage of the illness?
- How is she/he showing it?
- What has given you the greatest comfort in dealing with an event like this?
- What information do you need most right now?

Such questions probe the surface to enable the family members to reveal and reflect on their own stories. Such questions prompt the practitioner to pick up any sign of difficulty. Where these stories are shared it can help the family to understand each other's experience, strengthen positive coping systems, and surface and resolve any misconceptions or conflicts that may simmer beneath the surface.

Richard declines my offer of reflexology. I consider insisting but he says he wants Hettie to have one and she is keen. I blend lavender, geranium and bergamot essential oils into the reflexology base cream massage. These oils have the ability to ease stress and fatigue. Hettie loves the smell.

'I love lavender . . . I use it at home to help me sleep.'

She settles in the recliner, a blanket wraps her into a cocoon, and against the background noise of Richard's nebuliser she sleeps as I work her feet. Richard reads the paper. He becomes very relaxed during the treatment. His breathing and chest pain ease, so much, that he doesn't need to ask for his regular break-through oromorph. It seems to work both ways – if I treat the patient, the carer becomes very relaxed and *vice versa*. It is as if Hettie's energy field spreads through the whole room intermingling with other energy fields. As I centre energy and massage the physical foot, so I massage this wider energy field and help ease the tension.

Two weeks later, Monday March 15

I have not visited the hospice for two weeks. Richard hangs tenaciously onto life. The staff felt he was dying last Friday and then Saturday, then Sunday but still he hangs on. He moves his head in some deep recognition to my greeting but then slips back into his oblivion. I stay with him using therapeutic touch to move the heat out of his chest and body until he is cooler and breathes more easily.

Hettie and Sophie arrive. They are pleased but seem surprised to see me. I feel guilty, as if I had let them down. They stayed at Richard's bedside for two days until they became exhausted and frustrated with the waiting and had to retreat to find respite and sleep, both of which have been elusive. Ed has also deteriorated even though he has been visiting Richard. Ed's despair is sharpened by his own impending death, the whole family wilting in the face of this double tragedy.

Sophie has pain radiating up the right side of her neck. She accepts my offer to help. I mix marjoram, lavender and pettigrain in apricot kernel carrier oil. A delightful aroma. The oils will help with stress and ease her taught neck and shoulder muscles. She sits on a chair as I work the right side of neck and along her trapezius muscle. A large knot is the source of her pain radiating up into her neck.

'Ouch . . .'

as I slowly loosen the knot. Two lesser knots are similarly loosened. All the time she continues to speak with Kirsty, no pause just like her father! Yet slowly her talk lessens as she relaxes into the massage. Afterwards her pain has eased. She can move her head from side to side again. She feels lighter as her stress melted away. I suggest she add some of the mix into her bath. The oils will help ease her suffering mind so she can sleep.

I wish Richard well on his journey for I shall not see him alive again. I give Hettie a hug and my phone number if she or Sophie ever need my help. It is a deeply poignant moment for I have dwelt within this family and touched their suffering.

Reflection

Is my guilt a failure of responsibility that I wasn't available to the family who trusted me? Should I have created space to be available knowing how beneficial my connection and therapy were for this family? I am concerned I have broken a trust.

I take refuge in Milton Mayeroff's words (1971:45):

> In caring I commit myself to the other; I hold myself out as someone who can be depended on. If there is an acute break within this relation because of my indifference or neglect, I feel guilty, as if the other were to say – 'where were you when I needed you, why did you let me down?' This guilt results from my sense of having betrayed the other, and my conscience calls me back to it. The more important this particular other is to me, the more pronounced is my guilt.

Perhaps I am being too precious. I am just one carer amongst others who have greater continuity. Perhaps I assume too much responsibility and lost the balance between intimacy and distance. I know at times I get drawn into the other's suffering, despite my efforts to be mindful. My guilt informs me I lost my way. Guilt is self-destructive and alienating. It blunts compassion because it sucks my energy. Reflection helps me listen to my inner contradictory voices to find this balance.

Three days later, Thursday March 18

A blustery March day. Richard's name is missing from the name board. He died at 8 pm on Tuesday. In the evening, I write a poem:

Clay

The hard fecund earth beckons
I sense her vibration draw closer
I hear the thin wail of ancestors
Drift across the solemn distance
between this place and that
I hear the lisp of unspoken words
I hear the call of black birds as they
Sail on silver currents;
Maybe a raven's croak amidst the din
And gathering gloom of earthly life.

I am clay fashioned by spirit to be human,
Strings of carbon linked in complex chains
evolved into the body wrapped in spirit;
How many lives passed
and those yet to come?
Soon I will be clay again
Returned to the earth
Upon which tender feet will trip in play and dance
To nourish the harvest
So the wheat stands tall and fruitful.

I hold the moist clay in my hands,
These hands that heal and ease suffering
And shape the giving clay into a head,
Scoop sockets for eyes and lumps for ears;
The senses already formed,
And perhaps a mouth so the breath
can flow amongst all the breaths that flow
Moment by moment across the distance;
Pause now to sense the space
Where I sit before the tipi
Turning the earth
Feeling the soft sunrise in my eyes.

Yasmina

Agnes (care assistant) pulls me aside and asks if I can help Yasmina. She is an 18-year-old Muslim girl. Her brother is with her. She has pain in her neck due to constant retching and cannot get comfortable. She is emaciated as a consequence of her stomach and lung cancer. Her large brown eyes gaze out from hollows sunken in her face. Her face sinks into itself. Yet she is beautiful. She wears a black hooded top that covers her head. Agnes asks Yasmina if she minds if I gently massage her neck to help ease her pain. She looks at Nasrat, her brother. He does not object. His eyes reveal a deep sorrow for his dying sister.

I blow a small fuse inside, nothing drastic, maybe just two amperes but enough to divert my energy. Agnes has stolen my voice in suggesting the massage treatment. Would a massage be the most appropriate response? But she has set the scene and I do not want to make one at this vulnerable moment in time.

I make up a massage cream with black pepper and camomile to ease the ache, and with orange to help ease the nausea. Yasmina's vertebrae protrude from her skin in a dramatic line of humps. Gently, very gently, I move along each side of her neck. I feel the tension of my burnt fuse. It disconcerts me. I also quickly realise the folly of this approach and suggest that therapeutic touch may be more beneficial. I explain what this is and they agree.

I create therapeutic space by placing my hands over Yasmina's head and ask her to imagine a soft healing and loving light surround her. I suggest it is the love of God. I suggest she breathe in this light with each in-breath, filling her suffering body with this light. I suggest that feels good. Relax into the light and with each out-breath let go of fear and surrender to God's divine love. As I talk, Nasrat comes increasing closer to the bed until he takes her hand. I sense I am taking a risk talking about God and taking therapy into a religious domain of which I know little. Agnes is the other side alongside me. It is a special moment. There is suspense in the air. The tension lifts from me as I recover my energy and feel such a light about me.

Yasmina surrenders completely, even though her eyes remain half open. After about 15 minutes I stop. Yasmina is deeply relaxed. Nasrat thanks me. For a minute or two, I am breathless as if I have been holding my breath during the therapy. But I am also shaken at the power of such practice. Later, Agnes tells me that Yasmina has never felt so peaceful. It is an affirmation of my intuition to respond in this way to her.

I ask myself who is Yasmina . . . this strange dark gaunt young woman with hollow eyes and her brother, fearful, protective, distressed by her side? What does she feel and think as she hovers on the brink of death. Do I read her signs well enough? Does she know she is close to death? What must it be like to contemplate her death being so young? Do I give offence in my ignorance of Muslim ritual? Does she suffer? Can I begin to understand? Too late to explore with her what meaning her dying has for her or her belief in any God . . . yet perhaps God is a metaphor for meaning in life . . . that somehow there is something beyond this earthly life that gives meaning to being on earth . . . that God is the last refuge, a sanctuary beyond the toils of mortal life. No matter the questions my doubting reflection creates, I cannot dwell in fear or uncertainty. Like a warrior riding the windhorse I must have faith and courage, and being mindful my intuition leads me confidently through the uncertainty. Lets face it, every situation is one of uncertainty simply because it has never been faced before. Doubt drains my energy and makes me less available. As I gaze into the void of suffering I can only wonder and embrace the mystery with open arms yet mindful of the 'spiritual traps' that caught me floundering with Jane (see Figure 6.2, page 219).

Although I cannot know Yasmina I can be with her. To do so I must let go of any pretence that I can know or understand her experience. I can touch her suffering and flow with it with compassion, mindful of who I am. Goldstein (2002:89) describes mindfulness as:

the quality of mind that notices what is present, without judgement, without inter-ference. It is like a mirror that clearly reflects what comes before it.

In other words, being mindful guides me to see things as they truly are, rather than as a projection of myself. Being mindful is the ability to pay attention to self within each unfolding moment in such a way that one remains fully available to ease the suffering and guide the other towards where they need to go. If the body can be equated to an energy system controlled by a series of fuses, then how easily fuses blow over seemingly trite issues. How could I get wrapped up in self-concern in the face of Yasmina's suffering? When fuses blow equanimity is lost and energy is cut off with the consequence that I am less available.

The next morning a solitary red candle burns for Yasmina. I am told it was a peaceful death. She had no more pain or retching. I hope my healing touch helped her find peace. Perhaps she did surrender to God. I speculate but I wonder what she sensed as death wrapped her in its arms.

The kiss of the dark god[20]
Taken so young into the mystery
Wrapped in black gossamer
Your veil floating on the soft wind of death
You taste the kiss of the dark god;
Your spirit free from earthly chore
Your family weep
bereft that they still breathe
that your hollow eyes blink no more,
as you ride the windhorse home.

Tuesday March 30

Another red candle burns to honour a patient who had died in the early hours of the morning. A nurse turns to her colleague and says we need to clean the 'Rose Room' now the undertakers have taken the body. The 'Rose Room' – where people in transit to the undertakers are discreetly placed. 'Rose' softens the impression of a mortuary. The 'body' – talk that confirms the person's transition from life to death. Normal hospice talk, yet I would prefer to hear the nurses talk of 'Iris' or 'Mrs Thompson'. There is something incongruent with softening the mortuary name to 'Rose' and then calling a dead person 'a body'. It feels disrespectful. Perhaps I should have said something but I didn't and the moment passed. But would I have been right to challenge this behaviour? The dilemmas of everyday practice, yet at the root of my dilemma is my fear of conflict that undermines my integrity. Perhaps I might have said:

'You mean Iris?'

with a smile on my face. Role modelling that makes the point yet without direct confrontation. You might ask 'Does it make any difference that the staff talk about the body?' Perhaps not, I felt the contradiction. I feel the soft ground beneath my feet.

---

[20] The poem is inspired by Susan Boulet's painting *Kiss of the Dark God* painted in 1994.

Martha and Millie

I visit Martha. She is asleep. Outside the room, a woman chats with nurses. Eye contact, a smile. Shortly afterwards I bump into her in the small kitchen.

I say:

'You're Martha's daughter?'
'Yes, I'm Millie.'

I inform her I am the complementary therapist and had popped in to ask Martha if she would like any therapy.

Millie exclaims tearfully that she is unable to touch her mum; that she is frightened of the consequences. Yet, as a consequence she feels guilty. I instinctively touch her shoulder as if to reassure her that it's OK to hold such feelings. Yet as I do so, I immediately challenge myself whether this touch is appropriate. The spectre of Lisa's response haunts me (page 99). I feel the soft ground beneath my feet.

Millie visibly relaxes or perhaps crumples might be a better word. My touch holds her. I acknowledge how tough it can be to dwell with people, especially our mothers, as they die. It seems like a moment of reconciliation with herself.

Martha is awake. She has refused all treatment and now wishes to die. She has a urinary tract infection but has refused antibiotics. I inform her I am a complementary therapist but she mishears.

'I don't want physiotherapy.'

I reiterate what I can offer and she asks what I do. In response she says she was a healer and used Reiki – she asks me to see her later after she has spoken with her daughter. In the meantime, she agrees to an aroma-stone. I use sandalwood and lavender to combat the odour, to help with the urinary tract infection and to ease the anxiety in the room. Sandalwood is an oil I rarely use, yet I sense I have underestimated its value in helping people who are dying. Worwood (1999:249) notes that sandalwood is:

> A fragrance that stretches out to the universe, into the hallowed space between heaven and earth, to contact the divine presence. Sandalwood brings our wisdom into a meditative state, quieting us so we can hear and rejoice in the choral singing of the universal soul. It brings us into the great cosmic prayer, the infinite meditation.

I love this description of *quieting us so we can hear.* That is exactly what Martha wants and what Millie needs help with. Indeed it is true for all of us – the way our chatter, our stuff, our noise gets in the way of what is really important. Of course, this is the value of meditation and centring within complementary therapy practice.

How better could I help ease someone's dying than to use such an oil? I have questioned before how Worwood knows that essential oils have these spiritual qualities. Perhaps *knows* is the wrong word. Perhaps a better word is *intuits.* In one sense it doesn't matter, because the description of sandalwood is my healing intent. Her description strengthens my intentionality. Reading the description to the patient can also be very beneficial to implant the healing intent. Essential oils vibrate at high frequencies, and it is this quality that contributes most to healing, perhaps more than the oil's diverse chemical constituents that are linked to varying therapeutic claims. Martha smiles as I leave her as if we have a connection through our healing.

Yet I am bothered about the way I instinctively touched Millie. Was that appropriate despite the beneficial consequence? I am still haunted by my *faux pas* with Lisa, that somehow it is never appropriate to instinctively touch strangers, I must be more mindful of reading the signs, for even a mild lapse can cause suffering. Perhaps I did read them on a subconscious level and beat myself up for no reason.

Later I return to Martha's bedside. Millie smiles and seems at ease in the large armchair by her mother's side. Another smile from Martha. She is amenable to the idea of having therapeutic touch. Millie rises to leave but I suggest she stays for I know the energy will bond mother and daughter. And so, in the soft glow of the late sun illuminating the room I give Martha therapeutic touch, transporting us both into a universal dimension beyond suffering where she can *let go of her resistance* and ease her troubled spirit.

A week later, April 6

Another blustery cold day, one moment blue sky and the next a hailstone blizzard. Seems to me ideal hospice weather with its turbulent emotions and moments of deep peace, often shifting moment by moment. Martha is dead. I wonder if Millie touched her mother before she died. No one is going to Martha's funeral. Is that a reflection of the way staff felt about her? I feel strangely irritated at the staff's 'rejection' of Martha. I want to compensate by attending myself. However, attending a funeral is a question of personal choice outside normal caring yet should it be? I know from my experience of attending Kristin's funeral (page 156) how much the family valued my attendance, or at least the attendance of someone from the hospice they could identify with on an emotional level. My attendance was a reflection of my personal care rather than as a representative of hospice care. I sense a troubling distinction between what is personal and what is professional.

The following week I share my experience of Millie and Martha with the palliative care students. I speculate whether touching Millie gave her permission to touch her mother, raising the question – how can we best help daughters in such distress, for without doubt dying raises unsettling issues that have been taboo in everyday life.

Reflection

My experience with Martha and Millie surfaces many significant issues, illuminating that one mundane experience can, on reflection, reveal much about the nature of holistic practice, easing suffering and being available:

- The use and meaning of ritual using a candle to respect for someone who has died. The ritual challenges practitioners not to take death for granted, that each death is profound
- *Easing suffering – letting go of resistance*
- Patient's rights for withdrawal of treatment and negative staff attitudes
- Empathy – tuning into the other's wavelength/knowing the person and reading the signs
- *Dwelling with* the family
- Taboo of *touch* and the significance of past experience
- Use and efficacy of aromatherapy oils
- Knowing the impact of therapeutic touch
- Closure/attendance of funerals and bereavement support
- *The troubling distinction between what is personal and what is professional*
- Unresolved issues and interpersonal conflict within families as death approaches
- *Quietening us so we can hear* – the nature of mindful practice

Even so, my list is not exhaustive. What have I *not* paid attention to? I am sure the reader can identify other significant issues in relating to this experience in terms of your own experience. The list highlights how particular issues can be drawn out or foregrounded against the background of the 'whole experience'. The idea of *the soft ground beneath my feet* reflects the complexity of everyday practice, where everything is indeterminate, a mystery unfolding. To be an effective practitioner requires me to hold the vision and tread softly so I do not sink in the quagmire of suffering. The experience has, at its core, the intent to ease Millie and Martha's *suffering*, notably the idea of *letting go of resistance* so they can flow where they need to flow to. Issues such as *dwelling with* have been a thread through the narrative. Meeting people in palliative care is often fleeting and under traumatic conditions. Barely time to draw breath. The text draws attention to the significance of *quietening us so we can hear* – the art of mindfulness . . . creating a clearing for self and others within the moment to listen amidst the din of the unfolding drama.

Knowing the impact of therapeutic touch creates a healing field with the whole family is a profound insight into my practice. I had observed this phenomenon in previous experiences but had not so mindfully applied this insight into my practice.

The significance of *empathy* – whilst I might touch the edge of Martha and Millie's feelings I appreciate that I can never really know how they feel. In the immediacy of the moment, I interpret the surface ripple without deeper exploration and respond. Perhaps the next day I might have sat with Millie or Martha to explore their feelings. Maybe. But maybe the reasons for suffering can be unspoken. It is an intriguing aspect of care.

Understanding touch – just because I got it wrong with Lisa doesn't mean I always get it wrong. Perhaps given the situation again, I might not touch Millie, yet perhaps my touch was a response to an intuitive reading of signs.

Yet my experience with Lisa *does* constrain me. It *is* a boulder I carry about that I need to offload. I know that cognitively – but emotionally it isn't so easy. The boulder feels lighter when I share it with others.

Sensing *a troubling distinction between what is personal and what is professional* reflects my personal agency to hold particular values and act with integrity even if contrary to professional and organisational dogma. I claim autonomy but accept responsibility for what I do, but what if I was told I couldn't attend a funeral because of hospice policy as a condition of my tenure? I can identify at least six areas of responsibility. So – where does my primary responsibility lie?

I rank my order of responsibility as follows:

	Self-ranking	Organisation ranking	Doctor ranking
To myself for acting with virtue and integrity	1		
To my patients and families for responding with best practice	2		
To my colleagues for responding in collaborative ways (not for carrying out prescribed medical treatments)	3		
To my profession for acting within professional ethics	4		
To my organisation for acting within defined roles and policies	5		
To society for being a 'good nurse or therapist'	6		

Your reflection

Use this table to rank me and then yourself in response to your own experience. Imagine how your employer and medical colleagues might also rank your priority of responsibility within the same situation. If there is divergence between ranking then the troubling distinction lies smouldering with potential conflict within self and with others. The ranking order does not diminish the significance of lesser-ranked responsibilities. However, it does highlight the potential for troubling distinctions, especially when organisations are transactional and impose expectations on the way the practitioner should or should not act.

Revisit the 'Influences grid' (Figure 4.2, page 45) and consider the potential tension between 'expectations from self how I should act' and 'expectations from others'? Does this raise issues of integrity? I hear Friedson's (1970) words echo in my mind that bureaucratic organisations such as health care trusts are primarily concerned with their own smooth running and only secondary with patient care. Do you sense a grain of truth in this claim?

As a result of my inquiry into whether attending funerals was a significant therapeutic act, the hospice imposed a policy that only two nurses should attend a funeral and attend in uniform although no mandatory attendance was demanded – which meant that some funerals are attended and some not.

Is that equitable? Staff could not attend a funeral in their own time. In other words, knowing the patient is a professional affair. Now I really feel the troubling distinction as such policy gives offence to my personal agency. Reflect on your own policies – do they enhance or constrain holistic practice?

Indigo

Tuesday April 6

I have been told that Indigo is a very 'spiritual' woman. She is 60 years old and dying. Around her bed sit her sister, her niece and a man I am unable to identify. I feel an intruder hovering but the women welcome me to the bedside. I feel their anxiety as they watch Indigo struggle. Her pain management has been reviewed and changed yet I see she is not comfortable. I ask her if she is comfortable. She repeats the word comfortable but her consciousness is clouded. Indigo, even as she nears death, has such elegance. Between the lines and ravages of illness her beauty radiates.

I suggest to the family that therapeutic touch might help Indigo feel more peaceful. The man asks what is therapeutic touch, is it a proven treatment? I feel his anxiety burn in his challenge. My answers do not convince him but the women intercede and ask me to do it for Indigo. He retreats to a chair in the window overlooking the gardens. I set up an aroma-stone with neroli and frankincense essential oils. I say these oils will help to soften the tenseness and implant a sense of the sacred. After the TT I sit and hold Indigo's hand and sense she finds this comforting. In response, I gently massage her hands and in the quiet peace of the afternoon we find some stillness. The man stays in his chair staring at me as if I am a witch doctor, waving my hands and mixing my potions, making vague claims of easing suffering. Yet even he can see that Indigo is more comfortable and the anxiety of the women eased. We must have faith.

Two days later

Indigo lies on her bed. Her arm is tucked up behind her head, her eyes are closed. She makes little movements of her waxed lips. Shifts of her pelvis as if trying to get comfortable, little furrows of pain between her eyes. Her swollen abdomen incongruent with her emaciated body. The staff are struggling to keep on top of her pain, the diamorphine dose has reached 160 mg via the syringe driver.

A friend from church sits with her. The aroma-stone has gone. I find it in the clinical room 'in soak'. A care assistant carelessly says it went dry and they have not had time to replenish it. A flicker of irritation. It is not a question of 'time' – it is a question of 'attention'. The seemingly relentless struggle to establish aromatherapy within everyday practice is a persistent theme running through the narrative. Perhaps a more correct interpretation is to say my inability to adequately confront and change the neglect of aroma-stones is a persistent theme running through the narrative. Along the Noble Eight-Fold

Path, the step of 'perfect speech' is most challenging in a world that avoids straight talking and conflict. Lama Surya Das (1997:200) notes:

> Words can be gifts, words can be weapons, words can be magic; words can be prayer, poetry, or song. What is traditionally known as right speech is the third touchstone on the Eight-Fold Path. So speak the truth. Tell it like it is. There is no reason to do otherwise.

The key to speech is not to project my irritation. To do that requires being mindful of my irritation and melt it in the moment. If I fail then it is likely my words will be a weapon to attack the other person. People at war cannot work together well. I did not avoid the topic as I have done in previous situations scattered through the narrative. Perhaps I did project something of my irritation, enough for her to get the 'emotional' message. I subsequently informed the senior nurse (yet again) but nothing changes. Is it simply a fact of life, the way things are or could I do more to confront the situation using perfect speech? Therein is my challenge without fear of 'upsetting the applecart'. Indeed with perfect speech it is impossible to upset the applecart! As it is, I clean and replenish the stone.

Indigo opens her eyes and greets her friend with delight. It is a mutual delight. Her friend reads a scripture and I feel the words vibrate and lift me into a serene place. A moment of immense poignancy. Her friend leaves and thanks me for the aroma-stone – she knows the significance of burning oils and senses my care. As I give Indigo therapeutic touch I suggest to her that God is holding her. She opens her eyes and gazes at me. I hold her gaze and she smiles. My soul is touched by her presence. I am in awe sharing such a spiritual moment as her death closes in. Such is the profound nature of our practice. Perhaps I should have some large signs made:

Aroma-stone in use
Please be mindful and respect its use

Later I write clearly in Indigo's notes how beneficial the aroma-stone has been to ease Indigo's and her visitors' *suffering*. The word *suffering* feels powerful, emotional, even confrontational. Normally I would have written something like 'The aroma-stone has helped Indigo to feel more relaxed. More neutral, less emphatic.

Aroma-stones are clearly beneficial and appreciated by patients and families, so what messages do their neglect give? I would expect a nursing leadership to watch and search for deviations from good practice and take necessary corrective action as active transactional leadership. However, a passive leadership is evident that doesn't intervene even when standards are not met (Bass 1988). When I drew nursing leadership's attention to this neglect I received a sympathetic acknowledgement but nothing changed.

After the shift report, Kirsty (staff nurse) approaches me.

> 'I read your comment . . . I'm sorry about that. We need to try harder. I know it's important.'

I thank her but soften my tone.

'I don't want to make a fuss but it is frustrating . . .'

Yet I feel apologetic like a small child who has been telling tales. I feel like I am picking up the few apples that I have dislodged from the applecart. Actions have consequences.

Friday April 16

Walking in the woods, I witness nature's renewal as the new green leaves spring forth from the bare trees. I am mindful of how easy it is to get wrapped up in matters of the day, being complacent, of taking things like nature's unfolding for granted and of neglecting one's own spiritual growth. Walking in the woods wakes me up, renews me. Touched by beauty I write a poem dedicated to renewal.

Renewal

New leaf,
transparent green,
emerges from closed bud
upon the twig;
Innocence of renewal,
Yet what knowing lies within
the delicate leaf
evolved as it has
through countless years.

New catkin flower
Pollen lies thick along the stem
stains yellow
the quivering hand
that holds such beauty
in awe;
All about nature bursting
with new life
within the deep forest.

Do we pause to see
such life unfolding?
Do we pause to hear the birds
sing their songs
between the silence?
Do we feel our own hearts
burst with new life
If we could simply stop
the rot?

Renewal, the yearly quest
to shake and stir the roots,
to nourish new growth
and prune the decay
which, if neglected
gathers up each day
until you feel the strain
that inexorably suffocates
the aching senses.

In the deep forest
I pause to feel renewal
so love can radiate
through each cell
through each fibre of my being
freeing me to see and
dwell at ease within life's
    mystery
letting go of decay
opening to beauty.

Monday June 21

It feels a paradox that I write a poem on renewal and then don't reflect on my practice for two months. I sense the way stress slowly accumulates, drip by drip in the metaphoric water butt. Because it accumulates slowly, it is barely perceptible unless of course something dramatic happens. However, when left unattended the water butt slowly fills until it can no longer contain the stress. The water spills over the top creating an emotional mess that is uncomfortable for everyone to experience. People are uncomfortable with such mess so they scurry to mop it up as if it never happened. The water butt recedes to a manageable level but is never empty. Inexorably it begins to rise again.

Water butts have a tap that can drain off water and be used to water the garden. Through reflection, we can become mindful of our accumulating stress and learn to turn on our water taps and drain the butt. We can then dissipate this negative energy and turn it into positive energy to water our gardens so we can grow and blossom.

I didn't feel particularly stressed at the time of writing about Indigo but I had become jaded. I felt less available to patients and my colleagues. I sensed it in a growing lack of tolerance to small things like the aroma-stone. Something inside me triggered a need for renewal; a need to gather and nourish myself, to remind myself of who I am and what I do. Such recognition is a strength not a weakness. That's why the poem 'renewal' felt so significant.

Tommy

Summer solstice

The day is cold and gloomy with periodic bursts of heavy rain. Tommy is 41. I am informed he has an aortic mass possibly stemming from a seminoma that was diagnosed and treated 10 years previously. He is described as in pain, breathless, very agitated with frequent panic attacks. His two sisters are with him.

I ask Sharron (staff nurse) about his agitation – can we fathom his thoughts and emotions behind this label? Sharron, always opinionated, says that Tommy wants to die now, that he has had enough. He is not afraid of death itself – just the dying process. I always wonder when I hear this said – whether it's really true or not. Perhaps he does seek ultimate release from his pain especially when we struggle so hard to master it. Death itself must be such a mystery for anyone staring it in the face. Maybe I just project the way I might feel contemplating the imminence of my own death. I don't pursue it as Sharron is adamant. She feels that Tommy would not appreciate any complementary therapy. She speaks parentally for him and his family. I bow to her pressure and do not visit him or his sisters yet I am left feeling disconcerted with this conversation. No matter what difference of opinion we might have, we should be able to discuss and collaborate in making the best decision for the patient's well-being. Clearly that would involve Tommy and his family. Yet sometimes people are not prepared to listen. Better to smile than to snarl. A smile in itself will shift the wind.

I realise that this is not the moment to assert my autonomy. Sharron is *his* nurse this evening and she is fiercely protective of *her* patients that often blinds her to other perspectives and be defensive of her own. She marks and patrols her territory. I sense the way her anxiety makes her intolerant of interference as if interference is a threat. If I am drawn into confrontation I am at risk of becoming wrapped up in her anxiety that will spill out across the floor as unresolved conflict depleting our energy to be available with patients and with each other.

Better to yield. Yielding is not failure. It is being able to read the signs and be sensitive to the unfolding moment. Yielding is yielding to self, to tame one's ruffled ego; it is not primarily concerned with yielding to another although it may seem like that on the surface. Yielding is being mindful that conflict is a battle of egos that can only lead to destruction for all concerned despite the illusion of a winner. Mindfulness is seeing things for what they are, cutting through illusion. It isn't imperative I treat Tommy this evening. Perhaps tomorrow, depending on the circumstances I will not yield.

At home I work out my angst. If contained, it will simmer and harm me. The risk is that it leaks out as horizontal violence (Street 1992) whereby one's anxiety (for whatever reason) is unconsciously projected into others as *crooked arrows*. Hurt, practitioners lash out and hurt those closest to them being an easier target than the true antagonists. *Crooked* arrows are the arrows a person fires that reflect a hurt or wounded self. In contrast, *Straight* arrows are the arrows a person fires that reflect a healthy self (Blackwolf & Gina Jones 1995).

Crooked arrows	Straight arrows
Self-centredness	Come to self
Fear	Befriend self
Dependency	Accept self
Denial	Value self
Expectations (from self and others)	Become self
Stress	Love self
Depression	Celebrate self
	Share self

The imagery of crooked and straight arrows offers a powerful model to reflect on my self-esteem. The effort through reflection is to recognise the arrows we fire and work to diminish the crooked arrows and nurture the straight arrows.[21] Crooked arrows take our energy and blunt caring. In firing straight arrows the crooked arrows naturally weaken. Each of the straight arrows prepare you for the last arrow – *share self*. The straight arrow of *come to self* is the invitation to reflect as the path to know self. Listen to Blackwolf and Gina (1995:161–162):

---

[21] The reader is directed to Blackwolf and Gina's text for a description of each arrow.

Give it (self) now freely. Look to and learn from the robin. How stately, how unpretentious, how humble, how predictable, how friendly. The robin is a good model for us. It gives itself easily to all the world. Give your time, your Self, to others . . . Share your smiles. Share your joy as well as your sadness. Serve others to serve yourself. Enrich society and you will enrich yourself.

So my task is to share self – to be available to Sharron and others in the mutual caring quest. It is a call for caring.

I pick up my colouring pencils and draw a warshield to defend against the crooked arrows. I decorate my warshield with *Namaji*, a native American word that reflects the four qualities of respect, honour, dignity and pride (Blackwolf & Gina Jones 1995:130).

> Like the lily pads in the lake, Namaji unfolds at different levels. Some lilies get less sun, deep down in the water, on their strong vine. They are flooded with the brushing concerns of their world. Other lilies get more sun, close to the top of the water, and are able to look out to the other side and see what is possible. Some lily pads lay on top of the water and touch the wonder of a new state of being, while others transcend the water as flower stems, opening to the sunlight of wisdom. As you transcend the depths of your life, you experience Namaji – a higher state of consciousness.

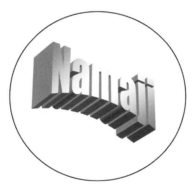

Reflection is my unfolding path through levels of consciousness towards Namaji. Namaji is a state of inner harmony and a vital attribute of the holistic practitioner. Sherwood (1997:30) notes that:

> Inner harmony can only be achieved when there is balance in relationships with others.

I am uncertain of the veracity of Sherwood's sentiment. I sense through my narrative, that a balance of relationship with others is a reflection of the state of balance within myself. Perhaps the more I am in inner harmony, or realise Namaji, then the more I find harmony with others. This makes sense, in that the more certain I am with myself then the more certain I am with others. I sense that the more I project Namaji then the more others respond positively to me. In other words, who I am has a significant influence on the practice environment for both colleagues and patients.

In contrast with an inner harmony, there is a shadow side of harmony that leads to dysfunctional relationships between colleagues. It is an illusionary harmony that we all get on well together reflected within the hospice culture of *niceness* as a collective mutual pretence to avoid dealing with conflict, as if conflict would pierce the container and all the suppressed existential angst would pour out and drown people.

I once wrote:

> The hospice is a nice place
> Full of nice people
> Nice is so sanitising
> So containing.

(Johns 2004b:61)

The culture of 'niceness' complements the culture of 'the good death' – the culture of the 'good nurse' that constrains the open expression and positive resolution of conflict – *Quiet voices please and brush away that conflict otherwise it tears the illusion that the hospice is a peaceful calm place.* The culture of niceness quietens the voices of conflict. In doing so it stifles integrity. No matter how mundane the situation, it is vital I act with integrity to facilitate dialogue to benefit patient well-being. Yet I sense my voice has often been quiet when perhaps it should have been heard. Not an easy confession. The narrative can be read as the quest to strengthen my voice to assert holistic values whenever threatened.

Yet, when conflict does burst from the container, people quickly clear the mess up to smooth the nice of harmony rather than deal with the conflict itself although the whispers are like acid.

> The warshield could equally be a drum. Beat the message of Namaji!

Reflection on being parental

In dialogue, practitioners are committed to working together toward shared vision. Vision is the background for everyday practice, but needs to be frequently projected into the foreground to affirm its meaning. As the being available template asserts, the more I hold a vision in my mind, the more likely I am to realise my vision as a reality. Working together, practitioners must listen to and respect what the other person is saying. This requires an openness of mind no matter if there is a clash of values or opinions.

The pattern of communication between Sharron and myself can be viewed using transactional analysis (TA) (Stewart & Joines 1987). Simply put, TA recognises that people communicate from different ego states; the child, adult and parent. The child ego is essentially irresponsible and seeks instant gratification. The adult ego is essential the voice of responsibility and reason.

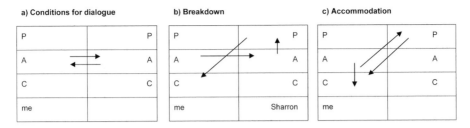

Figure 6.3 Transactional analysis patterns of communication.

The parent ego is essentially an authoritative and controlling mode. To ensure communication, patterns of communication need to be reciprocated. If not, breakdown occurs. To dialogue required both Sharron and myself to be in adult ego mode (Figure 6.3a). If one or both of us becomes fearful or anxious, then we would shift into parental or child mode.

Barber (1993) identifies that the parent ego is fearful of losing control, losing self-respect, and losing respect of others, whilst the child ego is fearful of persecution, rejection, and being overwhelmed.

In response to her fear of losing control, Sharron flipped into parental script. Initially her response resulted in crossed lines of communication and breakdown as I stayed in adult mode (Figure 6.3b). We could only recover communication if I accommodated her response either deliberatively, or in response to my fear of persecution, and becoming the compliant child (Figure 6.3c). Being mindful of Sharron's ego state. I was able to manage my own anxiety and yield rather than be drawn into a child mode or worse, reciprocate the parent. Imagine two parents battling for control of the hurt child (Tommy). As I say better to smile and yield than snarl and fight in that particular situation. We can dialogue or fight another day when the patient is not caught in the crossfire. Yet, clinical decisions need to be made **now** – **now** is the moment for dialogue.

Barber (1993:359) offers advice about staying in adult mode:

- Give myself permission to stay with your uncertainties
- Accept your emotions as energies rather than anxieties or symptoms to be locked away
- Witness your responses rather than indulge or swamp yourself in them
- Allow yourself to make mistakes
- Share your insights, observations, feelings with others
- Avoid win–lose situations
- Don't defend your views, just share your evidence
- Stay aware of your defences and work towards giving them up

This advice offers a useful way to reflect on and learn through experience, especially to confront the fears that characterise the flight into parental and child ego modes. I suppose I did sense a threat to my autonomy, a sense of locked horns over control that reflected a failure of dialogue. Yet I was also mindful of staying in adult mode and hence mindful of my defences and sliding into either competing parent or accommodating child modes.

The next day

In contrast with yesterday, it is a beautiful still warm morning. Blue skies with wisps of high cloud. It is joy to drive to the hospice through the lanes at 6.30 am. The winds have shifted. Tommy has picked up overnight. Sharron is not on duty. The new pain management regimen has done the trick using diamorphine 850 mg, ketamine 200 mg, ketorolac 90 mg alongside Nozinan 50 mg and midazolam 10 mg delivered via four syringe drivers. Some cocktail. He said to the night staff:

'Why didn't I have this before?'

He has slept, and this morning he is on the 'up'. Yesterday he was on the 'down' – the rollercoaster ride – hold tight! The sisters were told yesterday that the 'injection' (diamorphine) would probably be 'it'. A week ago they had been told that Tommy probably had two or three days. I wonder why doctors make these predictions and why nurses are not present when these messages are given. It is the nurses who pick up the consequences of these false prophecies. Do the family then cease to believe us? Do they lose trust in us?

Tommy wants to see his father yet his sisters are hostile towards their father because of family trauma that has not healed. Neither wants to put him up but agree they would be civil to him if he visited the hospice. How dying brings to the surface unresolved conflicts that have been hidden in the family attics. It now spills out and the caring team find themselves knee-deep in this angst. If it's Tommy's wish it must be respected especially now as he has 'picked up'. Who knows when the reaper will come calling? Perhaps he is waiting for his father to come.

The sisters are full of life; yet their life is on hold, uncertain what to do. Lora, the younger sister sports her England vest. They had all watched the game last evening (England vs Croatia), a useful distraction from the waiting and wondering. I casually offer my therapies to the sisters but they do not see themselves as the focus of care. Indeed they play down any sense of stress or tiredness.

Tommy has a severe cramp in his right hand and accepts my offer to massage it. I massage both hands and forearms. He finds this very relaxing. The cramp unfolds and disperses. Smiles all round yet 15 minutes later he has a panic attack resulting in severe cramps I cannot ease. I give way and let him have Valium to quell the rage.

Donald

Donald is going home today. He is 92 years old and has cancer of his oesophagus. He warmly greets me. He fears he has had more diarrhoea. Indeed as he says this we hear the telltale gurgle of the diarrhoea coming away from him. I say I will fetch help to sort him out. He is also anxious about getting ready to go home.

I pull the curtains to reveal the beautiful blue sky. The heron glistens in the sun. The ornamental tree is covered in new lime green leaves that blend exquisitely with the blue sky. My favourite room stirring. In that moment I could glimpse the impermanence of everything and shatter the thousand illusions that bind me.

Christine joins me. I mention the leaves against the sky and she murmurs her approval. First we disconnect his percutaneous endoscopic gastrostomy (PEG) tube feeding. He feels the feed is too much for him. I suggest he tells the dietician and not passively accept what he is prescribed. Sometimes dieticians only see the body and not the person suffering. Christine gives him an extra flush with water because he feels dry. He likes to suck ice so I fetch him some whilst we give him his medications via the PEG tube.

He has been having palliative radiotherapy to shrink the oesophageal tumour. Five years ago, he first noted he was losing weight. His GP had simply said 'Old people do lose weight'. However, Donald noted that his swallowing got snagged. He compensated by mashing his food more and more until then he couldn't swallow even that. He went back to his GP and was referred. By then any curative treatment was beyond him. He missed his last radiotherapy appointment but does not think he will have any more now. His swallowing is now easier. He can swallow some sips of water and even some ice. He is thankful for such small mercies.

I ask if he is a religious man. He says he believes but has no active faith.

'Does believing bring you any comfort with the thought of dying?'

He is unsure of this. He says:

'I was told not to expect the Queen's message but I may live another five years. I don't want to die.'

I catch his gaze and smile. His life expectancy is totally unrealistic. Yet perhaps it comforts him and his wife to believe in this possibility.

As we bath him, I prompt him to talk through his life. His great love is his garden. He shares how he spent 20 years sorting the garden out and the last six years enjoying the fruits of his labour. His wife Jocelyn potters about the flower beds and someone is hired to do the 'heavy stuff'. She came in yesterday and said how much she had enjoyed doing the garden this past week. He wants to persuade Jocelyn to move after he dies to a smaller garden she can manage more easily. Putting his house in order, trying to ensure those left behind can manage in the best way.

We reach his legs. I inquire:

'Did you play soccer?'

He reveals that playing soccer and playing the cornet in a band were the loves of his life. He was only 19 when he had an accident playing soccer that knocked out his two front teeth and ruined his cornet-playing career. He also gave up football and so that only left girls. His first marriage only lasted three years. He met another girl in 'munitions' and has been with her since. No children.

'My career became a married man.'

Jocelyn is 82 and rather frail.

'Even though we have carers four times a day she needed this break from caring for me.'

I apply some moisturising lotion to his dry legs and spend a few minutes massaging his feet, being careful of the dressing covering his heal pressure sore.

The diarrhoea is squashed up between his legs contained within the large 'nappy' pad he is wearing. We quickly clean him and leave him refreshed sitting in bed to await his transport. It is nearly ten o'clock – we have patiently and mindfully spent two hours with him. He is grateful for our attention but would now like to rest in preparation for going home. His night had been disturbed with the diarrhoea. Bathing someone creates this space to dwell and really to know someone. It has been a joy working with Christine again. Being with Christine nourishes my spirit whereas Sharron diminished it. Such stark contrast. To be available to our patients we need to be available to each other. We need to conserve energy for caring not to deplete it on petty squabble and grudges.

Eric

Eric was admitted yesterday for respite care. I introduce myself as the complementary therapist. I ask him how he feels about being here. He says:

'I didn't want to come in at first because I associated it with death – that people didn't come out again, but I'm pleased I did come. I can see it's very different from that . . . I wasn't eating for four days prior to admission but now I'm eating a fried breakfast!'

I don't ask if he feels he will come out again. On the surface, he seems relaxed about his cancer and the future. So much so that he can't see how I can help him?

'Do you have any specific problems?'

He says his right leg is very oedematous and left leg slightly oedematous. I suggest that maybe a gentle massage might help his circulation and help ease his oedema although I can't 'massage' the oedema away directly. I suggest I can bring him to a greater state of relaxation despite his doubts.

He doesn't answer directly but complains his ear irritates. He attributes this to getting water in his ear as the irritation commenced after a jacuzzi bath. However, he acknowledges that he has had this problem several times over the past month. I tweak his toes and the irritation has gone.

'How did you do that?'
'Magic . . . well not quite. I tweaked your ear reflex point.'

He is genuinely impressed, so much so that he requests a foot massage! He agrees it was deeply relaxing. However, ten minutes later the irritation returns. Perhaps I could teach him to tweak his own toes but he is immobile. He laughs.

'Maybe you can teach the missus.'

He likes the aroma of patchouli and frankincense in the massage cream so I set up an aroma-stone using the same oils.

After lunch, he is still tormented by his ear. He requests a cotton bud but to no avail. I suggest he holds his nose and blows – it works! Perhaps peppermint essential oil will help as it is reputed to clear the mind (Davis 1999). I put four drops onto some gauze. He inhales deeply and loves the smell. He feels his mind and ear clear immediately! I also add some to his aroma-stone mix. Later, when I go to say goodbye he enthuses to his gathered family about the treatments. His ear irritation has not recurred. Subtle things like the tweaking of toes, blowing your nose, and peppermint can make such a difference! All good science?

I sensed Eric is a practical person, and so I needed to show him if I could be useful to him. As fate would have it he provided me with the perfect showcase. Even though the result was not perfect he saw the possibilities of complementary therapies. Through responding to **him** he became interested in me and opened up the potential for working together.

Pauline

Pauline talks through her 'history' unfolding the story of her diagnosis and treatment. She is continuing with cycles of chemotherapy. Patterns of tiredness, her hair thinning. Until recently her hair had been down to her waist. She cut it off in anticipation of the hair loss. She has weakness in her left leg. Since being at the hospice she has commenced steroids to see if that will help relieve some of the pressure and improve her leg. Brain and bone scans booked. Has the cancer spread? Part of her is pessimistic that she will die. Part of her hopes she can be cured yet, in her words:

'Deep down I sense the worse.'

She is seemingly calm about this prospect although anxious about care for her husband who has had two strokes.

'I need to sort out my life so I can die with things sorted.'

These words feel like the plaintiff cry of a thousand voices.
She has no will so I suggest meeting Daphne, our social worker. She believes in God although has no active religious life. However, she wants to be burnt.

'I can't stand the thought of those worms.'

I say:

'It's just your body your spirit would have flown a long time before the worms get you.'

Macabre talk, yet it feels quite natural.

'I used to be eight stone. When I last weighed myself I was six stone eight pounds. I daren't weigh myself anymore.'

She doesn't have much appetite yet she would like to put on weight. I suggest high calorie drinks?

'I like Fortisips . . . strawberry is my favourite.'
'I will go foraging for you.'

Pauline thanks me.

'It's good to talk like this . . . there is no one I can really talk to.'

> Surrounded by silence,
> People do not know what to say to you
> and you cannot say it
> fearful of the signs.
> When you need to be understood and loved
> you feel alone.
> What does your husband think and feel?
> Does he also suffer in the silence?
> Open into this space
> where you can pour your tears and fears,
> where you can find the words.
> Strangers – yet our souls touch easily

Pauline waits with relish for her jacuzzi bath. I note her dry skin. She likes the idea of some oils in her bath. I add a few drops of lemon, geranium, juniper berry and lavender oils to the running bath. Lemon will help boost her immune system. The geranium is an adrenal gland booster and stimulates the lymphatic system and will be excellent for Pauline's dry skin. Juniper will help the body and mind rid itself of toxins. Lavender will help to bring the body into balance (Davis 1999:176). Pauline giggles with anticipation as if we are child conspirators. How quickly play lifts the gloom. Visions of Kristin. I suggest a facial and reflexology after her bath if she is agreeable?

'Yes please!'

In the small kitchen I discover a wide range of forti-juices but no strawberry! We have forest fruits, pineapple, apple and pear, blackcurrant, apricot. Her husband arrives whilst she is bathing so I suggest her therapy after lunch. The jacuzzi bath was wonderful and gives her a good appetite for lunch. She ponders the juices and chooses pineapple.

After lunch she eagerly awaits me. I commence the facial by gently resting my hands on her temples, holding her, until I am one with her. She is still even when a new patient arrives in the adjacent bed. She is deeply moved by the therapy. She says they have nourished her spirit. A nurse comments that the atmosphere in the room was serene during the treatment accompanied by the rainforest music and the delicious aroma of the essential oils I had used.

A moment of stillness that transforms suffering. Her spirit has been energised as if a black hole is now filled with light and colour . . .

> Your suffering like a black hole
> that sucks your spirit dry
> and draws you ever deeper into its oblivion
> your cry of anguish barely heard
> not a word of comfort
> to soften the descent;
> let me hold you
> a moment of stillness
> to fill your hole with light and colour.

Postscript

It is now November. The leaves, once green, have turned into hues of reds and yellows. Soon they will turn brown and fall in the cycle of seasons. And so my journey and journal continue into the new day and uncertain future. My faith has blossomed as I embrace and dwell in the mystery of caring. I can better appreciate the nature of suffering and am more able to realise the spiritual within myself and within others. Indeed, the two are a reflection of each other. Appreciating the spiritual lifts each mundane moment into something sacred, a gaze, a touch, washing someone's feet. It is the heart of my practice. I am certain that reading the text has triggered your reflection on your own experiences. Through reflection we can share our stories and learn from each other towards creating a more caring world where suffering is eased and people emerge into the light.

The gateway to becoming mindful is through reflection. Listen to my teachers Blackwolf and Gina Jones (1996:298):

> Practise reflecting through the day. Become aware of everything you do. Often we live without this awareness. As you walk down your path, return to healthy self-consciousness. Expand this to include others on your path and the path itself. Notice the way your foot steps down on the grass. Move with deliberate intention. Become aware of how your body feels, the wind on your face, your relaxed posture. Notice the colours around you, the earth beneath you, the clouds above you, the experience within you. Become aware of all that is you and surrounds you. Challenge yourself to notice the unnoticeable. See what you can see. Hear what is present. Expand your experience to include all that is present in the now! You will be astounded by all that you have been missing. There is much to honour as you journey through this life.

Appendix 1

Summary of therapies

Therapeutic touch	A technique to massage the etheric energy field usually found between three and four inches from the person's body in order to detect and smooth out disharmony in the body.
Reflexology	The process of gentle but firm manipulation of the feet and or hands to stimulate specific reflex points of the body. This is based on the principle that there are reflexes running along the body that terminate in the feet and the hands, and that the body's organs and systems are reflected onto the surface of the skin (Norman & Cowan 1989). Studies – for example Hodgson (2000) – have shown the therapeutic benefit for people with advanced cancer.
Aromatherapy	The use of specific oils obtained from organic sources for therapeutic benefit. These oils can be used in different ways. In the narrative, I describe using oils within massage and for inhalation using an aroma-stone.
Healing	I can only describe this as a sense of tuning into something beyond the mind. I sense it emanates from a collision of a deep faith within and cosmic forces without. It evolves a surrender of the therapist to flow with the healing force.
Massage	Manipulation of the soft tissues of the body using a variety of 'strokes' for therapeutic benefit, often combined with aromatherapy.
Indian head massage	A massage technique involving the upper back, neck, shoulders, head and face often combined with aromatherapy.

References

Autton, N. (1989) *Touch – an Exploration*. Dartmann, Longman & Todd, London.

Barber, P. (1993) Developing the 'person' of the professional carer. In Hinchliff, S., Norman, S. & Schober, J (eds) *Nursing Practice and Health Care* (2nd edition) Edward Arnold, London, pp344–373.

Bass, B.M. (1990) *Bass & Stodgill's Handbook of Leadership* (3rd edition) Free Press, New York.

Bauby, J.D. (1997) *The Diving-Bell and the Butterfly*. Fourth Estate, London.

Beck, C.Y. (1989) *Everyday Zen*. Thorsons, London.

Belenky, M.F., Clinchy, B.M., Goldberger, N.R. & Tarule, J.M. (1986) *Women's Ways of Knowing: The Development of Self, Voice and Mind*. Basic Books, New York.

Benner, P., Tanner, C. & Chesla, C. (1996) *Expertise in Nursing Practice*. Springer, New York.

Benner, P. & Wrubel, J. (1989) *The Primacy of Caring*. Addison-Wesley, Menlo Park.

Buddhadasa Bhikkhu (1997) *Mindfulness with breathing (revised edition)* Wisdom Publications, Boston.

Blackford, J. (2003) Cultural frameworks of nursing practice: exposing an exclusionary health care culture. *Nursing Inquiry* **10**(4): 236–244.

Bloom, W. (2001) *The Endorphin Effect*. Piatkus, London.

Bochner, A.P. (2001) Narrative's virtues. *Qualitative Inquiry* **7**(2): 131–157.

Bochner, A. & Ellis, C. (eds) (2002) *Ethnographically Speaking*. AltaMira Press, Walnut Creek, California.

Bohm, D. (1996) *On Dialogue* (ed Nichol, L.). Routledge, London.

Bolton, S. (2000) Who cares? Offering emotion work as a 'gift' in the nursing labour process. *Journal of Advanced Nursing* **32**(3): 580–586.

Borglum, D. (1997) The long shadow of good intentions. *Tricycle* **7**(1): 66–69.

Boyd, E. & Fales, A. (1983) Reflective learning: key to learning from experience. *Journal of Humanistic Psychology* **23**(2): 99–117.

Boykin, A. & Schoenhofer, S. (1991) Story as link between nursing practice, ontology, epistemology. *Image: Journal of Nursing Scholarship* **23**: 245–248.

Bradshaw, A. (1996) The spiritual dimension of hospice. *Social Science & Medicine* **43**: 409–419.

Cara, C. (1999) Relational caring inquiry: nurses' perspective on how management can promote a caring practice. *International Journal of Human Caring* **3**(1): 22–30.

Carper, B. (1978) Fundamental patterns of knowing in nursing. *Advances in Nursing Science* **1**(1): 13–23.

Carter, A. & Sanderson, H. (1995) The use of touch in nursing practice. *Nursing Standard* **9**(16): 11–17.

Cavanagh, S. (1991) The conflict management style of staff nurses and nurse managers. *Journal of Advanced Nursing* **16**: 1254–60.

Chang, S.O. (2001) The conceptual structure of physical touch in caring. *Journal of Advanced Nursing* **33**: 820–827.

Charmaz, K. (1983) Loss of self: a fundamental form of suffering in the chronically ill. *Sociology of Health and Illness* **5**(2): 168–195.

Chödrön, P. (1997) *When Things Fall Apart: Heart Advice in Difficult Times*. Shambhala, Boston.

Chödrön, P. (2003) *The Wisdom of No Escape*. Element, London.

Cixous, H. (1996) Sorties: Out and point: attacks/ways out/forays. In Cixous, H. & Clement, H.C. *The Newly Born Woman*. Tauris, London.

Clandinin, D.J. & Connelly, F.M. (2000) *Narrative Inquiry: experience and story in qualitative research*. Jossey-Bass, San Francisco.

Clarke, M. (1986) Action and reflection: practice and theory in nursing. *Journal of Advanced Nursing* **11**: 3–11.

Coles, R. (1989) *The Call of Stories: teaching and moral imagination*. Houghton Mifflin, Boston.

Cohen, A. (2002) *Living Enlightenment: a call for evolution beyond ego*. Moksha Press, Lennox, MA.

Cope, M. (2001) *Lead Yourself*. Momentum Books, London.

Corley, M.C. & Goren, S. (1998) The dark side of nursing: impact of stigmatizing responses on patients. *Scholarly Inquiry for Nursing Practice: an International Journal* **12**(2): 99–118.

Cowling, W.R. (2000) Healing as appreciating wholeness. *Advances in Nursing Science* **22**(3): 16–32.

Cox, M. (1988) *Structuring the Therapeutic Process* (revised edition). Jessica Kingsley Publishing, London.

Davidhizar, R. & Giger, J. (1997) When touch is not the best approach. *Journal of Clinical Nursing* **6**(3): 203–206.

Davis, P. (1999) *Aromatherapy A–Z*. CW Daniel Co., Saffron Walden.

Delmar, C. (2004) Development of ethical expertise: a question of courage. *International Journal of Human Caring* **8**(3): 8–12.

Dewey, J. (1933) *How We Think*. J.C. Heath, Boston.

Dickson, A. (1982) *A Woman in Your Own Right*. Quartet Books, London.

Dossey, L. (1993) *Healing Words: The Power of Prayer and the Practice of Medicine*. Harper, New York.

Dreyfus, H. & Dreyfus, S. (1996) The relationship of theory and practice and the acquisition of skill. In Benner, P., Tanner, C. & Chesla, C. (eds) *Expertise in Nursing Practice*. Springer, New York.

Duhamel, F. and Dupuis, F. (2003) Families in palliative care: exploring family and health-care professionals/beliefs. *International Journal of Palliative Nursing* **9**(3): 113–119.

Edwards, S. (1998) An anthropological interpretation of nurses' and patients' perceptions of the use of space and touch. *Journal of Advanced Nursing* **28**: 809–17.

Eifried, S. (1998) Helping patients find meaning: a caring response to suffering. *International Journal of Human Caring* **2**(1): 33–39.

Erikson, E. (1982) *The Life Cycle Completed*. Norton, New York.

Evans, J. (2002) Cautious caregivers: gender stereotypes and the sexualisation of men nurses' touch. *Journal of Advanced Nursing* **40**(4): 441–448.

Fagerhaugh, S. & Strauss, A. (1977) *Politics of Pain: Staff Patient Interaction*. Addison-Wesley, London.

Fay, B. (1987) *Critical Social Science*. Polity Press, Cambridge.

Flemons, D. & Green, S. (2002a) Stories that conform/stories that transform. A Conversation in Four Parts. Part 1: Autoethnographies: constraints, openings, onto-logies, and findings. In Bochner, A. & Ellis, C. (eds) *Ethnographically Speaking*. AltaMira Press, Walnut Park, California, pp87–94.

Flemons, D. & Green, S. (2002b) Stories that conform/stories that transform. A Conversation in Four Parts. Part 4: Healing and Connecting. In Bochner, A. & Ellis, C. (eds) *Ethnographically Speaking*. AltaMira Press, Walnut Park, California, pp187–190.

Frank, A. (2000) Illness and autobiographical work: dialogue as narrative destabilization. *Qualitative Sociology* **23**(1): 135–156.

Frank, A. (2002) Relations of caring; demoralization and remoralization in the clinic. *International Journal of Human Caring* **6**(2): 13–19.

Frederiksson, L. (1999) Modes of relating in a caring conversation: a research synthesis on presence, touch and listening. *Journal of Advanced Nursing* **30**(5): 1167–76.

Friedson, E. (1970) *Professional Dominance*. Aldine Atherton, Chicago.

Gadamer, H.-G. (1975) *Truth and Method*. (Trans. Barden, G. & Cumming, J.) Seabury Press, New York.

Gerber, R. (1988) *Vibrational Healing*. Bear & Company Publishing, Santa Fe.

Georges, J. (2004) The Politics of suffering: implications for nursing science. *Advances In Nursing Science* **27**(4): 250–256.

Greene, M. (1988) *The Dialectic of Freedom*. Teachers College Press, Columbia University, New York.

Goethe, J.W. van (1999) *Maxims and Reflections*. Penguin Classics New Edition, London.

Goldstein, J. (2002) *One Dharma: The emerging Western Buddhism*. Rider, London.

Gully, E. (2005) Creating sacred space: a journey to the soul. In Johns, C. & Freshwater, D. (eds) *Transforming Nursing Through Reflective Practice* (2nd edition) Blackwell Publishing, Oxford.

Hall, L. (1964) Nursing – what is it? *Canadian Nurse* **60**(2): 150–154.

Halldórsdóttir, S. (1996) Caring and uncaring encounters in nursing and health care – developing a theory. *Medical Dissertations* No. 493. Department of Caring Sciences, Linköping University, Sweden.

Halldórsdóttir, S. (1999) Suffering . . . *International Journal for Human Caring* **3**(1).

Harrison, E. (2000) Intolerable human suffering and the role of the ancestor: literary criticism as a means of analysis. *Journal of Advanced Nursing* **32**(3): 689–694.

Hem, M. & Heggen, K. (2003) Being a professional and being human: one nurse's relationship with a psychiatric patient. *Journal of Advanced Nursing* **43**(1): 101–108.

Heyse-Moore, L.H. (1996) On spiritual pain in the dying. *Mortality* **1**(3): 297–315.

Hoad, T.F. (1986) *The Concise Oxford Dictionary of English Etymology*. Oxford University Press, Oxford.

Hodgson, H. (2000) Does reflexology impact on cancer patients' quality of life? *Nursing Standard* **14**(31): 33–38.

Howard, J. (1995) *The 38 Flower Remedies*. Wigmore Publications, London.

Jacobson, M. (1998) *Whiteness of a Different Colour: European immigrants and the alchemy of race*. Harvard University Press, Cambridge, MA.

James, N. (1989) Emotional labour: skill and work in the social regulation of feeling. *Sociological Review* **37**: 15–42.

Jarrett, L. & Johns, C. (2005) Constructing the reflexive narrative. In Johns, C. & Freshwater, D. (eds) *Transforming Nursing Through Reflective Practice* (2nd edition) Blackwell Publishing, Oxford, pp162–179.

Johns, C. (1991) The Burford Nursing Development Unit Holistic Model of Nursing Practice. *Journal of Advanced Nursing* **16**: 1090–1098.

Johns, C. (1994) *The Burford NDU Model: Caring in Practice*. Blackwell Science, Oxford.

Johns, C. (1995) Framing learning through reflection within Carper's fundamental ways of knowing. *Journal of Advanced Nursing* **22**: 226–234.

Johns, C. (1998) *Becoming an effective practitioner through guided reflection.* PhD thesis. Open University, Milton Keynes.

Johns, C. (2000a) *Becoming a Reflective Practitioner.* Blackwell Science, Oxford.

Johns, C. (2000b) Working with Alice. *Complementary Therapies in Nursing & Midwifery* **6**(4): 199–203.

Johns, C. (2002) *Guided Reflection: Advancing Practice.* Blackwell Publishing, Oxford.

Johns, C. (2004a) *Becoming a Reflective Practitioner* (2nd edition). Blackwell Publishing, Oxford.

Johns, C. (2004b) *Being Mindful, Easing Suffering: reflections on palliative care.* London, Jessica Kingsley Publishing.

Johns, C. (2005) Balancing the winds. *Reflective Practice* **6**(1): 67–84.

Johns, C. & Hardy, H. (2005) Voice as a metaphor for transformation through reflection. In Johns, C. & Freshwater, D. (eds) *Transforming Nursing through Reflective Practice.* Blackwell Publishing, Oxford, pp85–98.

Johns, C. & McCormack, B. (1998) Unfolding the conditions where the transformative potential of guided reflection (clinical supervision) might flourish or flounder. In Johns, C. & Freshwater, D. (eds) *Transforming Nursing Through Reflective Practice* (1st edition) . (eds C. Johns & D., Freshwater). Blackwell Science, Oxford, pp62–77.

Johnson, M. & Webb, C. (1995) Rediscovering unpopular patients: the concept of social judgment. *Journal of Advanced Nursing* **21**: 466–475.

Jones, Blackwolf & Jones, G. (1995) *Listen to the Drum.* Commune-A-Key Publishing, Salt Lake City.

Jones, Blackwolf & Jones, G. (1996) *Earth Dance Drum.* Commune-A-Key Publishing, Salt Lake City.

Jourard, S. (1971) *The Transparent Self.* Van Nostrand, Norwalk, CT.

Kearney, M. (1992) Palliative medicine – just another speciality? *Palliative Medicine* **6**: 39–46.

Kearney, M. (1997) *Mortally Wounded: Stories Of Soul Pain, Death and Healing.* Touchstone, New York.

Kelly, M.P. & May, D. (1982) Good and bad patients: a review of the literature and a theoretical critique. *Journal of Advanced Nursing* **7**: 147–156.

Klass, D., Silverman, P. & Nickman, S. (1996) *Continuing Bonds: New Understandings in Grief.* Taylor & Francis, London.

Knable, J. (1981) Handholding: one means of transcending barriers of communication. *Heart and Lung* **10**(6): 1106–10.

Kralik, D., Koch, T. & Telford, K. (2001) Constructions of sexuality for midlife women living with chronic illness. *Journal of Advanced Nursing* **35**(2): 180–187.

Kramer, M. (1990) Holistic nursing: implications for knowledge development and utilisation. In Chaska, N. (ed) *The Nursing Profession: Turning Points.* C.V. Mosby, St. Louis.

Kuhn, T. (1970) *The Structure of Scientific Revolutions.* University of Chicago Press, Chicago.

Lama Surya Das (1997) *Awakening the Buddha Within.* Bantam Books, London.

Lather, P. (1986a) Research as praxis. *Harvard Education Review* **56**(3): 257–277.

Lather, P. (1986b) Issues of validity in open ideological research: between a rock and a soft place. *Interchange* **17**(4): 63–84.

Lawler, J. (1991) *Behind the Screens: Nursing, Somology and the Problems of the Body.* Churchill Livingstone, Melbourne.

Lawless, J. (2002) *The Encyclopedia of Essential Oils.* Thorsons, London.

Lawton, J. (2000) *The Dying Process: patients' experiences of palliative care.* Routledge, London.

Leeuwen, R.Van & Cusveller, B. (2004) Nursing competencies for spiritual care. *Journal of Advanced Nursing* **48**(3): 234–246.

Lemieux, L., Kaiser, S., Pereira, J. & Meadows, L.M. (2004) Sexuality in spiritual care: patient perspectives. *Palliative Medicine* **18**: 630–637.

Logstrup, K.E. (1997) *The Ethical Demand*. University of Notre Dame Press, Notre Dame, Indiana.

Longaker, C. (1997) *Facing Death and Finding Hope*. Arrow Books, London.

Lunghi, M. (2004) Playing the endgame: reflections on waiting. *International Journal of Palliative Nursing* **10**(8): 374–377.

Margolis, H. (1993) *Paradigm and Barriers: how habits of mind govern scientific beliefs*. University of Chicago Press, Chicago.

Marris, P. (1986) *Loss and Change*. Routledge & Kegan Paul, London.

Matthew, I. (1995) *The Impact of God: Soundings from St John of the Cross*. Hodder & Stoughton, London.

Maury, M. (1989) *Marguerite Maury's Guide to Aromatherapy*. CW Daniel, Saffron Walden.

Mayeroff, M. (1971) *On Caring*. Harper Perennial, New York.

McNamara, B., Waddell, D. & Colvin, M. (1994) The institutionalisation of the good death. *Social Science & Medicine* **39**(11): 1501–1508.

Menzies-Lyth, I. (1988) A case study in the functioning of social systems as a defence against anxiety. In *Containing Anxiety in Institutions: Selected Essays*. Free Association Books, London.

Meta, A. & Ezer, H. (2003) My love is hurting: the meaning spouses attribute to their loved ones' pain during palliative care. *Journal of Palliative Care* **19**(2): 87–94.

Mezirow, J. (1981) A Critical theory of adult learning and education. *Adult Education* **32**(1): 3–24.

Miller, H. (1963) *Black Spring*. Grove Press, New York.

Milligan, M., Fanning, M., Hunter, S., Tadjali, M. & Stevens, E. (2002) Reflexology audit: patient satisfaction, impact on quality of life and availability in Scottish hospices. *International Journal of Palliative Nursing* **8**(100): 489–496.

Moncrieff, R. (1970) *Odours*. London: Heinemann Medical.

Morse, J. (1991) Negotiating commitment and involvement in the nurse-patient relationship. *Journal of Advanced Nursing* **16**: 552–558.

Naden, D. & Eriksson, K. (2002) Encounter: a fundamental category of nursing as art. *International Journal of Human Caring* **6**(1): 34–40.

Nagapriya (2004) *Exploring Karma and Rebirth*. Windhorse Publications, Birmingham.

Neihardt, J.G. (1988) *Black Elk Speaks*. A Bison Book, University of Nebraska Press, Lincoln, NE.

Newman, M. (1994) *Health as Expanded Consciousness*. National League for Nursing, New York.

Newman, M. (1999) The rhythm of relating in a paradigm of wholeness. *Image: Journal of Nursing Scholarship* **31**(3): 227–230.

Nhat Hanh, Thich. (1987) *Being Peace*. Parallax Press, Berkeley, CA.

Nhat Hanh, Thich. (1993) *The Blooming of a Lotus*. Beacon Press, Boston, MA.

Nhat Hanh, Thich. (2005) *Thich Nhat Hanh 2005 Calendar*, Brush Dance, San Rafael, CA.

National Health Service Management Executive (1993) *A Vision for the Future*. HMSO, London.

Noddings, N. (1984) *Caring – a Feminine Approach to Ethics and Moral Education*. University of California Press, Berkeley.

Norman, L. & Cowan, T. (1989) *The Reflexology Handbook*. Piatkus, London.

Nursing & Midwifery Council (2002) *Code of Professional Conduct*. NMC, London.

O'Donohue (1997) *Anam Cara*. Bantam Press, London.

Okri, B. (1997) *A Way of Being Free*. Phoenix House, London.

Oliver, M. (1990) *House of Light*. Beacon Press, Boston, MA.

Paramananda (2001) *A Deeper Beauty*. Windhorse, Birmingham.

Pearl, E. (2001) *The Reconnection: Heal Others, Heal Yourself*. Hay House Inc, Carlsbad, CA.

Pearson, A. (1983) *The Clinical Nursing Unit*. Heinemann, London.

Perbedy, S. (2000) Spiritual care of dying people. In Dickenson D. & Johnson, M. (eds) *Death, Dying and Bereavement*. The Open University and Sage Publications, London.

Perry, B. (1996) Influence of nurse gender on the use of silence, touch and humour. *International Journal of Palliative Nursing* **2**(1): 7–14.

Petrone , M. (1999) *Touching the Rainbow*. Health Promotion Department, East Sussex, Brighton and Hove Health Authority.

Petrone, M. (2003) *The Emotional Cancer Journey*. MAP Foundation (www.mapfoundation. org).

Pickrel, J. (1989) Tell me your story: using life review in counselling the terminally ill. *Death Studies* **13**: 127–135.

Pinar, W.F. (1981) 'Whole, bright, deep with understanding': issues in qualitative research and autobiographical method. *Journal of Curriculum Studies* **13**(3): 173–188.

Prashant, L. (2002) The art of holding space: degriefing part 3. *Massage and Bodywork*. **June/July**: 67–73.

Price, S. & Price, L. (1999) *Aromatherapy for Health Professionals* (2nd edition). Churchill Livingstone, Edinburgh.

Prigogine, I. (1980) *From Being to Becoming*. W.H. Freeman, San Francisco.

Puzan, E. (2003) The unbearable whiteness of being (in nursing). *Nursing Inquiry* **10**(3): 193–200.

Radbruch, L. (2002) Reflections on the use of sedation in terminal care. *European Journal of Palliative Care* **9**(6): 237–239.

Rael, J. (1993) *Being and Vibration*. Council Oak Books, Oklahoma.

Randall, F. & Downie, R.S. (1999) *Palliative Care Ethics* (2nd edition). Oxford University Press, Oxford.

Reiman, R.N. (1996) *Kitchen Table Wisdom: Stories that Heal*. Riverhead Books, New York.

Rinpoche, S. (1992) *The Tibetan Book of Living and Dying*. Rider, London.

Roach, Sr. S. (1992) *The Human Act of Caring*. Canadian Hospital Association Press, Ottawa.

Rogers, C. (1969) *Freedom to Learn: a view of what education might be*. Merrill, Columbus, OH.

Roper, N., Logan, W. & Tierney, A.J. (1980) *The Elements of Nursing*. Churchill Livingstone, Edinburgh.

Rossiter-Thornton, J. (2002) Prayer in your practice. *Complementary Therapies in Nursing & Midwifery* **8**(1): 21–28.

Roth, G. (1997) *Sweat your Prayers: movement as spiritual practice*. Newleaf, Dublin.

Rumi (2001) *Hidden Music*. Trans Maryam Mafi & Azima Melita Kolin. Thorsons, London.

Sahajananda, J.M. (2003) *You are the Light*. O Books, Winchester.

Salzberg, S. (1995) *Loving Kindness: the revolutionary art of happiness*. Shambhala, Boston.

Salzberg, S. (2002) *Faith: Trusting your own deepest experience*. Riverhead Books, New York.

Sangharakshita (1990) *Vision and Transformation*. Windhorse, Birmingham.

Sangharakshita (1997) *The Taste of Freedom* (2nd edition). Windhorse, Birmingham.

Sangharakshita (1999) *The Bodhisattva Ideal*. Windhorse, Birmingham.

Schön, D. (1983) *The Reflective Practitioner*. Avebury, Aldershot.

Schön, D. (1987) *Educating the Reflective Practitioner*. Jossey-Bass, San Francisco.

Schwarcz, V. (1997) The pane of sorrow: public uses of personal grief in modern China. In Kleinman, A., Das, V. & Lock, M. (eds). *Social Suffering*. University of California Press, Berkeley, CA.

Seedhouse, D. (1988) *Ethics: the heart of health care*. John Wiley, Chichester.

Senge, P. (1990) *The 5th Discipline: the art and practice of the learning organisation*. Century Business, London.

Sherwood, G. (1997) Patterns of caring: the healing connection of interpersonal harmony. *International Journal of Human Caring* 1(1): 30–38.

Smith, J. & Deemer, D. (2000) The problem of criteria in the age of relativism. In Denzin, N. & Lincoln, Y. (eds) *Handbook of Qualitative Research* (2nd edition). Sage, London, pp887–896.

Stewart, I. and Joines, V. (1987) *TA Today: a new introduction to Transactional Analysis*. Lifespace Publishing, Nottingham & Chapel Hill.

Stockwell, F. (1972) *The Unpopular Patient*. Royal College of Nursing, London.

Street, A. (1992) *Inside Nursing: a critical ethnography of clinical nursing*. State University of New York Press, Albany.

Stroebe, M. & Schut, H. (1999) The dual process of coping with bereavement: rationale and description. *Death Studies* 23: 197–224.

Surya Das, L. (1997) *Awakening the Buddha Within*. Bantam Books, London.

Susuki, S. (1999) *Zen Mind, Beginner's Mind: informal talks on Zen meditation and practice*. (1st revised edition) Weatherhill, New York.

Thomas, K. & Kilmann, R. (1974) *Thomas Kilmann Conflict Mode Instrument*. Xicom, Toledo, OH.

Tolle, E. (2001) *The Power of NOW*. Hodder & Stoughton, London.

Toombs, S. (1995) The Lived Experience of Disability. *Human Studies* 18: 9–23.

Tong, E., McGraw, S., Dobihal, E., Baggish, R., Cherlin E. & Bradley E. (2003) What is a good death? Minority and Non-minority perspectives. *Journal of Palliative Care* 19(3): 168–175.

Trueman, I. & Parker, J. (2004) Life review in palliative care. *European Journal of Palliative Care* 11(6): 249–253.

Trungpa, C. (1984) *Shambhala: The Sacred Path of the Warrior*. Shambhala, Boston.

Trungpa, C. (2002) *Cutting Through Spiritual Materialism*. Shambhala, Boston.

Tufnell, M. & Crickmay, C. (2004) *A Widening Field: Journeys in Body and Imagination*. Dance Books, Alton.

Walter, T. (1999) *On Bereavement: the culture of grief*. Open University Press, Buckingham.

Walter, T. (2002) Spirituality in palliative care: opportunity or burden? *Palliative Medicine* 16: 133–139.

Wheatley, M. (1999) *Leadership and the New Science: Discovering Order In A Chaotic World*. Berrett-Koehler publishers, San Francisco.

White, K., Wilkes, L., Cooper, K. & Barbato, M. (2004) The impact of unrelieved patient suffering on palliative care nurses. *International Journal of Palliative Nursing* 10(9): 438–444.

Wholihan, D. (1992) The value of reminiscence in hospice care. *American Journal of Hospice Palliative Care* 9: 33–35.

Wilber, K. (1998) *The eye of spirit: an integral vision for a world gone slightly mad.* Shambhala, Boston.

Woolf, V. (1945) *A Room of One's Own.* Penguin Books, Harmondsworth.

World Health Organization (2003) Defintion of palliative care. www.who.int/cancer/palliative/definition/en

Winterson, J. (2001) *The Powerbook.* Vintage, London.

Winterson, J. (2004) *The Passion.* Vintage, London.

Winterson, J. (2005) *Lighthousekeeping.* Harper Perennial, London.

Worwood, V. (1999) *The Fragrant Heavens: the spiritual dimension of fragrance and aromatherapy.* Doubleday, London.

Wright, M. (2002) The essence of spiritual care: a phenomenological enquiry. *Palliative Medicine* **16**: 125–132.

Young, M. & Cullen, L. (1996) *A Good Death: Conversations with East Londoners.* Routledge, London.

Younger, J. (1995) The alienation of the sufferer. *Advances in Nursing Science* **17**(4): 53–72.

Discography

Bliss: *Bliss – the Journey* (1997) Diviniti Publishing.

Rusty Crutcher: *Serpent Mound* (1996) *Ocean Eclipse* (1992) *Chaco Canyon* (1990) all Emerald Green Sound (www.emeraldgreensound.com).

Enya: *Watermark* (1988) WEA Records.

Hilmar Örn Hilmarsson and Sigur Ros: *Angels of the Universe* (2001) Fat Cat Records.

Kate Rusby: *Falling*, from *Underneath the Stars* (2003) Pure Records.

Suzanne Vega: *Cracking*, from Suzanne Vega (1985) A&M Records.

Index

Page entries for figures are denoted in *italic*.
Page entries for boxes are denoted in **bold**.

action-oriented reflection, 7–8
aesthetic response, 31–2
agitation
    Callum, 160, 161, 163–4
    Carol, 109, 112
    as soul pain, 166–7, 168
    Tommy, 253, 258
Ain-dah-ing, 229
aloneness, 39, 40, 43–4, 51, 223–4
alternative, *see* complementary medicine
ancestral roots, connecting with, 237–8, 239,
        240
Andrea (patient), 126–32, 137
    anger at misdiagnosis, 126–7
    brave face, 128
    compassion for, 130, 131
    complementary/medical therapies,
        tension between, 128, 129
    healing crisis, 127
    nausea, 128, 129, 131, 132
    poem for, untitled, 130
    valley of love, 127
Angels of the Universe, film music, 233
anger about dying, 126–7, 198, 213, 214
Anne (patient)/Gay, 158–60
    remembrance through, 160
antidepressant, grapefruit as, 146
anxiety
    facing/harnessing, 53
    Gerard, 89, 90
    Hugh, 225–6
    Jackie, 78, 80, 82
    Penny, 175
    therapist's, 53, 159, 160
aroma stones/aromatherapy, **265**; *see also*
        essential oils
    Andrea, 129, 132
    Anne, 159, 160

Carol, 110, 111
Edith, 228
Gerard, 88, 89, 99, 104
Jackie, 73–4, 77
Jim, 70, 71
Kristin, 145, 146, 153, 154
Linda, 133, 134, 136, 137, 139
Louise, 186
Martha, 246
Martin, 198, 199
Morgan, 115, 117
Penny, 169
Peter, 123–4
placebo effect, 234
Richard, 230
role in creating reverence/serenity, 202
role in easing suffering, 251
Ruby, 189
staff failure to maintain, 250, 251
Trevor, 142
The Art of Holding Space paper, 77, 78
assertiveness mantra, 186
attention, paying, 188; *see also* mindfulness
Avril, 205–7, 208
    despair, 205
    essential oils, spiritual qualities, 205, 206
    faith, 206–7
    poem, *Falling*, 206
    silent scream, 206

Bach Flower Remedies, 227
bathing patients, 192, 193, 259, 260
Beck, Yoko, 20
Being, 223
being available template, 21, *22*, 35, 49, 57
being heard, 54
being in-place, *8*, 8–9
Being Mindful, easing Suffering, 56, 61
Being and Vibration, 187
being with mentality, 125
Billie, 204–5, 208

Bimadisawin, 3
Bliss (group), 214, 232
Bloom, William, 74
Blue poem, 105
boundaries
    personal/professional, 177, 201, 247, 249, 250
    therapeutic, 154, 158
The breath poem, 215
The breath of love poem, 239
breath work, 37–8
breathing
    cheyne-stoke, 107
    role of massage, 211–12
bringing the mind home, 37–8
brokenness of the other, sensitivity to, 27, 28
Buddhism, 3, 5
    essential phowa, 67, 85, 107, 154, 199
    noble truths, **23**
Burford Nursing Development Unit (NDU) model, 12, 19
    ensuring model realises effective practice, 15–16
    explicit assumptions, 12–13
    leadership, 19
    learning organisation, 12, 13, 16–18, 19
    mental models, 18
    personal mastery, 18–19
    reflective systems, 13–16
    structural view of reflective framework, *13*
    systems thinking, 18
burn-out, 33
butterfly effect, 9–10

The call home poem, 200
Callum (patient)/Rachel, 160–68
    agitation, 160, 161, 163–4, 166, 167
    chaos, 163
    compassion for, 164, 165, 166
    complementary medicine, attitudes towards, 164
    delayed diagnosis, 165
    dependence/regression, 161–2
    despair, 161
    fall into grace, 167, 168
    family conflicts, 165
    fear of death, 167
    handholding, 164
    mindfulness of discomfort, 165–6
    sedative/neuroleptic medication, 163, 164, 165, 168

soul pain, 166–7, 168
    touch, 162, 163
caregiver/receiver relationship, 20–21
caring
    as dance, 3–4, 66, 72, 125
    environment, *34*, 34–5
    holistic vision, 7–8
    investing with meaning, 10
    loss of, 33
    making visible, 7–8
    spiritual realm, 222–4
Caring in Practice, *see* Burford Nursing Development Unit (NDU) model
Carl (patient), 61
Carol (patient)/Amanda, 108–14
    agitation, 109, 112
    hallucinations/visits from the dead, 108–9
    holism, 113
    sedation dilemma, 109, 112
    symptom management approach, 112–13
    watching your own daughter die, 110–11
case study vs. chronological approach, 56
centering rituals, 188
Chaco Canyon, 146, 230
chaos, 6–7, 9–10, 57–8, 163
cheyne-stoke breathing, 107
Cindy (patient), 190–92
    facial expressions during therapy, 190
Clay poem, 243
closure ritual, 87
Code of Professional Conduct (NMC), 201
coherence, 60–1
comfort zone, 54
commitment, 9, 53, 60, 242
communication, staff, 15, 256–7, *257*
compassion, 27–9
    brokenness of other, sensitivity to, 27, 28
    non-attachment, 29
    for patients, 130, 164, 165, 166, 195
    reflection on, 131, 177
    touching, spiritual, 29
    trap, 218, *219*, 220
complementary therapy/ies
    attitudes towards, 128, 129, 164
    marginalisation of, 186
    over-learning of techniques, 189–90
    and refusal of conventional, 88, 89, 94, 97
    resistance to, 230, 231, 240
    summary of, **265**
confession of suffering, 201
conflict, managing, *71*

connection with the other person, 72, 78
consciousness
    dwelling, 24
    expanded, 6
    levels of, 54, 99, 188, *255, 256*
constructed voice, 125, *126*
contradiction, dealing with, 5–6
control, being in, 167, 168, 183, 227; *see also*
    good death
crisis
    healing, 127
    recognition, 6
critical consciousness levels, 54
crooked/straight arrows, 254–5
Crutcher, Rusty, 80, 89, 133, 137, 146, 230,
    236
cues for action, 47–8

dance
    caring, 3–4, 66, 72, 125
    five rhythms of, **66**
    synchronised talk, 229
dead, visits from, 76–7, 108–9
death, *see* dying
A Deeper Beauty, 214
The Deer poem, 214
depression, Edith, 228, 236, 237
despair, 161, 205, 235
diagnosis, delayed/wrong, 126–7, 165
dialogue, *see* levels of dialogue; narrative
    dialogue
dignity, 114, 120, 143, 148, 172
discipline, 9, 59–60
distance/intimacy, 158, 121–2
divine light, 67, 85, 86, 107
Donald (patient), 258–60
    bathing, 259, 260
    life story, 259
    putting house in order, 259
dreams, 237
    unfulfilled, 25
dwelling consciousness, 24
dying/facing death, 21, 24–5; *see also* fear of
    death; good death
    acceptance, 72, 79, 81, 167, 168
    complacency towards, 201
    euphemisms for, 245
    false prophecies of time of, 258
    feelings about, 68, 198
    mystery of, 68, 179, 197, 204
    reverence for, 30
    social death, 151, 180

    talking about, 240
    waiting for, 152, 153
    watching your own daughter die, 110–11
    what is it like, 25, 30, 205

ear reflex point, 261
Edith (patient), 228–9, 236, 237, 238
    Ain-dah-ing, 229
    depression, 228, 236, 237
    Indian head massage, 228–9
    synchronised talk dance, 229
Edward (patient), 65–9
    essential phowa, Buddhist practice, 67
    family conflicts, 66, 67
    feelings about death, 68
ego integrity, 210
Elizabeth (patient), 181–5
    being in control, 183
    niceness, hospice culture of, 181–2, 183
    palliative perspective, use of medical
        resources, 184
    respecting patient's decisions, 184, 185
Emotional Cancer Journey, 41
emotional labour/care, 104, 193–4
empathy, 33, 248
empowerment based on understanding, 7
The Endorphin Effect, 74
energy, healing, 45, 187, 188, *188*, 223, 233,
    246–7
The English Patient film, 142
Enya, 77, 99, 147, 156, 158, 199, 203, 226
Eric (patient), 260–61
essential oils
    benzoin, 115, 117, 142, 211
    bergamot, 88, 125, 205
    eucalyptus, 189
    frankincense, 73, 89, 142, 145, 154, 159,
        169, 230
    geranium, 262
    grapefruit, 146, 228
    juniper berry, 159, 169, 263
    lavender, 88, 104, 189, 205, 228, 241, 263
    lemon, 262
    marjoram, 104
    neroli, 99
    patchouli, 73, 89, 159, 169, 228, 230
    peppermint, 129, 132
    pettigrain, 137, 205, 234
    remembrance through, 160
    rose, 228
    sandalwood, 145, 246
    spiritual qualities, 99, 205, 206, 246

tea tree, 104
vetiver, 136–7, 142
ylang ylang, 133, 134, 135
essential phowa, Buddhist practice, 67, 85, 107, 154, 199
ethical action, 46–7
evidence-based practice, 11, 46
experience
   learning from, 47
   practical wisdom, 10–11
   reflection-on, 4, 5
expert-based practice, 11, 32, 130
expertise, reflection on, 130–32

facials, 145–6, 263
Faith, 206
faith, 239; *see also* God; spirituality
   avoiding imposition of, 26–7
   loss of, 216–19
   patient's, 206–7
   practitioner's, 217, 263
fall into grace, 167, 168, 176
Falling poem, 206
false consciousness, 5–6
family conflicts, 66, 67, 165, 258
fear of death
   Billie, 204, 205
   Callum, 167
   Edith, 229
   Hugh, 227
   Jane, 217, 220
   Kristin, 145
   Tommy, 253
feminist perspectives, 58–9
Finding stillness within poem, 38
foot massage, *see* reflexology; massage
four quadrant model, 50, *51*, 60
framing
   perspectives, 48–9, **49**
   theoretical, 46
funerals, 86–7, *87*, 105–6, 156–7, 247–50

Gerard (patient), 88–107
   anxiety, 89, 90
   autonomy, personal/professional, 92, *92*
   Blue poem, 105
   cancer spread/realism, 92, 93–5
   family grief, 98
   funeral, 105–6
   good death, 103
   healing space, 99

The heron & the tree poem, 104
   humour, 89, 99
   music, 89, 99, 106
   opioid therapy, 96
   presence, 98
   refusal of conventional medicine, 88, 89, 94, 97
   spiritual/religious, 93
   stench of wound, 88, 89, 92, 104
Gill (patient), 233
God, *see also* faith; spirituality
   blaming, 213, 214, 216–19
   grace of, 197
good death, 60, 180–81; *see also* dying
   culture, 200, 256
   as easing suffering, 181
   expectation of, 218, 221
   quest for, 80, 81, 83, 84, 103
   and sedation, 180
   ten domains of, *113*, 113–14
good intention, long shadow of, 219
goodbye, saying, 74–5
grace
   fall into, 167, 168, 177
   of God, 197
grief, 21
   family, 82, 87–8, 98
   for Kristin, 155, 157, 158
   for Martin, 200
   reflection on, 225
ground beneath your feet, feeling, 216
growth, as mutual process of realisation, 12
guidance, need for, 52–4
Guided Reflection: advancing practice, 56

hallucinations/visits from the dead, 108–9
handholding, 164; *see also* touch
Hanh, Thich Nhat, 97, 201
healing, **265**
   and compassion, 27–9
   energy, 45, 187, 188, *188*, 223, 233, 246–7
   love, 238
   space, 77–8, 99
health, 6, 20, 21
Hebs (patient), 207–8
Henry (patient), 208–10
   ego integrity, 210
   life review, 209–10
The heron & the tree poem, 41, 65, 86, 87, 104
   imagery, 80, 81, 82–3
   narrative approach, 36

Hettie poem, 235
holistic vision of caring, 7–8, 20, 113
holographic reflection, 9–10, *10*
hospice, 65
    culture of niceness, 181–2, 183, 256
    talk, 245
hovering-in-the-moment, 73
Hugh (patient), 225–8
    anxiety, 225–6
    Bach Flower Remedies, 227
    fear of death/losing control, 227
    guilt/pain of spouse, 226
humour, 72, 78, 89, 99

idiot compassion, 218, *219*
Indian head massage, 228–9, **265**
Indigo (patient), 250–53
    poem, *Renewal*, 252, 253
    step of perfect speech, 251
    stress accumulation, water butt
        metaphor, 252–3
influences grid, *45*
information needed, to nurse
    patient/family, 13–15, 102, 123, 210
intimacy/distance, 158, 121–2
*Intolerable human suffering: the role of the
    ancestor*, 237
intuition, 32, 132, 189

Jackie (patient), 41, 72–88
    acceptance of death, 72, 79, 81
    anxiety, 78, 80, 82
    connection with the other person, 72,
      78
    divine light, 85, 86
    essential phowa, Buddhist practice, 85
    family grief, 82, 87–8
    funeral, 86–7, *87*
    good death, quest for, 80, 81, 83, 84
    guided meditation, 75–6
    The heron & the tree poem, 86, 87
    humour, 84
    mindfulness of healing space, 77
    music, 77, 80, 82, 87
    presence in the moment, 76, 78, 85
    reverence, 85
    saying goodbye, 74–5
    sedation, 80, 82, 83
    silence, 72, 84
    smiling, 74
    visits from the dead, 76–7
    withdrawal from the world, 82

Jane (patient), 216–21
    compassion trap, 220
    expectation of good death, 218, 221
    faith, loss of, 216–19
    fear of death, 217, 220
    feeling the ground beneath your feet,
      216
    long shadow of good intention, 219
    pain under control of patient, 221
    sedation, resisting, 220, 221
    soul pain, 221
    spiritual traps, 218, *219*, 244
Jim (patient), 70–71
Jones, Blackwolf and Gina, 3, 4, 69, 148, 154,
    155, 158, 229, 254, 255, 264
journal writing, 39–41
The Journey, 214, 215, 232
Joyce (patient), 189–90

The kiss of the dark god poem, 244
knowing
    desirable practice, 20–21, 35
    the person, 14, 29–31, 131, 230, 233
    reflective, 11
    self, 33
    sources of, 46–50
    tacit, 32
Kristin (patient), 143–58, 182
    death, 154
    dignity, 148
    essential phowa, Buddhist practice, 154
    facial, 145–6
    fear of death, 145
    funeral, 156–7
    grief, 155, 157, 158
    healing, 146, 147
    intimacy and distance, 158
    love, 155, 156, 158
    music therapy, 147
    pathologising selfhood, 150
    poems, *A love story / The waiting room*, 152,
      154, 156
    power of touch, 148
    sexuality, 146, 150, 151
    social death/withdrawal, 151
    spirituality, 157
    suffering, space/distance from, 155
    therapeutic boundaries, 154, 158

labels, difficult patient, 134–5, 136, 140
Lady Marmalade, 157
leadership, 19

learning
  from experience, 47
  holograph of reflective, *10*
  organisation, creating, 12, 13, 16–18, 19
  team, 17–18
Len (patient), 210–12
  authority, perceptions of, 210–11
  essential oils to help breathing, 211
  massage, important role in pulmonary therapy, 211–12
letting go, 167, 168, 248
levels of dialogue, 36
  with other sources of knowledge, 50–1
  with self, 37–41
  with story text, 41–5
  between text and guides/peers, 52–5
  between text and other sources of knowing, 46–50
  to weave narrative, 55–61
life stories, *see* stories
light, divine, 67, 85, 86, 107
Linda (patient), 132–41
  difficult patient labels, 134–5, 136, 140
  music, 133, 134
  sexuality, 133, 135, 136, 138–9, 140–41
listening, mindful, 30, 188
Logstrup, Knud Ejler, 28, 29
Louise (patient), 185–7
  assertiveness mantra, 186
love
  expressing, 195, 199
  and fear of death, 229
  healing, 238
  Kristin, 155, 156, 158
  Penny, 170
  Russell, 214
  unconditional, 27–9
  valley of, 127, 174
A love story poem, 156
Luke (patient), 177–9
  finding meaning, 179
  mystery of death, 179
  relatives, therapy for, 178, 179

managing conflict grid, *71*
Martha (patient)/Millie, 246–50
  funeral attendance, 247, 248, 249, 250
  personal/professional boundaries, 247, 249, 250
  touch, taboo/understanding, 246, 247, 248

Martin (patient), 192–201
  anger about dying, 198
  anguish, unrecognised by nurses, 199
  bathing a patient, 192, 193
  compassion, 195
  confusion, 196
  drug toxicity, 194, 195, 196
  emotional labour/care, 193–4
  essential phowa, 199
  grief, 200
  love, expressing, 195, 199
  pain control problems, 192, 194, 195
  patient confidentiality rights, 192–3
  poem, *The call home*, 200
  sedation, request for, 199
  symptom management, 192, 200
massage, **265**
  arm, 221
  foot, *see* reflexology
  Indian head, 228–9
  pulling out pain/nausea through, 203, 218, 230, 242
  role in pulmonary therapy, 211–12
Maureen (patient), 201–2
meaning, 68
  finding, 116, 179, 238
  of health/illness for this person, 14, 123, 210
  investing caring with, 10
medical model, 14, 31
meditation, 37–8, 75–6, 97, 215
mental models, 18
methodological influences grids, 53, *56*, 249
Michael's wife, 139
mindfulness, 4–5, 25, 132, 188, 244–5
  of discomfort, 165–6
  essential oils to improve, 211
  of healing space, 77
  listening, 188
  and over-learning of techniques, 189–90
  of self, 4, 9, 33
  through reflection, 264
Mindfulness of Breathing meditation practice, 215
misdiagnosis, 126–7, 165
model for structured reflection (MSR), 42, *42, 49*, 49–50
models, mental, 18
Mona (patient), 122–3
mooring metaphor, 238

Morgan (patient), 114–18
facing illness/finding meaning, 116
sedatives, 117, 118
motivation, 53
motor neurone disease (MND), 114, 115
MSR (model for structured reflection), 42, *42*, *49*, 49–50
multiple sclerosis, 132, 140
music for
Billie, 205
Gerard, 89, 99, 106
Jackie, 77, 80, 82, 87
Kristin, 147
Linda, 133, 134
Muslim culture/religion, 107–8, 244
mystery of death, 68, 179, 197, 204
myth of the hero, 167

Namaji/higher state of consciousness, *255*, *256*
narrative dialogue, 36–7, 51; *see also* levels of dialogue; stories
adequacy/coherence, 56, 60–1
case study vs. chronological approach, 56
disruption/destabilisation narratives, 61
editing/culling entries, 56
plot, 57
reflective text, constructing, *55*, 56
reflexivity, 57–8
self-inquiry, 57
weaving, 52, 55–61
National Institute for Clinical Excellence (NICE) guidelines, 223
nature, connection with, 187
nausea, relief through massage, 218
NDU model, *see* Burford Nursing Development Unit (NDU) model
niceness, hospice culture of, 181–2, 183, 256
noble eight-fold path of suffering, 25–7, *26*, *27*, 119, 250, 251
noble truths, Buddhist philosophy, **23**
non-attachment, 29
notes, patient's, 186
now, 76, 78, 85
nurses, *see also* practitioners
bad nurse labels, 140
disempowerment of, 34–5
insensitivity, 199
male, 101–2
non-engagement, 70, 71
oppression of, 7, 8

parental behaviour towards patients, 253, 256–8
suffering, effect on, 200
Nursing Development Unit (NDU) model, *see* Burford Nursing Development Unit (NDU) model

Ocean Eclipse music, 137, 236
odour/perfuming, 123–4; *see also* aroma-stones; aromatherapy
Okri, Ben, 51
Oliver, Mary, 214, 215
opioid therapy, 96
organisational culture, *34*, 34–5
Outing, 207

pain
anticipating, 205
control problems, 192, 194, 195
drawing out through massage, 203, 230, 242
Penny, 175
relief, 202, 203
soul, 99, 166–7, 168, 221
of spouse, 226
under control of patient, 221
palliative
care, vision for, 22
perspective, use of medical resources, 184
WHO definition of, **23**
panic attacks, 253, 258
Paramanandra, 214
parental behaviour, nurses, 253, 256–8
The Passion, 59
patients, *see also* Andrea; Anne; Callum; Carl; Carol; Cindy; Donald; Edith; Edward; Elizabeth; Eric; Gerard; Gill; Hebs; Henry; Hugh; Indigo; Jackie; Jane; Jim; Joyce; Kristin; Len; Linda; Louise; Luke; Martha; Martin; Maureen; Mona; Morgan; Paula; Pauline; Penny; Peter; Rachel; Ralph; Richard; Ron; Ruby; Russell; Saved; Susan; Tommy; Tony; Trevor; Veronica; Yasmina
confidentiality rights, 192–3
difficult patient labels, 134–5, 136, 140
empowerment, 187
feelings, paying attention to, 43–4
information needed to nurse, 13–15
knowing, 29–31, 131, 230, 233
negative feelings towards, 123

respecting decisions/wishes, 172, 184, 185
seeing beauty in, 214, 223, 224
standing alongside/dwelling with, 24
pattern of situation, 131
Paula (patient), 179–80
Pauline (patient), 261–3
cremation wish, 262
facial, 263
poems, untitled, 262, 263
Pearl, Eric, 188–9, 190–91
peers, guidance from, 52–5
Penny (patient), 168–77
anxiety, 175
dignity, 172
love for, 170, 174
making a will, 173
pain, 175
poems, untitled/*Sometimes*, 171, 172, 176
relationships with children, 173, 174
respect for wishes, 172
sacred, 170, 177
unease/resistance, 169
visualisation, healing light, 169
perfect effort steps, 119
perfuming, 123–4
Peter (patient)/Sam, 123–6
Petrone, Michele Angelo, 41
phronesis, 10
placebo effect, aromatherapy, 234
playfulness, 59–60
poems/poetry, 40, 41; *see also The heron & the tree*
on being alone, 224
Blue, 105
The breath, 215
The breath of love, 239
The call home, 200
Clay, 243
The Deer, 214
Falling, 206
Finding stillness within, 38
Hettie, 235
The journey, 214, 215, 232
The kiss of the dark god, 244
A love story, 156
Renewal, 252, 253
Sometimes, 171
untitled, 130, 143, 172, 176, 204, 222, 262–3
The waiting room, 152, 154
poignancy, 67

The Powerbook, 42–3
practitioner/s, *see also* nurses
assertiveness, 240
availability, 12, 111–12
burn-out, 33
communication patterns, 256–7, *257*
containment of despair, 235
faith, 217, 263
guilt, 241, 242
personal mastery, 18–19
presence in the moment, 76, 78, 85
professional/personal
autonomy, 92, *92*
boundaries, 177, 201, 247, 249, 250
professionalist stance, 33
proprioception of thought, 36
pulmonary therapy, *see* breathing
putting one's house in order, 259

quieting us so we can hear, 246, 248

Rachel (patient), 202–4
pain relief, 202, 203
poem for, 204
Rael, Joseph, 187, 188
Ralph (patient)/Maisey, 118–22
dignity, 120
going home to die decision, 119, 120
perfect effort steps, 119
touch/hugs, 120, 121
realism, 92, 93–5, 259
The Reconnection, 188
reflection, 3–4
action-oriented, 7–8
being in-place, *8*, 8–9
contradiction, 5–6
harnessing energy, *6*, 6–7
holographic reflection, 9–10, *10*
mindfulness, 4–5
practical wisdom, 10–11
qualities, 9
reflection-on-experience, 4, 5
triggers for, 6
reflections inspired by
Andrea, 130–32
Avril, 206–7
Callum, 165–6
Carol, 111–14
Edward, 67–9
Gerard, 96–7, 100–03, 104
Jackie, 73, 75, 78, 81, 87
Kristin, 158

reflections inspired by (*cont'd*)
  Linda, 134–5
  Luke, 179
  Martha, 247–50
  Martin, 200–01
  Mona, 123
  Morgan, 118
  Penny, 176–7
  Peter, 125, *126*
  Ralph, 121–2
  Richard, 237–9, 240, 242
  Saved, 108
  Tommy, 253, 256–8
  Veronica, 225
reflective
  framework, structural view, *13*
  knowing, 11
  model for clinical practice, *see* Burford
    Nursing Development Unit (NDU)
    model
  practice, 3–4, 11
  systems, 13–16
  text, constructing, *55*, 56
reflexivity, 12–13, 54, 57–8
reflexology, *see also* massage
  Andrea, 127, 128, 129, 132
  Eric, 261
  Gerard, 89–91, 94, 97–9
  Hugh, 226, 227
  Jackie, 78, 80, 83, 84
  Kristin, 147
  Jane, 218
  Linda, 134
  Luke, 178, 179
  Martin, 195
  Morgan, 115, 116
  Penny, 169, 170, 173
  Richard, 230, 232, 236, 240
relationship, caregiver/receiver, 20–21
  assertiveness in, 253–4, 256, 257–8
  non-attachment, 29
relatives, therapy for, 178, 179
  Amanda, 108–14
  Gay, 158–60
  Hettie, 235, 240
  Maisey, 118–22
  Michael's wife, 139
  Millie, 246–50
  Rachel, 160–68
  Sam, 123–6
relaxation, 37–8, 51
religion, 68; *see also* faith; God; spirituality

Muslim, 107–8 , 244
remembrance through aroma, 160
remoralisation, 173
Renewal poem, 252, 253
responsibility, ranking areas of, *249*
reverence, 85
Richard (patient)/Hettie, 229–33, 233–5,
    236–43
  caring commitment, 242
  comfort, need for, 231
  containing despair, 235
  deterioration, 231
  dreams/visualisations, 237
  knowing him, 230, 233
  poems, *The breath of love/Clay/Hettie*, 235,
    239, 243
  relief of pain through massage, 230, 242
  resistance to complementary therapy,
    230, 231
  suffering of spouse, 235, 240
  talking about dying, 240
ritual
  centering, 188
  closure, 87
  funeral, 106
roller coaster metaphor, 235, 258
Ron (patient), 114
A Room of One's Own, 58
Roth, Gabrielle, 66
Ruby (patient), 189
Rusby, Kate, 206
Russell (patient), 212–15
  anger, 213, 214
  beauty, 214
  love, 214
  poems, *The Breath/The Journey*, 214, 215,
    232

sacred, 170, 177
  space, 202
  vibration, 187, *188*
Sahajananda, 197
Saint John of the Cross, quotation from, 58,
    164, 174
sati, 4
Saved (patient), 107–8
  divine light, 107
  essential phowa, Buddhist practice, 107
  Muslim culture, 107–8
sedation
  Callum, 163, 164, 165, 168
  Carol, 109, 112

Jackie, 80, 82, 83
  Morgan, 117, 118
  request for, Martin, 199
  resisting, Jane, 220, 221
  as social death, 180
self
  dialogue with, 37–41
  knowing, 33
  mindfulness of, 4, 9, 33
  sharing, 254–5
  storied, 39–41
  true nature of, 223
  understanding in context, 7
self-inquiry, 57
selfhood, pathologising, 150
Serpent's mound music, 80, 133
sexuality
  Kristin, 146, 150, 151
  Linda, 133, 135–6, 138–9, 140–41
silence, 72, 84
smells, pleasure of, 207–8; *see also* aroma-
    stones/aromatherapy
smiling, 74
social death, 82, 151, 180
soft ground beneath my feet, 245, 246, 248
Sometimes, 171
soul
  dark night of, 174
  pain, 99, 166–7, 168, 221
sound/vibration
  sacred, 187, *188*
  transmission, healing as, 188, 223, 233,
    246–7
space
  healing, 77–8, 99
  sacred, 202
spiritual touching, 29
spirituality, 67–9; *see also* faith
  Buddhist perspective, 69
  Gerard, 93
  Indigo, 251
  Jackie, 84
  Jim, 71
  Kristin, 157
  Maureen, 202
  realm of care, 222–4
  and religion, 68
  responding to patient needs, 44
  traps, 218, *219*, 244
spouses, *see* relatives
step of perfect speech, 251
stillness, 37–8

storied self, 39–41
stories
  change through, 61
  Donald, 259
  Henry, 209–10
  knowing patient's, 131
  listening to, 30
story text, dialogue with, 41–5
  drawing out significance, 42–3
  influences grid, *45*
  influencing factors, 44–5, *44*
  paying attention to feelings, 43–4
  responding to patient spiritual needs, 44
stress accumulation, water butt metaphor,
    252–3
suffering
  acknowledging, 22
  cause, 24
  confession of, 201
  easing, 12, 22, 24–5, 237, 251
  effect on nurses, 200
  empathising with, 33
  expressing, 238, 239
  finding meaning in, 238
  intolerable, 237, *238*
  noble eight-fold path, 25–7, *26*, *27*, 119,
    250, 251
  noble truths, Buddhist philosophy, **23**
  reflection on, 237–9, 240
  space/distance from, 155
  spirituality and, 71
  of spouse, 235, 240
  unrelieved, 103
supervision, clinical, 54–5
Susan (patient), 137–8
swampy lowlands metaphor, 32, 54
*Sweat your Prayers; movement as spiritual
    practice*, 66
symptom management model, 112–13, 192,
    200, 223
synchronised talk dance, 229
systems thinking, 18

TA (transactional analysis), 256–7, *257*
taboo, touching as, 246, 247, 248
talk dance, synchronised, 229
team learning, 17–18
therapeutic touch (TT)
  Anne, 159
  Callum, 165
  Cindy, 190, 191
  Elizabeth, 183, 184

therapeutic touch (TT) (*cont'd*)
  Gerard, 89, 90, 91, 94, 99
  Indigo, 250
  Jackie, 77
  Joyce, 189
  Kristin, 147, 149, 151, 153–4
  Martha, 247, 248
  Martin, 194, 195, 196, 197, 199
  Mona, 123
  Penny, 176
  Rachel, 203
  Richard, 241
  Yasmina, 244, 245
therapies, *see* complementary therapies
therapists, *see* practitioners
time, giving/having, 73, *73*
Tommy (patient), 253–8
  agitation/panic attacks, 253, 258
  assertiveness, relations with nursing staff, 253–4, 256, 257–8
  crooked/straight arrows, 254–5
  false prophecies of time of death, 258
  family conflicts, 258
  fear of process of dying, 253
  inner harmony, 255–6
  Namaji/higher state of consciousness, *255, 256*
  niceness, hospice culture, 256
  roller coaster metaphor, 258
  sharing self, 254–5
Tony (patient), 180, 181
touch/touching, 112, 162, 163
  power of, 148
  Ralph, 120, 121
  socially acceptable, 100–03, 106, 121, 247
  spiritual, 29
  as taboo, 246, 247, 248
  therapeutic, *see* therapeutic touch
Touching the Rainbow, 41
transactional analysis (TA)/patterns of communication, 256–7, *257*
Trevor (patient), 141–3
  dignity, 143
  poem for, 143
trust, attributes of, 52, **53**
truth, 7, 8, 197
  commitment to, 60
  noble, Buddhist philosophy, **23**

TT, *see* therapeutic touch
Tufnell, Miranda, 41

unconditional love, 27–9

valley of love, 127, 174
Veronica (patient), 39–47, 50, 221–5
  aloneness, 223, 224
  arm massage, 221
  beauty of patient, seeing, 223, 224
  poems, untitled, 222, 224
  spirituality/spiritual realm of care, 222–4
vibration
  sacred, 187, *188*
  transmission, healing as, 188, 223, 233, 246–7
vision, caring, 16–17, *17*, 21–3, 130–31
  operationalising within the unfolding moment, 13–15
  for palliative care, 22
  realising, 25
  shared, 256
  transforming, 7
  WHO definition, **23**
Vision for the Future document (NHSME 1993), 54
visits from the dead, 76–7, 108–9
visualisation, healing light, 169
voice, constructed, 125, *126*

waiting for death, 152, 153
The waiting room poem, 152, 154
Watermark album, 77, 156, 158
WHO definition of palliative care, **23**
The Widening Field, 41
will, making a, 173
windhorse imagery, 97, 125, 244
Winterson, Jeannette, 42–3, 51, 59, 223
wisdom, practical, 10–11, 69
withdrawal, social, 82, 151, 180

Yasmina (patient), 243–5
  mindfulness, 244–5
  Muslim culture/religion, 244
  poem, *The kiss of the dark god*, 244
yin and yang, *125*
You are the Light, 197